Lung Epithelial Biology: Pathogenesis and Treatment of Pulmonary Diseases

Lung Epithelial Biology: Pathogenesis and Treatment of Pulmonary Diseases

Editor: Tabatha Colby

AMERICAN
MEDICAL PUBLISHERS
www.americanmedicalpublishers.com

AMERICAN
MEDICAL PUBLISHERS
www.americanmedicalpublishers.com

Cataloging-in-Publication Data

Lung epithelial biology : pathogenesis and treatment of pulmonary diseases / edited by Tabatha Colby.
p. cm.
Includes bibliographical references and index.
ISBN 979-8-88740-234-5
1. Lungs--Diseases. 2. Lungs--Diseases--Pathogenesis. 3. Lungs--Diseases--Treatment.
4. Epithelial cells. 5. Respiratory organs--Diseases. 6. Respiratory infections. I. Colby, Tabatha.
RC756 .L86 2023
616.24--dc23

American Medical Publishers,
41 Flatbush Avenue,
1st Floor, New York,
NY 11217, USA

ISBN 979-8-88740-234-5 (Hardback)

Contents

Preface

Lung epithelial biology is focused on the study of epithelial cells present in the lungs. These cells are located in the interface between the organism and the environment, and perform various significant functions like fluid balance, barrier protection, surfactant and mucus production, as well as inducing immune responses. The respiratory epithelium acts as a functional and physical barrier responsible for safeguarding against infectious agents. The alveolar surface is stacked with membranous pneumocytes called granular pneumocytes, type I alveolar epithelial cells (AEC I) and type II alveolar epithelial cells (AEC II). AEC I are thin, squamous and large cells that contribute in gaseous exchange. These cells also create a barrier to detect microbial products for initiating inflammatory responses. AEC II are cuboidal cells responsible for epithelium reparation upon injury and ion transport. These are also involved in lung defense through the secretion of antimicrobial products, like complement, lysozyme, and surfactant proteins (SP). This book is a valuable compilation of topics, ranging from the basic to the most complex advancements in the study of lung epithelial biology. Researchers and students engaged in the treatment of pulmonary diseases will be assisted by it.

Significant researches are present in this book. Intensive efforts have been employed by authors to make this book an outstanding discourse. This book contains the enlightening chapters which have been written on the basis of significant researches done by the experts.

Finally, I would also like to thank all the members involved in this book for being a team and meeting all the deadlines for the submission of their respective works. I would also like to thank my friends and family for being supportive in my efforts.

Editor

1

GM-CSF and IL-33 Orchestrate Polynucleation and Polyploidy of Resident Murine Alveolar Macrophages in a Murine Model of Allergic Asthma

Katharina M. Quell [1,†], Kuheli Dutta [1,†], Ülkü R. Korkmaz [1], Larissa Nogueira de Almeida [1], Tillman Vollbrandt [2], Peter König [3,4], Ian Lewkowich [5,6], George S. Deepe, Jr. [7], Admar Verschoor [8], Jörg Köhl [1,4,5] and Yves Laumonnier [1,4,*]

1 Institute for Systemic Inflammation Research, University of Lübeck, 23538 Lübeck, Germany; katharina.quell@web.de (K.M.Q.); kuheli.dutta14@gmail.com (K.D.); RabiaUelkue.Korkmaz@uksh.de (Ü.R.K.); LarissaNogueirade.Almeida@uksh.de (L.N.d.A.); joerg.koehl@uksh.de (J.K.)
2 Cell Analysis Core Facility, University of Lübeck, 23538 Lübeck, Germany; Tillman.Vollbrandt@uksh.de
3 Institute of Anatomy, University of Lübeck, 23538 Lübeck, Germany; koenig@anat.uni-luebeck.de
4 Airway Research Center North, Member of the German Center for Lung Research (DZL), 23538 Lübeck, Germany
5 Division of Immunobiology, Cincinnati Children's Hospital, Cincinnati, OH 45229, USA; Ian.Lewkowich@cchmc.org
6 Department of Pediatrics, University of Cincinnati, Cincinnati, OH 45229, USA
7 College of Medicine, University of Cincinnati, Cincinnati, OH 45229, USA; Deepegs@ucmail.uc.edu
8 Department of Infectious Diseases and Microbiology, University of Lübeck, 23538 Lübeck, Germany; Admar.Verschoor@uksh.de
* Correspondence: yves.laumonnier@uksh.de
† They contributed equally to this study.

Abstract: Allergic asthma is a chronical pulmonary disease with high prevalence. It manifests as a maladaptive immune response to common airborne allergens and is characterized by airway hyperresponsiveness, eosinophilia, type 2 cytokine-associated inflammation, and mucus overproduction. Alveolar macrophages (AMs), although contributing to lung homeostasis and tolerance to allergens at steady state, have attracted less attention compared to professional antigen-presenting and adaptive immune cells in their contributions. Using an acute model of house dust mite-driven allergic asthma in mice, we showed that a fraction of resident tissue-associated AMs, while polarizing to the alternatively activated M2 phenotype, exhibited signs of polynucleation and polyploidy. Mechanistically, in vitro assays showed that only Granulocyte-Macrophage Colony Stimulating Factor and interleukins IL-13 and IL-33, but not IL-4 or IL-5, participate in the establishment of this phenotype, which resulted from division defects and not cell-cell fusion as shown by microscopy. Intriguingly, mRNA analysis of AMs isolated from allergic asthmatic lungs failed to show changes in the expression of genes involved in DNA damage control except for *MafB*. Altogether, our data support the idea that upon allergic inflammation, AMs undergo DNA damage-induced stresses, which may provide new unconventional therapeutical approaches to treat allergic asthma.

Keywords: allergic asthma; alveolar macrophages; division defect; polynucleation; mouse model

---

1. Introduction

Asthma is a widespread disease affecting 300 million people around the world and estimations predict that 100 million more will be affected by 2050 [1]. It is characterized by airway hyper-responsiveness, narrowing of the airways, inflammatory cell recruitment, and increased mucus production [2]. Further, allergic asthma is characterized by an allergen-triggered eosinophilic infiltration; the presence of type 2 cytokines such as interleukin (IL)-4, IL-5, and IL-13; and the presence of Immunoglobulin IgE [2]. By suppressing inflammatory responses through the secretion of anti-inflammatory cytokines such as IL-10 and IL-12, Alveolar macrophages (AMs) are associated, at steady state, with the maintenance of immunological homeostasis of the lungs [3]. During the sensitization phase, resident AMs maintain homeostasis, until high levels of cytokines such as IL-4, IL-13, and interferon (IFN)-γ are reached and the phenotype of AMs changes to a more pro-inflammatory one [3]. In addition, macrophages derived from peripheral blood-recruited monocytes infiltrate the lungs where they secrete additional pro-inflammatory mediators [3]. However, as the inflammatory response matures, resident AMs develop an anti-inflammatory phenotype, which ultimately tames and resolves the inflammation and assists in tissue remodeling [4].

Interestingly, one unique feature of macrophages is their ability to form multinucleated giant cells (MNGCs). Although their functions remain elusive, these MNGCs are thought to be responsible for engulfing large particles like foreign material, intracellular bacteria, parasites, and fungi [5]. In addition, they participate in physiological processes including the formation of osteoclasts, which resorb bone tissue; or the formation of foreign body giant cells, which degrade and resorb foreign materials [6]; and promote tissue repair and remodeling [7]. However, while these functions are often considered anti-inflammatory, MNGCs are also found in pathophysiological conditions, in particular in granuloma-associated diseases [5] and promote the progression/resolution of various diseases [8].

To date, multinuclear or polynuclear AMs have solely been identified in bronchoalveolar lavage of patients with asbestos exposure-induced interstitial lung disease [9,10], while polynucleation has been reported in a murine model of allergic asthma [11]. Although MNGCs in bones form in response to Th2-related inflammation, in particular upon IL-4 exposure [12,13], no mechanism has been proposed to explain the formation of MNGCs or polynucleated macrophages in allergic inflamed lungs. Currently, MNGCs arise either from cell-cell fusion mechanisms [6] or DNA damage and division defects in tuberculosis (TB)-associated granuloma [14].

Here we show that following the induction of allergic lung inflammation, driven by repeated exposure to house dust mite extract (HDM), a fraction of the MHCII$^+$ alveolar macrophages (AMs) exhibits a polynuclear phenotype. These macrophages can be identified by flow cytometric analysis from lung cell isolates and by histology. Furthermore, in vitro studies demonstrate that activation of steady state primary AMs with growth factor such as Granulocyte Macrophage-Colony Stimulating Factor (GM-CSF), and cytokines such as IL-13 and IL-33, but not IL-4 or IL-5, are instrumental to drive polynucleation and polyploidy of AMs. Further, in vitro assays, mRNA analysis, and visual examination of polynuclear macrophages suggest that they arise principally from cell division defects rather than cell-cell fusion.

2. Results

2.1. Allergic Asthma-Driven Inflammatory Conditions Trigger an M2 Activation of Alveolar Macrophages

Activation of alveolar macrophages is associated with allergic asthma-driven inflammation. Intratracheal (HDM) exposure induced (Figure S1A) robust airway hyperresponsiveness (AHR) and strong inflammation of the airways, characterized mainly by an infiltration of eosinophils and T cells (Figure 1A) in BALB/c mice. Furthermore, SiglecF$^+$CD11c$^+$ tissue-associated alveolar macrophages (tAMs) showed an upregulation of MHCII expression in HDM-treated mice, compared to the PBS-treated control, 72 h after the final HDM exposure (Figure 1B). This led to a heterogeneous population of tAMs characterized by high and low MHCII expression. To further evaluate the characteristics of MHCII$^+$ versus MHCII$^-$ populations, we examined the expression of additional specific macrophage markers. In both HDM-triggered MHCII$^+$ and MHCII$^-$ cells, we observed similar levels of MerTK and CD64 (Figure 1C), while they remained low for CD11b and negative for F4/80 (Figure 1C), confirming their resident AM phenotype. Moreover, RT-PCR analysis of FACS-purified MHCII^{+} and MHC^{-} populations from both PBS- and HDM-exposed animals demonstrated that HDM-exposure was uniquely associated with a shift towards an M2 macrophage phenotype characterized by high levels of *Arg1* and low levels of *Nos2* (Figure 1D). Both MHCII^{+} and MHCII^{-} populations demonstrated similar skewing (Figure 1D). Further, both MHCII^{+} and MHCII^{-} AMs showed a low expression level of *Ccr2* mRNA (Figure 1D), and HDM sensitization of *Ccr2*$^{-/-}$ mice did not result in changes in the frequency of MHCII^{+} tAMs (Figure 1E), suggesting that they did not derive from blood-recruited monocytes.

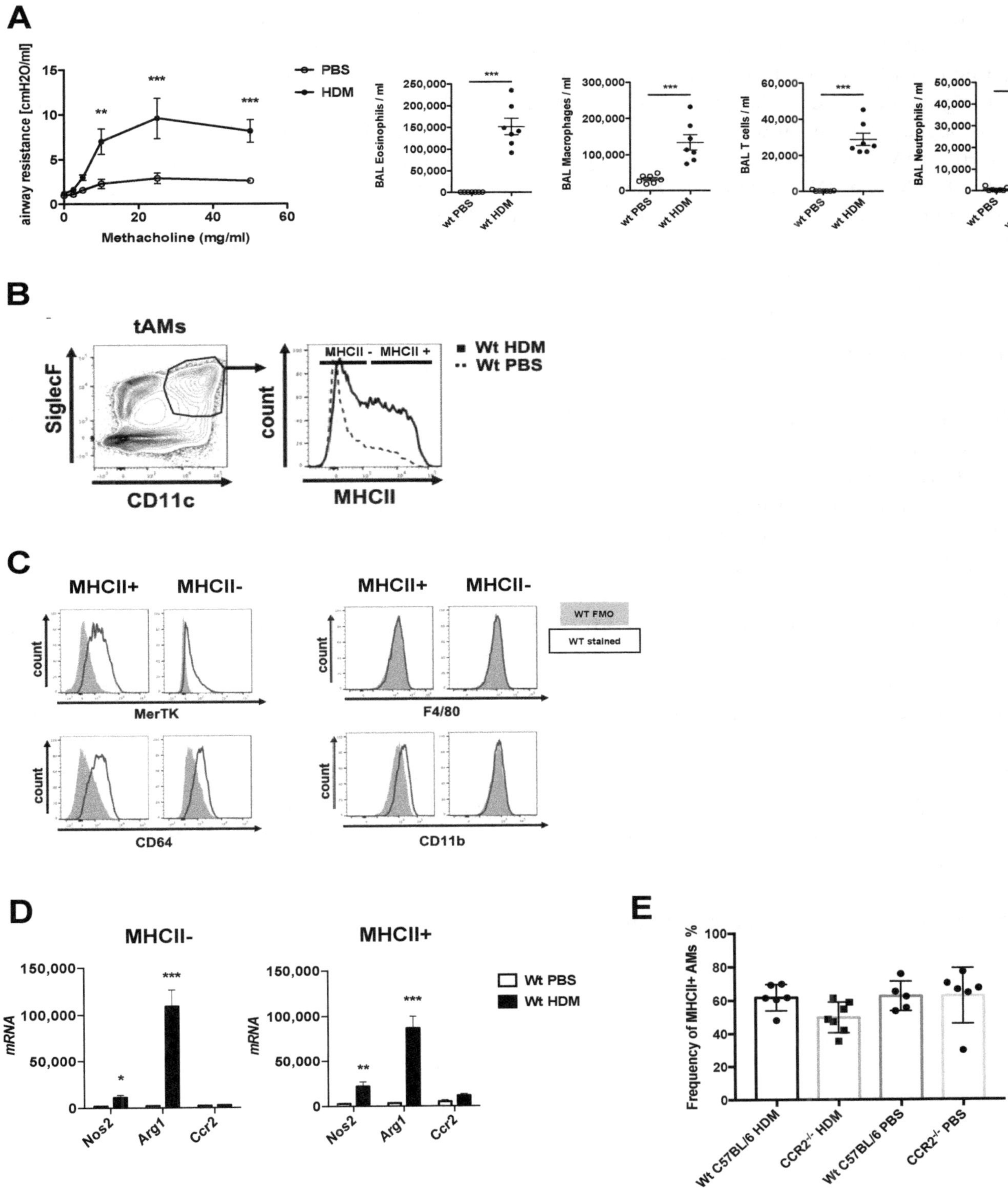

Figure 1. Allergic asthmatic inflammatory conditions drive a heterogenous expression of MHCII in tissue resident alveolar macrophages. (**A**) Characterization of the allergic asthma phenotype of mice exposed

to house dust mite extract (HDM) compared to non-asthmatic control (PBS). Upon HDM exposure, mice show increased airway hyperresponsiveness (AHR) upon methacoline exposure, as shown by increased airway resistance and strong inflammatory cell influx consisting mostly in eosinophils, T cells and to a lower extent neutrophils. Data show mean value ± SEM; $n = 7–8$ per group. Statistical significance in the AHR dose response curves was assessed using a two ways ANOVA. Statistical significance of the cellular recruitments in the airways was assessed using a t-test. ** $p < 0.01$; *** $p < 0.001$. (**B**) $CD11c^{+}SiglecF^{+}$ resident tissue-associated alveolar macrophages (tAMs) express different levels of MHCII complex upon HDM-driven allergic asthma inflammation. (**C**) Flow cytometric assessment of different markers of MHCII+ and MHCII− tAMs of HDM-treated mice, based on the gating provided in (B). Histograms show FMO control (grey) and MHCII signal (black) in the two subpopulations. The markers tested at the surface of $CD11c^{+}SiglecF^{+}$ tAMs were MerTK, CD64 and classical macrophages surface markers such as CD11b and F4/80. (**D**) RT-PCR analysis of MHCII+ and MCHII− tAMs for mRNA levels of *Nos2*, *Arg1* and *Ccr2* upon allergic inflammation. Data show mean value ± SEM of mRNA abundance reported to *S14* mRNA in sorted MHCII+ and MCHII− tAMs; $n = 4–7$ per group. Statistical significance between PBS and HDM samples was assessed using a t-test; * $p < 0.05$; ** $p < 0.01$; *** $p < 0.001$. (**E**) Frequency of MHCII+ AMs in lungs of C57BL/6 WT and $Ccr2^{-/-}$ mice upon HDM-driven allergic asthma. Data show mean value ± SEM; $n = 5–6$ animals.

2.2. *HDM-Driven $MHCII^{+}$ Activated tAMs Exhibit Signs of Polynucleation*

We stained and sorted $MHCII^{-}$ and $MHCII^{+}$ tAMs from allergic inflamed lung tissue and examined their morphological appearance by May-Giemsa staining. As expected, $MHCII^{-}$ tAMs showed characteristic macrophage morphology (Figure 2A). In contrast, examination of $MHCII^{+}$ tAMs revealed that, in addition to such morphologically classical cells, several macrophages harbored more than two nuclei. However, these cells did not show distinct multinuclear and large expansion of the cell body, which is typical for large giant cells [15] (Figure 2A). These data suggested that upon induction of allergic inflammation, tAMs might form polynucleated cells although not MNGCs. Staining of DNA with Hoechst 33342 in both $MHCII^{-}$ and $MHCII^{+}$ populations showed an increase in the amount of DNA in HDM-treated cells compared to the PBS (Figure 2C), suggesting either polynucleation or polyploidy was present in HDM-treated tAMs. Of note, while polynuclear cells with high DNA content were observed in lung tissue preparations, we could observe neither polynucleated (data not shown) nor tAMs with high DNA content (polypoid) in bronchoalveolar lavages of allergic asthmatic mice (Figure 2C). To ensure that the polynucleated tAMs identified did not arise from an artifact related to lung digestion, isolation procedure and/or FACS sorting, we examined 50 μm lung histology sections of HDM-treated WT stained with H&E staining. Interestingly, we identified two to four nuclei polynucleated cells, located around the alveoli (Figure 2D). Altogether, these findings suggested that polyploid and polynuclear cells might develop, in vivo, from $SiglecF^{+}CD11c^{+}$ tAMs during the effector phase of allergic asthma.

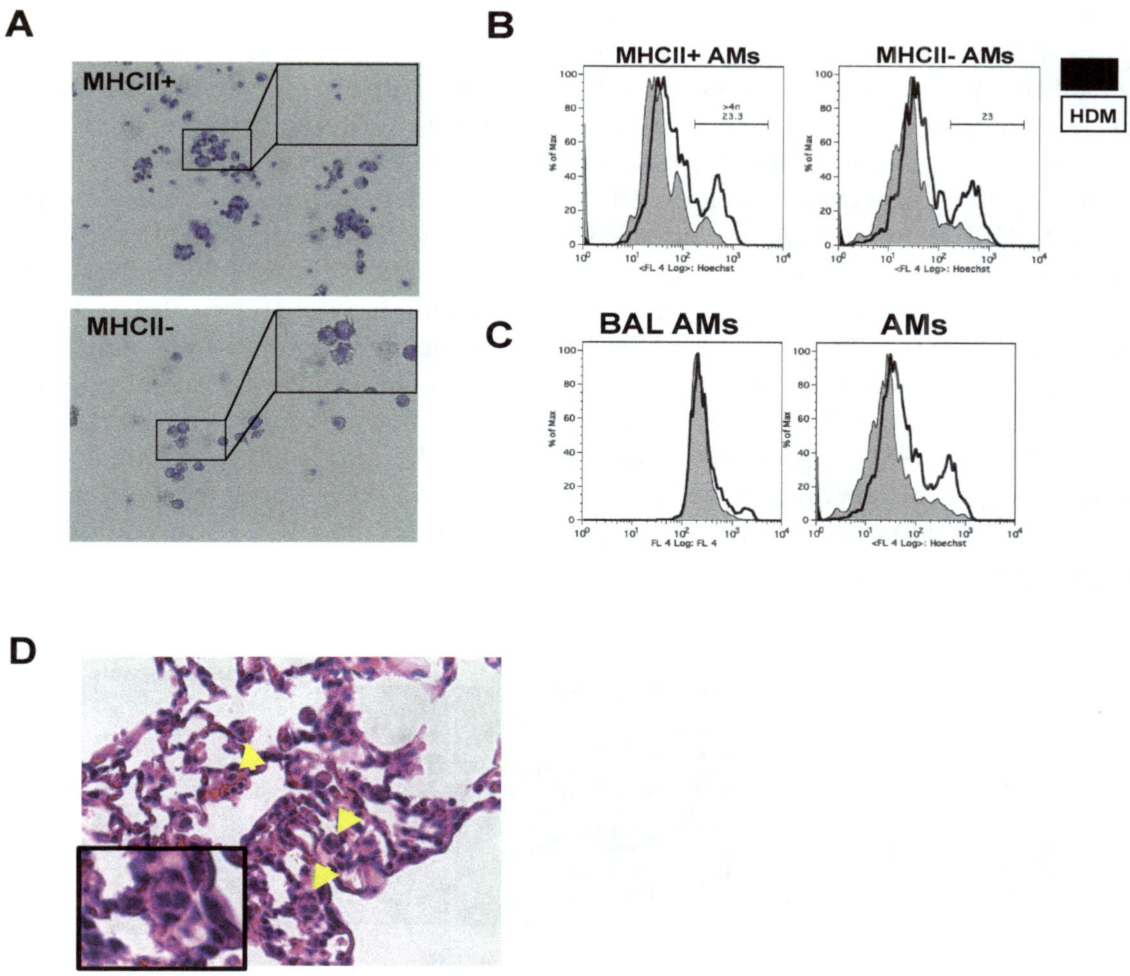

Figure 2. MHCII$^+$ tAMs subpopulation shows signs of polynucleation upon allergic asthma (**A**) CD11c$^+$SiglecF$^+$MHCII$^+$ resident tAMs from HDM-triggered asthmatic lungs but not the MCHII- subpopulation; showing cells with four to six nuclei. Data shown are representative of at least three independent experiments. Pictures were taken with a 20× objective. (**B**) CD11c$^+$ SiglecF$^+$ tAMs from HDM-induced asthma show increased DNA content by Hoechst 33342 staining. Data are representative of at least two independent experiments. (**C**) DNA content increase is observed in tissue tAMs but not in bronchoalveolar macrophages as shown by Hoechst 33342 staining. Data are representative of at least two independent experiments. (**D**) Histology section of HDM-treated mouse. Arrows indicate the presence of polynucleated cells in the alveolar compartment. Pictures were taken using a 20× objective.

2.3. In Vitro, GM-CSF Drives tAMs Polynucleation While IL-13 and IL-33 Polyploidy

To delineate the molecular mechanisms involved in the formation of polynucleated cells and to confirm their resident alveolar macrophage origin, we developed an in vitro assay to test the ability of type 2 cytokines and alarmin to induce tAM to polynuclear transformation. In addition to the reported expression of receptors for GM-CSF [16], IL-4 [17] and IL-5 [18,19], we found that steady state macrophages expressed the receptor for IL-33 (ST2) and IL-13 (IL-13Rα), but not Thymic stromal lymphopoietin (TSLP) receptor or the IL-17RB protein, the latter being a components of the IL-25 receptor (Figure 3A). Therefore, naïve tAMs from steady state lungs were FACS sorted based on their expression of Siglec F and CD11c, and stimulated in vitro for 7 days either with type 2 cytokines (IL-4, IL-5, IL-13) or IL-33, a well-known alarmin released upon allergen exposure by damaged epithelial cells. Further, we used GM-CSF, a major regulator of AMs differentiation that, similar to IL-4, has been shown to trigger the formation of multinucleated giant cell (MNGC) [15,20,21]. After fixation and staining cells with 4′,6-diamidino-2-phenylindole (DAPI) and FITC-labeled wheat germ agglutinin, we observed striking differences in cell density between medium controls, IL-4 or IL-5 stimulation on the one hand, and in cells stimulated with GM-CSF, IL-33 and to a lesser extent IL-13 on the other hand (Figure 3B). In addition to higher proliferation rates, GM-CSF-, IL-13- or IL-33-stimulated cells showed a healthier phenotype, characterized by strong adhesion and spreading of cellular dendrites. In contrast, cells kept in the media control or stimulated with IL-4 and IL-5 exhibited a rounded phenotype (Figure 3C). In the presence of GM-CSF, we observed binucleated (BiN) cells with nuclei frequently arranged symmetrically (Figure 3B,D), and the frequency of BiN cells was significantly increased in GM-CSF-stimulated tAMs compared to all other conditions (Figure 3D). BiN cells did not harbor a fragmented nucleus, and thus, did not appear apoptotic (Figure S1D). Although IL-4 drove bone marrow (BM)-derived macrophages into multinucleation in vitro (Figure 3E), it did not induce BiN tAMs formation, and the frequency of polynuclear macrophages upon IL-4 was similar to medium alone (Figure 3D). Intriguingly, neither IL-13 nor IL-33 triggered a clear increase in polynucleation frequency in vitro, although IL-33 given intra-tracheally to mice promoted a clear polynucleation phenotype in MHCII$^+$ tAMs (Figure 3F). However, both IL-13- and IL-33-stimulated cells harbored significantly enlarged nuclei compared to medium, IL-4-, and IL-5-stimulated cells, and to a lesser extent to GM-CSF treated cells (Figure 3G), suggesting that IL-13 or IL-33 stimulation may trigger tAMs polyploidy rather than poynucleation.

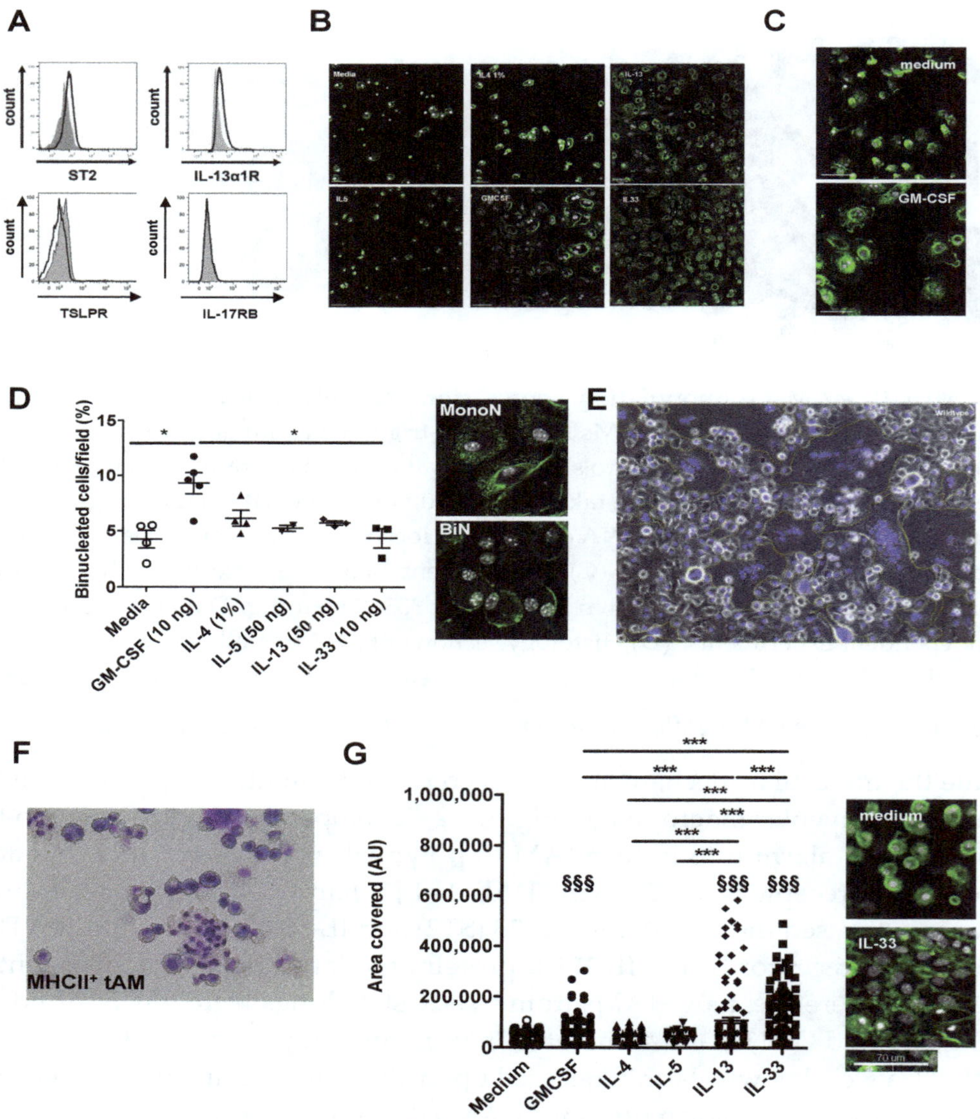

Figure 3. Tissue resident macrophages undergo binucleation upon GM-CSF treatment in vitro. (**A**) Resident tAMs express a receptor for IL-33 (ST2) and IL-13 (IL-13Ra), but not for IL-25 (IL-17RB)

and TSLP as shown by flow cytometry. Histograms show signal (black line) compared to Fluorescence minus one (FMO) controls (grey histogram). Data are representative of at least two independent stainings. (**B**) Visual examination of cultures of sorted Siglec F^+ $CD11c^+$ tAMs after 7 days of culture with medium alone, IL-4 (1%), IL-13 (50 ng/mL), IL-5 (50 ng/mL), IL-33 (50 ng/mL) or GM-CSF (10 ng/mL). Slides were stained with FITC-wheat germ agglutinin (green) and counterstained with DAPI (white). Data are representative of at least three independent experiments. Pictures were taken using a ×20 oil-immersion objective. (**C**) Close-up view of cells cultivated in medium alone or upon GM-CSF. Cells stimulated with GM-CSF exhibited dendrites and better adherence compared to cells in medium alone. Pictures were taken using a ×40 objective. (**D**) Evaluation of the frequency of polynucleated macrophages upon various stimulii. Data are mean value ± SEM; $n = 2–5$. Pictures show a representative example of mono and binucleated cells observed with a 40× objective, * $p < 0.05$. (**E**) BM-derived macrophage fusion induced by the presence of 1% IL-4 conditioned medium in the cell culture medium. Cells were stained with Hemacolor and the picture was taken in bright field microscopy using a ×20 objective. Data are representative of two experiments. (**F**) $CD11c^+SiglecF^+$ $MHCII^+$ resident tAMs from IL-33-triggered asthmatic lungs show cells with four to six nuclei after sorting, cytospinning and staining with diff-quick reagent. Data shown are representative of at least three independent experiments. Pictures were taken using a ×20 objective. (**G**) Area covered by the nuclei of tAMs cultured 7 days with the above-mentioned cytokines and growth factor (media change with cytokines at day 2, 3 and 5). The areas were measured after staining and microscopic evaluation, using Image J software. Pictures show a representative example of medium-treated and IL-33-treated cells using a 40× objective. Data are mean values ± SEM. Statistical significance was assessed using ANOVA. Asterisk refers to significance between the treatments, while § refers to significance compared to the medium control; §§§ and *** $p < 0.001$.

2.4. *GM-CSF-Driven Polynucleation of tAMs Resulted from Division Defects Rather Than Cell-Cell Fusion*

While the formation of polynuclear macrophages is typically thought to be driven by cellular fusion [20], recent data have indicated that polyploid granuloma-resident macrophages in *Mycobacterium Tuberculosis* (TB) infection are formed via altered cell division events and mitotic defects such as endoreplication and cytokinesis failure [14]. Therefore, we tested if the observed polynuclear cells, in our in vitro cultures, were generated by fusion or cell division defects. First, we purified naïve tAMs by FACS, labeled them either with PKH26 or carboxyfluorescein succinimidyl ester (CFSE) (Figure S1B) and combined the differently labeled tAMs in the presence of GM-CSF to induce BiN cell formation. After 5 days of co-culture, we identified BiN cells that were either $PKH26^+$ or $CFSE^+$, however only a few of them were $PKH26^+CFSE^+$ (Figure 4A). Although this may indicate that polynuclear macrophages were formed by fusion, we also observed mononucleated cells with a double positive signal, suggesting either phagocytosis of dying tAMs or cell fusion followed by nuclear fusion. However, careful examination of GM-CSF-treated tAMs in vitro cultures revealed that cells actively proliferated (Figure 4B), and micronuclei were observed (Figure 4C). Furthermore, tAMs present in the lung of allergic asthmatic mice exposed repeatedly to HDM over 4 weeks and cultured with GM-CSF for 24 h showed a symmetrical distribution of nuclei in the cells (Figure 4D), similar to polynuclear cells generated upon GM-CSF treatment of naive tAMs (Figure 3D). Altogether, our data suggested that cell division defects were the main mechanism involved in the formation of polynuclear tAMs.

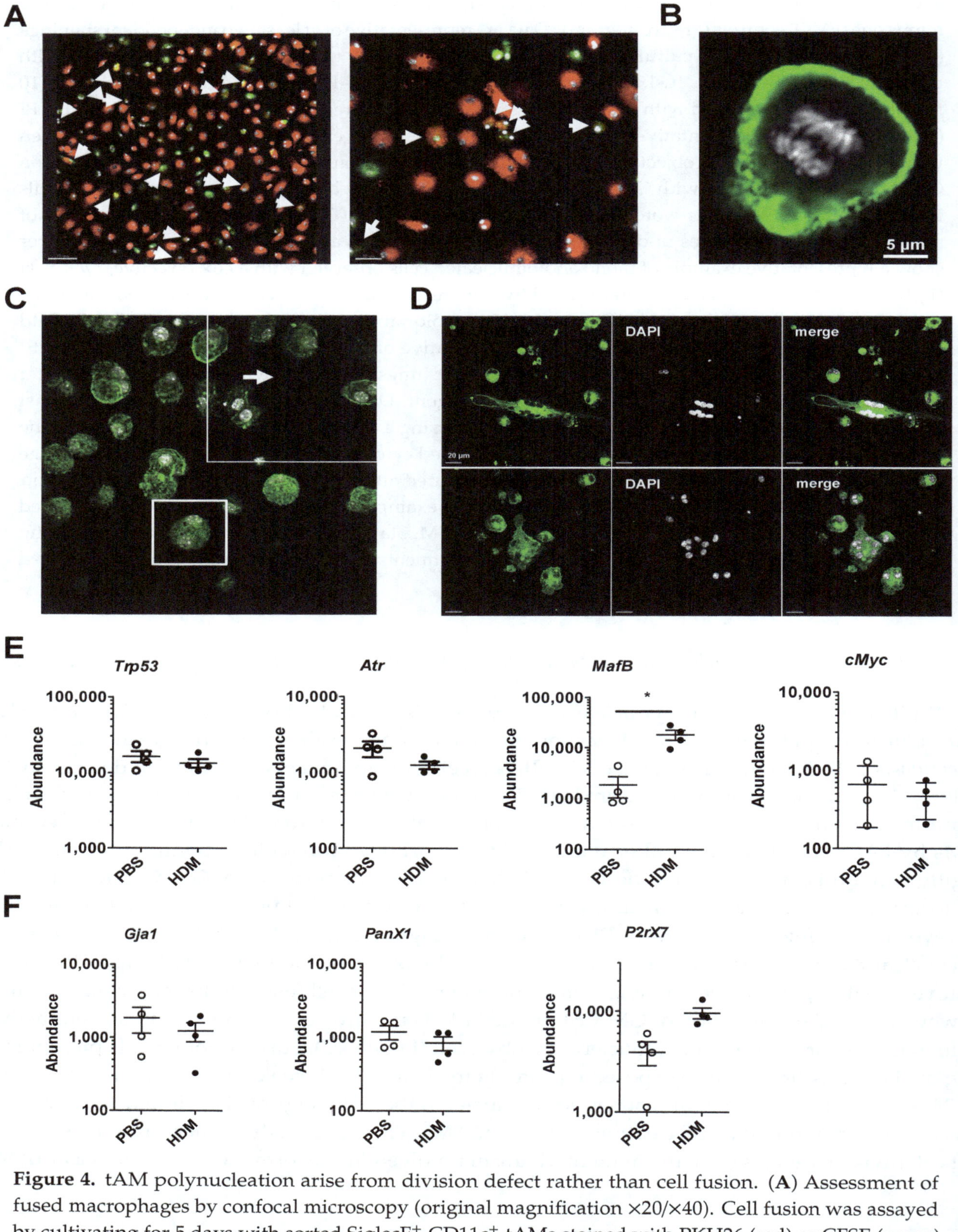

Figure 4. tAM polynucleation arise from division defect rather than cell fusion. (**A**) Assessment of fused macrophages by confocal microscopy (original magnification ×20/×40). Cell fusion was assayed by cultivating for 5 days with sorted SiglecF^{+} CD11c^{+} tAMs stained with PKH26 (red) or CFSE (green) and counterstained with DAPI (white). Bars represent 70/30 µm. Arrows show cells positive for both red and green staining. (**B**) SiglecF^{+} CD11c^{+} tAMs cultivated with GM-CSF show signs of proliferation. Cells were stained with FITC-WGA (green), counterstained with DAPI (white) and examined by fluorescence microscopy (original magnification ×60). (**C**) Evidences of division defect of tAMs by confocal microscopy (original magnification ×40). tAM cultivated with GM-CSF shows the presence of

micronucleus (shown by an arrow). Cells were stained with FITC-WGA (green) and counterstained with DAPI (white). (**D**) tAMs sorted from four-steps HDM-triggered asthmatic lungs were kept for 24 h in presence of GM-CSF. Cells show symmetrical polynucleation. Cells were stained with FITC-WGA (green) and counterstained with DAPI (white). Data are representative of two independent experiments. Picture were taken using a ×40 objective. (**E**) Cells from PBS or HDM treated mice for 4 weeks were isolated and analyzed for RNA content. Data show abundance of *Trp53, Atr, C-myc,* and *Mafb* mRNA reported to *S14* level, in SiglecF$^+$ CD11c$^+$ MHCII+ tAMs. Values shown are the mean ± SEM from $n = 4$ isolations. Statistical significance was assessed using a t-test. * $p < 0.05$. (**F**) Expression level of *Gja1, P2rx7,* and *Panx1* in the same samples were evaluated. Data show abundance of mRNA reported to *S14* level, in MHCII+ tAMs. Values are the mean ± SEM from $n = 4$ isolations.

2.5. HDM-Activated MHCII$^+$ tAMs Express Higher Levels of MafB

Since in TB-associated granuloma formation, polynucleation and polyploidy are associated with alterations in DNA damage control and changes in expression of *Mafb, C-myc, Trp53,* and *Atr* [14], we assessed the mRNA expression of these genes in the MHCII$^+$ subpopulations of HDM-triggered tAMs, by semi-quantitative real time PCR. Intriguingly, while the expression of *Mafb* was significantly increased in the HDM-treated mice in relation to the PBS treated mice, neither *Atr, Trp53* nor *C-myc* expression were altered upon HDM treatment in both the tAMs subpopulations compared to PBS controls (Figure 4E). However, in vitro, we observed that GM-CSF decreased the phosphorylation status of p53 in sorted AMs after 3 days of stimulation compared to non-stimulated controls (Supplementary Figure S2). In order to appreciate a contribution of cell fusion to the formation of polynuclear tAMs under allergic asthma conditions, we also delineated the expression of several genes associated to cell-cell fusion, such as *Gja1*, encoding Connexin 43, *P2x7* and *Panx1*. None of these genes increased in MHCII$^+$ cells upon HDM compared to PBS controls (Figure 4F).

3. Discussion

Multinucleated or polynucleated giant cells are a common cell type encountered in various physiological and pathological situations, ranging from bone osteoclast differentiation to granuloma formations in tuberculosis (TB) [14,22], histoplasma [23], sarcoidosis [24], Takayasu and giant cell arteritis [25], and in airways of asbestos-exposed workers [10]. By contrast, evidence for their formation during allergic asthma is limited. Although some were identified in an OVA-driven allergic asthma model [11], polynucleation of macrophages has not been reported in fatal allergic asthmatic human lungs. Here, we show that upon allergen-induced lung inflammation in a mouse model, a significant fraction of tissue-associate alveolar macrophages (tAMs) underwent polynucleation and polyploidy, although we did not find either polynucleation or polyploidy in BAL alveolar macrophages from asthmatic animals. Mechanistically, GM-CSF was the main trigger for polynucleation while IL-33 and IL-13 were involved in polyploidy. Neither IL-4 nor IL-5 drove these processes. In addition, cell division defects were the main cause for the formation of polynucleated tAMs in vitro and in vivo.

We observed that not all cytokines present in the asthma-associated pro-inflammatory milieu were equal in driving polynucleation of tAMs. Indeed, while GM-CSF was a potent driver, IL-33 was not as active in vitro, although its in vivo effect was stronger. GM-CSF is a master regulator of AMs differentiation and functions [26,27] and participates, with IL-4, in the MNGC formation in vitro [20]. Interestingly, although we confirm IL-4-induced polynucleation of BM-derived macrophages [15], IL-4 did not induce polynucleation of tAMs. This apparent discrepancy may be linked to the very peculiar phenotype of AMs. Indeed, in contrast to "classical" macrophages, such as BM-derived macrophages differentiated either with Macrophage-Colony Stimulating Factor (M-CSF) or GM-CSF, peritoneal and visceral adipose tissue-associated AMs express neither F4/80 nor CD11b but Siglec F [28,29]. Further, unlike other macrophages, tAMs do not express the anaphylatoxin receptor C3aR [28], suggesting that the difference between AMs/tAMs and other macrophages is great in terms of functionality. Supporting the idea that different macrophages show different responses to IL-4, a recent study showed that F4/80^{+} macrophages respond differently to IL-4 trigger compared to CD68^{+} and CD11b^{+} macrophages [30]. GM-CSF is a crucial growth factor for the development and homeostasis of alveolar macrophages [29,31,32]. Interestingly, while M-CSF is a well-known trigger of monocyte/macrophage multinucleation by fusion [33], GM-CSF plays a more accessory role in these processes [21,34]. However, GM-CSF is secreted by TB mutinuclear cells in vitro [35] and may fuel the formation of polynuclear granuloma besides TLR-2 signaling [14]. Further, similar to our observations that GM-CSF drives alveolar macrophage proliferation, increased GM-SCF drives AMs accumulation in smokers [36]. Besides the release of GM-CSF, allergen exposure directly triggers the secretion of various alarmins such as IL-33, TSLP or IL-25 [37] by damaged epithelial cells, or upon HDM exposure, after transient release of GM-CSF itself [38]. However, while tAMs from naive mice express the receptor for GM-CSF [19], IL-13, and IL-33, we did not observe the expression of TSLPR or IL-17RB (the specific receptor chain involved in the formation of the IL-25 receptor) in steady state alveolar macrophages, therefore limiting our study to IL-13 and IL-33. Intriguingly, IL-13 has been reported to act as an inducer of fusion-driven MNGC formation [5] and contributes to macrophage polarization in sarcoidosis-associated granuloma formation in vitro [39]. However, in tAMs, our data suggest that IL-13 drives polyploidy. This could be the result of an alternative use of IL-13Ra2/STAT3 signaling rather IL-13Ra1/STAT6 in tAMs. Indeed, IL-13Ra2 has been shown to contribute to allergic asthma [40] and plays a unique role in the function of conventional pulmonary dendritic cells [41]. In contrast, although IL-33 influences polarization of alveolar macrophages [42], there is limited evidence for a role of IL-33 in the formation of giant cells, although it may be a decisive pro-inflammatory cytokine contributing to the pathology of Giant Cell Arteritis [43]. Conversely, granulomas have been reported to be a source of IL-33 in pulmonary sarcoidosis [44].

Mechanistically, we showed that division defect seems to be the main reason for the polynucleation of tAMs rather than cell fusion. In particular, we observed a symmetrical distribution of nuclei in cells as well as the presence of features such as micronuclei. Both result from migration delays of the chromatids [45] and occur singly or in a recurrent manner [14]. Interestingly, the presence of micronuclei has been shown to activate STING and cGAS pathways [46] and may be a cause for type I Interferon production by AMs [47], a phenomenon previously observed in activated AMs [48,49]. Congruent with a lack of involvement of cell fusion in vitro using PKH26 and CFSE-labeled cells, we did not observe changes in the expression of genes reported to be involved in such mechanisms in vivo, such as connexin 43, associated with syncytial trans-epithelial alveolar communication [50], or PanX1 and P2X7R, receptors contributing to the cell fusion mechanisms [21,51] and participating in allergic asthma pathology [52]. Intriguingly, although tAMs showed clear signs of DNA damage, we did not evidence changes in genes controlling the response to such insults, such as *Trp53*, *C-myc* and *Atr* expression. However, *Trp53* expression does not necessarily reflect a modulation of p53 functions through its phosphorylation level [53]. In line with that, we observed a decrease in the phosphorylation status of p53 in tAMs stimulated in vitro with GM-CSF, suggesting that upon GM-CSF exposure, the cells are permissive to cell division although DNA damage might be present. Similarly, ATR expression and function may be uncoupled from its mRNA expression via modulation of its phosphorylation status, in particular in the control of DNA damage associated with cell death [54] or its isomeric status [55]. In contrast, *MafB* expression increased upon in vivo HDM exposure. Interestingly, in humans, MafB immunostaining in AMs correlates with altered spirometry in smokers [56]. Further, MafB also regulates type I IFN production through recruitment of coactivators to IFN regulatory factor [57], and double-strand DNA break-induced type I IFN has been shown to enhance DNA damage response in macrophages [58]. In addition, our observation of an allergic asthma-driven increased expression of *MafB* in tAMs may be in line with reports that Mafb upregulates the expression of M2 polarization markers such as MRC1 and CD163 [59]. Nonetheless, a classical function of IL-4-induced large MNGCs (with more than 10 nuclei/cell) is the phagocytosis of large and complement-opsonized materials, which is more effective than their unfused M2 macrophage precursors [15]. Although clearance of apoptotic cells by macrophages in the airways plays a vital role in the resolution of airway inflammation [60,61], it is unclear whether polynuclear tAMs play a similar role.

Finally, epidemiologic associations between atopies and protection against cancer development have been observed [62,63]. In that context, IgE has been reported to play a key role [63], possibly due to an IgE-driven macrophage rewiring [64]. However, besides this atopic protective effect, the fact that polynuclear macrophages arise from division defect, a major mechanism in tumorigenicity, suggests that some allergic inflammation and cancer mechanisms may overlap at the molecular levels. Therefore, pharmacological targeting of allergic lungs by anti-cancer drugs may (i) provide a new approach to clarify the functions of macrophage polynucleation in the development and/or severity of allergic asthma, and (ii) might be an interesting therapeutical approach in human allergic asthma.

4. Material and Methods

4.1. Animals

Mice on a BALB/c background were bred and housed in the specific-pathogen-free animal facility of the University of Lübeck. They were handled in accordance with the appropriate institutional and national guidelines. Experimental model studies were reviewed and approved as 86-7/17 and 44-5/18, by local authorities of the Animal Care and Use Committee (Ministerium für Landwirtschaft, Energiewende, Umwelt und ländliche Räume, Kiel, Germany). Genetically deficient *Ccr2* mice and their C57Bl/6 counterpart were bred and handled in the specific-pathogen-free animal facility of the University of Cincinnati (IACUC protocol #05-01-12-02, approved 2016) in accordance with the appropriate institutional and national guidelines.

4.2. Antibodies and Reagents

Anti-mouse Siglec F (clone E50-2440) labeled with Brilliant Violet (BV)421 was from BD Bioscience (San Jose, CA, USA). Anti-mouse CD64 (clone X54-5/7.1) labeled with Fluorescein isothiocyanate (FITC), anti-mouse IL17RB (clone 9B10) in Phycoerythrin (PE), anti-F4/80 (clone BM8) in BV510, and unlabeled anti-mouse TSLPR (clone 22H9) were from Biolegend (San Diego, CA, USA). Anti-TSLPR antibody was stained by a secondary anti-rat F(ab)$_2$ antibody labeled with Allophycocyanin (APC) (Cell Signaling Technology, Leiden, The Netherlands). Anti-mouse CD11b (clone M1/70) labeled with BV510, anti-mouse CD11c (clone N418) labeled with APC, anti-IL13Ra1 (13MOKA) in PE, anti-mouse MerTK (clone DS5MMER) labeled with PE-Cy7, anti-mouse MHCII (Clone M5/114.15.2) labelled with APC-eFluor 780, and unlabeled blocking anti-mouse CD16/CD32 antibodies were purchased by eBioscience (Thermofisher, Darmstadt, Germany). The anti-ST2 antibody (clone DJ8) labeled with APC was purchased from mdbbiosciences (Zürich, Switzerland). In addition, 4′,6-diamidino-2-phenylindole (DAPI) and FITC-labeled wheat germ agglutinin (WGA) protein were purchased from Invitrogen (Thermofisher, Darmstadt, Germany). Flow cytometry histograms show either fluorescence/counts or fluorescence/percentage of maximum (% of Max). The latter was used to provide a better comparison when the numbers of events measured in different samples differed widely. Flow cytometry data analysis were performed using FlowJo X (Flowjo, Ashland, OR, USA).

4.3. House Dust Mite (HDM)-Driven Allergic Asthma Model

In BALB/c mice, allergic asthma was induced by intratracheal (i.t.) application of HDM, carried out once a week for 4 consecutive weeks. BALB/c mice were anaesthetized (0.2% Xylazin & 5 mg/mL ketamine in 100 μL total) and HDM (Greer Laboratories, Lenoir, NC, USA) (100 μg/50 μL PBS) or PBS given i.t. Mice were sacrificed 72 h after the last challenge (Figure S1A). In C57Bl/6 mice (and $Ccr2^{-/-}$ on a C57Bl/6 background), HDM-triggered allergic asthma was established by intra-peritoneal injections of HDM (10 μg in PBS) twice on week 1 and 2, followed by intra-tracheal application of HDM (100 μg/50 μL PBS) on week 3 and 4. Lungs were harvested 72 h after the last challenge (Figure S1B).

4.4. Assessing the Allergic Asthma Phenotype

To measure the airway hyperresponsiveness (AHR), mice were anaesthetized and AHR measured upon mechanical ventilation using a FlexiVent (SciReq, Montreal, QC, Canada) system as described [65]. Aerosolized Acetyl-β-Methyl-Choline (methacholine) (0, 2.5, 5, 10, 25, and 50 mg/mL; Sigma-Aldrich, Steinheim, Germany) was generated by an ultrasonic nebulizer and delivered in-line through the inhalation port for 10 s. Airway resistance was measured 2 min later.

To assess the cellular infiltration in the airways, BAL fluid samples were obtained by cannulating the trachea, injecting 1 mL of ice-cold PBS, and by subsequently aspirating the BAL fluid. After red blood cell lysis, BAL fluid cells were washed once in PBS and counted using a Neubauer chamber (VWR International, Darmstadt, Germany). Frequencies of BAL fluid cells were determined by flow cytometry using the respective markers: Siglec F/Autofluorescence (macrophages), Siglec F (eosinophils), Ly6G (neutrophils), and CD3 and CD4 (T cells). Cell numbers were calculated using the cell-specific frequency of total and total cell counts/mL.

4.5. Lung Single Cell Suspension and Alveolar Macrophages Isolation

Lung harvests were performed as described previously [28]. Briefly, after flushing the airways with 1 mL PBS, lung lobes were taken out, placed in a 40 μm strainer, cut into small pieces, and incubated with 0.25 mg/mL liberase TL (Roche, Rotkreuz, Switzerland) and 0.5 mg/mL DNAse I (Sigma-Aldrich, Steinheim, Germany) in RPMI (Life Technology, Carlsbad, CA, USA). for 45 min. at 37 °C under gentle agitation. Then, lungs and cell suspension were pressed using a syringe plunger and washed with 10 mL wash media before centrifugation (350× *g*, 10 min.), and the excess of red blood cells present in the isolation was removed by red blood cell lysis. After washing, pulmonary cell suspension was blocked with an anti-CD16/32 antibody (eBioscience, Darmstadt, Germany) and stained. The tAM population was sorted by Fluorescence activated cell sorting (FACS) as live $SiglecF^+$ $CD11c^+$ cells, using an Aria III cell sorter (BD Bioscience, San Jose, CA, USA) [28]. In some cases, MHCII was added to discriminate tAM subpopulations. For simple measurements, cells were washed after staining and measured using an LSRII analyser (BD Bioscience, San Jose, CA, USA).

4.6. RNA Isolation and cDNA Synthesis, Real Time Semi-Quantitative Polymerase Chain Reaction

To assess the effect of HDM on the expression level of different genes by RT-PCR, freshly sorted $SiglecF^+$ $CD11c^+$ $MHCI^-$ or $MHCII^+$ tAMs were lysed using 150 μL Trizol (Invitrogen, Thermofisher, Darmstadt, Germany) and total RNA isolated using Direct-zol™ RNA Mini-Prep kit (Zymo Research, Freiburg, Germany) according to the manufacturer's instructions. Finally, freshly isolated RNAs were reverted into complementary (c)DNAs using PrimeScript RT Reagent kit, according to the manufacturer's instructions (TAKARA Bio, Saint-Germain-en-Laye, France). Quantitative PCR was done using iQ Syber green (Bio-rad Laboratories, Münich, Germany) on a CFX96 real-time PCR system (Bio-rad Laboratories, Münich, Germany) using the specific primers (Eurofins, Ebersberg, Germany). Raw data were analyzed using CFX Maestro™ Software (Bio-rad Laboratories, Münich, Germany). As a housekeeping gene, *S14* mRNA, encoding for the ribosomal protein, which is a part of the 40S ribosomal subunit, was used [66]. The primers used are described in Table 1. Finally, the relative abundance of target genes was calculated as mRNA abundance = $(1.8^{(cp\ S14-CP\ gen)}) * 100{,}000$.

Table 1. Primer list and description.

Primer Name	Sequence (5′–3′)
mP2rx7_F	GACAAACAAAGTCACCCGGAT
mP2rx7_R	CGCTCACCAAAGCAAAGCTAAT
mPanx1_F	CCACCGAGCCCAAGTTCAA
mPanx1_R	GGAGAAGCAGCTTATCTGGGT
mTrp53_F	CTCTCCCCCGCAAAAGAAAAA

Table 1. *Cont.*

Primer Name	Sequence (5′–3′)
mTrp53 R	CGGAACATCTCGAAGCGTTTA
*mAtr*_F	GAATGGGTGAACAATACTGCTGG
mAtr R	TTTGGTAGCATACACTGGCGA
*mMafb*_F	TTCGACCTTCTCAAGTTCGACG
mMafb R	TCGAGATGGGTCTTCGGTTCA
*mGja1*_F	ACAGCGGTTGAGTCAGCTTG
mGja1 R	GAGAGATGGGGAAGGACTTGT
*mMyc*_F	ATGCCCCTCAACGTGAACTTC
mMyc R	CGCAACATAGGATGGAGAGCA
*S14*_R	TGGCAGACACCAAACACATT
*S14*_F	GAGGAGTCTGGAGACGACGA

4.7. Primary Cell Culture for Immunofluorescence Microscopy

In order to evaluate the effect of cytokines on the ploidy of tissue-associated alveolar macrophages (tAMs), freshly sorted primary SiglecF$^+$ CD11c$^+$ tAMs (100–150 × 10^3 cells) were seeded with or without GM-CSF (10 ng/mL), IL-5 (50 ng/mL) (Peprotech corporation, Rocky Hill, USA), IL-13 (50 ng/mL), IL-33 (50 ng/mL) (eBioscience Thermofisher, Darmstadt, Germany), or IL-4 (1%), for 7 days on paramount slides in RPMI complete media supplemented with Penicillin/Streptomycin, L-Glutamin (all from Life Technology, Calsbad, CA, USA) and 10% FCS (PAA, Thermofisher, Darmstadt, Germany), 37 °C, 5% CO_2. Media was changed (including the cytokines) on day 2, 3 and 5. After 7 days, slides were washed with PBS, fixed with 2% formalin and stained with DAPI and wheat agglutinin protein (WGA, 1:100) for 15 min at RT in the dark. Finally, slides were washed to get rid of the excess of fluorochromes, covered with fluroshield and glass cover and examined using Laser Scanning Microscope FV1000 (Olympus corporation, Tokyio, Japan) (Figure S1C). For evaluation, five pictures per well were taken (four from each of the corners and one from the middle of the well) under 20× oil, 40×, 60× oil objectives. Raw data interpretation was performed using IMARIS (Bitplane, Concord, CA, USA) allowing the evaluation of the percentage of binucleated or polynucleated cells, hence giving a binucleation index. Of note, multinucleated cells were not confused with apoptotic cells (Figure S1D). To assess the activity of IL-4 in driving cell fusion, bone-marrow-derived macrophages were differentiated with *Macrophage Colony-Stimulating Factor* for 4 days before being kept for an additional 3 days in fresh medium containing 1% IL-4 conditioned medium coming from IL-4 secreting cells as described previously [15]. Furthermore, using Image J (NIH, USA), pictures were mathematically processed to calculate the area of nuclei, and the area below 5000 AU was removed from analysis after visual validation, as possible debris from dead cells. For cell-cell fusion assay, sorted SiglecF$^+$ CD11c$^+$ tAMs were divided into two pools, stained either with PKH26 (Sigma-Aldrich, Steinheim, Germany) or Carboxyfluorescein succinimidyl ester (CFSE) (Thermofisher, Darmstadt, Germany) according to manufacturer's recommendations (Figure S1E). After staining, cells were mixed at a 1:1 ratio and seeded on permanox slides 100–150 × 10^3 cells/well and cultivated with GM-CSF for 5 days with changes on day 2 and 3. Cells were counterstained with DAPI, washed and mounted before visual examination.

4.8. Statistical Analysis

Statistical analysis was performed using GraphPad Prism (version 8.0.1; GraphPad Software, Inc., LaJolla, USA). The graphs are presented as scatter plots with bars showing the individual samples and the mean ± standard error of the mean (SEM) respectively. Normal distribution of data was tested, when meaningful, using the Kolmogorov–Smirnov and D'Agostino–Pearson tests. Statistical differences between two groups were assessed by unpaired *t* test. Comparisons involving multiple groups were first evaluated by an analysis of variance (ANOVA) followed by Tukey's multiple comparison test. When groups were not normally distributed, they were analyzed using a Mann–Whitney U (two groups), or ANOVA on ranks (multiple groups) followed by a Dunn's multiple comparison test. A p value < 0.05 was considered statistically significant * $p < 0.05$; ** $p < 0.01$; §§§ *** $p < 0.001$).

Author Contributions: K.M.Q. and Y.L.; Methodology, K.M.Q., A.V., and Y.L.; Validation, K.M.Q., K.D. and Y.L.; Formal Analysis, K.M.Q., K.D. and Y.L.; Investigation, K.M.Q., K.D., Ü.R.K., A.V., T.V., P.K. and L.N.d.A.; Resources, T.V., I.L., P.K., G.S.D.J., and J.K.; Data Curation, K.M.Q., Y.L.; Writing—Original Draft Preparation, K.M.Q., K.D.; Writing—Review & Editing, K.M.Q., Y.L.; Visualization, K.M.Q., Y.L.; Supervision, Y.L.; Project Administration, Y.L.; Funding Acquisition, Y.L. All authors have read and agreed to the published version of the manuscript.

Acknowledgments: We thank G. Köhl and J. Ritter for their excellent technical assistance, as well as Prof. T. Goldmann for his suggestions.

Abbreviations

tAM	tissue-associated alveolar macrophage
BAL	bronchoalveolar lavage fluid
BiN	binucleated
BM	Bone marrow
CD	cluster of differentiation
GM-CSF	Granulocyte Macrophage-Colony Stimulating Factor
HDM	house dust mite
IFN	interferon
IL	interleukin
M-CSF	Macrophage-Colony Stimulating Factor
MFI	mean fluorescence intensity
MHC	major histocompability complex
MNGC	multinuclear giant cell
TB	tuberculosis
TSLP	Thymic stromal lymphopoietin
WGA	wheat germ agglutinin
WT	wild type

References

1. Yukselen, A.; Kendirli, S.G. Role of immunotherapy in the treatment of allergic asthma. *World J. Clin. Cases* **2014**, *2*, 859–865. [CrossRef] [PubMed]
2. Quirt, J.; Hildebrand, K.J.; Mazza, J.; Noya, F.; Kim, H. Asthma. *Allergy Asthma Clin. Immunol.* **2018**, *14*, 50. [CrossRef] [PubMed]
3. Lumeng, C.N. Lung Macrophage Diversity and Asthma. *Ann. Am. Thorac. Soc.* **2016**, *13* (Suppl. 1), 31–34.
4. Byrne, A.J.; Mathie, S.A.; Gregory, L.G.; Lloyd, C.M. Pulmonary macrophages: Key players in the innate defence of the airways. *Thorax* **2015**, *70*, 1189–1196. [CrossRef] [PubMed]
5. Brodbeck, W.G.; Anderson, J.M. Giant cell formation and function. *Curr. Opin. Hematol.* **2009**, *16*, 53–57. [CrossRef]
6. Brooks, P.J.; Glogauer, M.; McCulloch, C.A. An Overview of the Derivation and Function of Multinucleated Giant Cells and Their Role in Pathologic Processes. *Am. J. Pathol.* **2019**, *189*, 1145–1158. [CrossRef]
7. Quinn, M.T.; Schepetkin, I.A. Role of NADPH Oxidase in Formation and Function of Multinucleated Giant Cells. *J. Innate Immun.* **2009**, *1*, 509–526. [CrossRef]
8. Miron, R.J.; Bosshardt, D.D. Multinucleated Giant Cells: Good Guys or Bad Guys? *Tissue Eng. Part B Rev.* **2018**, *24*, 53–65. [CrossRef]

9. Agustí, C.; Xaubet, A.; Arriols, R.; Marín, A.; Montserrat, J.M.; Agustí-Vidal, A. Multinuclear Giant Cells in Bronchoalveolar Lavage in Interstitial Lung Diseases. *Respiration* **1987**, *51*, 307–311. [CrossRef]
10. Takemura, T.; Rom, W.N.; Ferrans, V.J.; Crystal, R.G. Morphologie Characterization of Alveolar Macrophages from Subjects with Occupational Exposure to Inorganic Particles. *Am. Rev. Respir. Dis.* **1989**, *140*, 1674–1685. [CrossRef]
11. Melgert, B.N.; Oriss, T.B.; Qi, Z.; Dixon-McCarthy, B.; Geerlings, M.; Hylkema, M.N.; Ray, A. Macrophages: Regulators of sex differences in asthma? *Am. J. Respir. Cell Mol. Biol.* **2010**, *42*, 595–603. [CrossRef] [PubMed]
12. Aghbali, A.; Rafieyan, S.; Mohamed-Khosroshahi, L.; Baradaran, B.; Shanehbandi, D.; Kouhsoltani, M. IL-4 induces the formation of multinucleated giant cells and expression of beta5 integrin in central giant cell lesion. *Med. Oral Patol. Oral Cir. Bucal.* **2017**, *22*, e1–e6. [PubMed]
13. Moreno, J.L.; Mikhailenko, I.; Tondravi, M.M.; Keegan, A.D. IL-4 promotes the formation of multinucleated giant cells from macrophage precursors by a STAT6-dependent, homotypic mechanism: Contribution of E-cadherin. *J. Leukoc. Biol.* **2007**, *82*, 1542–1553. [CrossRef] [PubMed]
14. Herrtwich, L.; Nanda, I.; Evangelou, K.; Nikolova, T.; Horn, V.; Sagar; Erny, D.; Stefanowski, J.; Rogell, L.; Klein, C.; et al. DNA Damage Signaling Instructs Polyploid Macrophage Fate in Granulomas. *Cell* **2016**, *167*, 1264–1280.e18. [CrossRef]
15. Milde, R.; Ritter, J.; Tennent, G.A.; Loesch, A.; Martinez, F.O.; Gordon, S.; Pepys, M.B.; Verschoor, A.; Helming, L. Multinucleated Giant Cells Are Specialized for Complement-Mediated Phagocytosis and Large Target Destruction. *Cell Rep.* **2015**, *13*, 1937–1948. [CrossRef]
16. Martinez-Moczygemba, M.; Doan, M.L.; Elidemir, O.; Fan, L.L.; Cheung, S.W.; Lei, J.T.; Moore, J.P.; Tavana, G.; Lewis, L.R.; Zhu, Y.; et al. Pulmonary alveolar proteinosis caused by deletion of the GM-CSFRα gene in the X chromosome pseudoautosomal region 1. *J. Exp. Med.* **2008**, *205*, 2711–2716. [CrossRef]
17. Nieuwenhuizen, N.E.; Kirstein, F.; Jayakumar, J.; Emedi, B.; Hurdayal, R.; Horsnell, W.G.; Lopata, A.L.; Brombacher, F. Allergic airway disease is unaffected by the absence of IL-4Rα–dependent alternatively activated macrophages. *J. Allergy Clin. Immunol.* **2012**, *130*, 743–750.e8. [CrossRef]
18. Schneider, C.; Nobs, S.P.; Heer, A.K.; Hirsch, E.; Penninger, J.M.; Siggs, O.M.; Kopf, M. Frontline Science: Coincidental null mutation of Csf2rα in a colony of PI3Kγ-/- mice causes alveolar macrophage deficiency and fatal respiratory viral infection. *J. Leukoc. Biol.* **2016**, *101*, 367–376. [CrossRef]
19. Nishinakamura, R.; Nakayama, N.; Hirabayashi, Y.; Inoue, T.; Aud, D.; McNeil, T.; Azuma, S.; Yoshida, S.; Toyoda, Y.; Aral, K.-I.; et al. Mice deficient for the IL-3/GM-CSF/IL-5 βc receptor exhibit lung pathology and impaired immune response, while βIL3 receptor-deficient mice are normal. *Immunity* **1995**, *2*, 211–222. [CrossRef]
20. Helming, L.; Gordon, S. Molecular mediators of macrophage fusion. *Trends Cell Biol.* **2009**, *19*, 514–522. [CrossRef]
21. Lemaire, I.; Falzoni, S.; Zhang, B.; Pellegatti, P.; Di Virgilio, F. The P2X7 Receptor and Pannexin-1 Are Both Required for the Promotion of Multinucleated Macrophages by the Inflammatory Cytokine GM-CSF. *J. Immunol.* **2011**, *187*, 3878–3887. [CrossRef] [PubMed]
22. Blauenfeldt, T.; Petrone, L.; Del Nonno, F.; Baiocchini, A.; Falasca, L.; Chiacchio, T.; Bondet, V.; Vanini, V.; Palmieri, F.; Galluccio, G.; et al. Interplay of DDP4 and IP-10 as a Potential Mechanism for Cell Recruitment to Tuberculosis Lesions. *Front. Immunol.* **2018**, *9*. [CrossRef] [PubMed]
23. Gailey, M.P.; Keeney, M.E.; Jensen, C.S. A cytomorphometric analysis of pulmonary and mediastinal granulomas: Differentiating histoplasmosis from sarcoidosis by fine-needle aspiration. *Cancer Cytopathol.* **2014**, *123*, 51–58. [CrossRef] [PubMed]
24. Okamoto, H.; Mizuno, K.; Horio, T. Monocyte-derived multinucleated giant cells and sarcoidosis. *J. Dermatol. Sci.* **2003**, *31*, 119–128. [CrossRef]
25. Kermani, T.A. Takayasu arteritis and giant cell arteritis: Are they a spectrum of the same disease? *Int. J. Rheum. Dis.* **2018**, *22* (Suppl. 1), 41–48. [CrossRef]
26. Berclaz, P.Y.; Shibata, Y.; Whitsett, J.A.; Trapnell, B.C. GM-CSF, via PU.1, regulates alveolar macrophage Fcgamma R-mediated phagocytosis and the IL-18/IFN-gamma -mediated molecular connection between innate and adaptive immunity in the lung. *Blood* **2002**, *100*, 4193–4200. [CrossRef]
27. Trapnell, B.C.; Whitsett, J.A. Gm-CSF regulates pulmonary surfactant homeostasis and alveolar macrophage-mediated innate host defense. *Annu. Rev. Physiol.* **2002**, *64*, 775–802. [CrossRef]

28. Quell, K.M.; Karsten, C.M.; Kordowski, A.; Almeida, L.N.; Briukhovetska, D.; Wiese, A.V.; Sun, J.; Ender, F.; Antoniou, K.; Schröder, T.; et al. Monitoring C3aR Expression Using a Floxed tdTomato-C3aR Reporter Knock-in Mouse. *J. Immunol.* **2017**, *199*, 688–706. [CrossRef]
29. Guilliams, M.; De Kleer, I.; Henri, S.; Post, S.; Vanhoutte, L.; De Prijck, S.; Deswarte, K.; Malissen, B.; Hammad, H.; Lambrecht, B. Alveolar macrophages develop from fetal monocytes that differentiate into long-lived cells in the first week of life via GM-CSF. *J. Exp. Med.* **2013**, *210*, 1977–1992. [CrossRef]
30. Hachim, D.; Lopresti, S.T.; Rege, R.D.; Umeda, Y.; Iftikhar, A.; Nolfi, A.L.; Skillen, C.D.; Brown, B.N. Distinct macrophage populations and phenotypes associated with IL-4 mediated immunomodulation at the host implant interface. *Biomater. Sci.* **2020**. [CrossRef]
31. Whitsett, J.A.; Wert, S.E.; Weaver, T.E. Alveolar surfactant homeostasis and the pathogenesis of pulmonary disease. *Annu Rev. Med.* **2010**, *61*, 105–119. [CrossRef] [PubMed]
32. Kawasaki, T.; Ito, K.; Miyata, H.; Akira, S.; Kawai, T. Deletion of PIKfyve alters alveolar macrophage populations and exacerbates allergic inflammation in mice. *EMBO J.* **2017**, *36*, 1707–1718. [CrossRef]
33. Lampiasi, N.; Russo, R.; Zito, F. The Alternative Faces of Macrophage Generate Osteoclasts. *BioMed Res. Int.* **2016**, *2016*, 1–9. [CrossRef] [PubMed]
34. Lemaire, I.; Yang, H. Colony Stimulating Factors Induce Alveolar Macrophage Differentiation and Giant Cell Formation. *Ann. N. Y. Acad. Sci.* **1996**, *796*, 173–181. [CrossRef] [PubMed]
35. Iljine, D.A.; Arkhipov, S.A.; Shkurupy, V.A. In Vitro Expression of IL-1α, GM-CSF, and TNF-α by Multinucleated Macrophages from BCG-Infected Mice. *Bull. Exp. Biol. Med.* **2013**, *155*, 663–666. [CrossRef] [PubMed]
36. Suzuki, T.; McCarthy, C.; Carey, B.C.; Borchers, M.; Beck, D.; Wikenheiser-Brokamp, K.A.; Black, D.; Chalk, C.; Trapnell, B.C. Increased Pulmonary GM-CSF Causes Alveolar Macrophage Accumulation. Mechanistic Implications for Desquamative Interstitial Pneumonitis. *Am. J. Respir. Cell Mol. Biol.* **2020**, *62*, 87–94. [CrossRef]
37. Zhang, J.; Chen, J.; Robinson, C. Cellular and Molecular Events in the Airway Epithelium Defining the Interaction between House Dust Mite Group 1 Allergens and Innate Defences. *Int. J. Mol. Sci.* **2018**, *19*, 3549. [CrossRef]
38. Llop-Guevara, A.; Chu, D.K.; Walker, T.D.; Goncharova, S.; Fattouh, R.; Silver, J.S.; Moore, C.L.; Xie, J.L.; O'Byrne, P.M.; Coyle, A.J.; et al. A GM-CSF/IL-33 Pathway Facilitates Allergic Airway Responses to Sub-Threshold House Dust Mite Exposure. *PLoS ONE* **2014**, *9*, e88714. [CrossRef]
39. Locke, L.W.; Crouser, E.D.; White, P.; Julian, M.W.; Caceres, E.G.; Papp, A.C.; Le, V.T.; Sadee, W.; Schlesinger, L.S. IL-13–regulated Macrophage Polarization during Granuloma Formation in an In Vitro Human Sarcoidosis Model. *Am. J. Respir. Cell Mol. Biol.* **2019**, *60*, 84–95. [CrossRef]
40. Chen, W.; Sivaprasad, U.; Gibson, A.M.; Ericksen, M.B.; Cunningham, C.M.; Bass, S.A.; Kinker, K.G.; Finkelman, F.D.; Wills-Karp, M.; Hershey, G.K.K. IL-13 receptor α2 contributes to development of experimental allergic asthma. *J. Allergy Clin. Immunol.* **2013**, *132*, 951–958.e1. [CrossRef]
41. Roy, S.; Liu, H.Y.; Jaeson, M.I.; Deimel, L.P.; Ranasinghe, C. Unique IL-13Ralpha2/STAT3 mediated IL-13 regulation detected in lung conventional dendritic cells, 24 h post viral vector vaccination. *Sci. Rep.* **2020**, *10*, 1017. [CrossRef] [PubMed]
42. Kurowska-Stolarska, M.; Stolarski, B.; Kewin, P.; Murphy, G.; Corrigan, C.J.; Ying, S.; Pitman, N.; Mirchandani, A.; Rana, B.; Van Rooijen, N.; et al. IL-33 Amplifies the Polarization of Alternatively Activated Macrophages That Contribute to Airway Inflammation. *J. Immunol.* **2009**, *183*, 6469–6477. [CrossRef] [PubMed]
43. Desbois, A.-C.; Cacoub, P.; Leroyer, A.S.; Tellier, E.; Garrido, M.; Maciejewski-Duval, A.; Comarmond, C.; Barete, S.; Arock, M.; Bruneval, P.; et al. Immunomodulatory role of Interleukin-33 in large vessel vasculitis. *Sci. Rep.* **2020**, *10*, 1–11. [CrossRef] [PubMed]
44. Kempf, W.; Zollinger, T.; Sachs, M.; Ullmer, E.; Cathomas, G.; Dirnhofer, S.; Mertz, K.D. Granulomas are a source of interleukin-33 expression in pulmonary and extrapulmonary sarcoidosis. *Hum. Pathol.* **2014**, *45*, 2202–2210. [CrossRef] [PubMed]
45. Soto, M.; García-Santisteban, I.; Krenning, L.; Medema, R.H.; Raaijmakers, J.A. Chromosomes trapped in micronuclei are liable to segregation errors. *J. Cell Sci.* **2018**, *131*, jcs214742. [CrossRef] [PubMed]
46. Harding, S.M.; Benci, J.L.; Irianto, J.; Discher, D.E.; Minn, A.J.; Greenberg, R.A. Mitotic progression following

DNA damage enables pattern recognition within micronuclei. *Nat. Cell Biol.* **2017**, *548*, 466–470. [CrossRef] [PubMed]

47. Morales, A.J.; Carrero, J.A.; Hung, P.J.; Tubbs, A.T.; Andrews, J.; Edelson, B.T.; Calderon, B.; Innes, C.L.; Paules, R.S.; Payton, J.E.; et al. A type I IFN-dependent DNA damage response regulates the genetic program and inflammasome activation in macrophages. *eLife* **2017**, *6*, e24655. [CrossRef]
48. Divangahi, M.; King, I.L.; Pernet, E. Alveolar macrophages and type I IFN in airway homeostasis and immunity. *Trends Immunol.* **2015**, *36*, 307–314. [CrossRef]
49. Kumagai, Y.; Takeuchi, O.; Kato, H.; Kumar, H.; Matsui, K.; Morii, E.; Aozasa, K.; Kawai, T.; Akira, S. Alveolar macrophages are the primary interferon-alpha producer in pulmonary infection with RNA viruses. *Immunity* **2007**, *27*, 240–252. [CrossRef]
50. Westphalen, K.; Gusarova, G.A.; Islam, M.N.; Subramanian, M.; Cohen, T.S.; Prince, A.S.; Bhattacharya, J. Sessile alveolar macrophages communicate with alveolar epithelium to modulate immunity. *Nat. Cell Biol.* **2014**, *506*, 503–506. [CrossRef]
51. Lemaire, I. Purinergic signaling in giant cell formation. *Front. Biosci.* **2012**, *4*, 41. [CrossRef]
52. Li, R.; Shang, Y.; Hu, X.; Yu, Y.; Zhou, T.; Xiong, W.; Zou, X. ATP/P2X7r axis mediates the pathological process of allergic asthma by inducing M2 polarization of alveolar macrophages. *Exp. Cell Res.* **2020**, *386*, 111708. [CrossRef] [PubMed]
53. Hastak, K.; Paul, R.K.; Agarwal, M.K.; Thakur, V.S.; Amin, A.R.M.R.; Agrawal, S.; Sramkoski, R.M.; Jacobberger, J.W.; Jackson, M.W.; Stark, G.R.; et al. DNA synthesis from unbalanced nucleotide pools causes limited DNA damage that triggers ATR-CHK1-dependent p53 activation. *Proc. Natl. Acad. Sci. USA* **2008**, *105*, 6314–6319. [CrossRef] [PubMed]
54. Liebl, M.C.; Hofmann, T.G. Cell Fate Regulation upon DNA Damage: p53 Serine 46 Kinases Pave the Cell Death Road. *BioEssays* **2019**, *41*, e1900127. [CrossRef] [PubMed]
55. Makinwa, Y.; Musich, P.R.; Zou, Y. Phosphorylation-Dependent Pin1 Isomerization of ATR: Its Role in Regulating ATR's Anti-apoptotic Function at Mitochondria, and the Implications in Cancer. *Front. Cell Dev. Biol.* **2020**, *8*, 281. [CrossRef]
56. Sato, M.; Shibata, Y.; Kimura, T.; Yamauchi, K.; Abe, S.; Inoue, S.; Kishi, H.; Oizumi, H.; Kubota, I. Immunohistochemical staining for transcription factor MafB in alveolar macrophages is correlated with spirometric measures of airflow limitation in smokers. *Respirology* **2010**, *16*, 124–130. [CrossRef]
57. Cuevas, V.D.; Anta, L.; Samaniego, R.; Orta-Zavalza, E.; De La Rosa, J.V.; Baujat, G.; Domínguez-Soto, Á.; Sánchez-Mateos, P.; Escribese, M.M.; Castrillo, A.; et al. MAFB Determines Human Macrophage Anti-Inflammatory Polarization: Relevance for the Pathogenic Mechanisms Operating in Multicentric Carpotarsal Osteolysis. *J. Immunol.* **2017**, *198*, 2070–2081. [CrossRef]
58. Horn, V.; Triantafyllopoulou, A. DNA damage signaling and polyploid macrophages in chronic inflammation. *Curr. Opin. Immunol.* **2018**, *50*, 55–63. [CrossRef]
59. Kim, H. The transcription factor MafB promotes anti-inflammatory M2 polarization and cholesterol efflux in macrophages. *Sci. Rep.* **2017**, *7*, 1–15. [CrossRef]
60. Woolley, K.L.; Gibson, P.G.; Carty, K.; Wilson, A.J.; Twaddell, S.H.; Woolley, M.J. Eosinophil apoptosis and the resolution of airway inflammation in asthma. *Am. J. Respir. Crit. Care Med.* **1996**, *154*, 237–243. [CrossRef]
61. Vandivier, R.W.; Henson, P.M.; Douglas, I.S. Burying the dead: The impact of failed apoptotic cell removal (efferocytosis) on chronic inflammatory lung disease. *Chest* **2006**, *129*, 1673–1682. [CrossRef] [PubMed]
62. Cui, Y.; Hill, A.W. Atopy and Specific Cancer Sites: A Review of Epidemiological Studies. *Clin. Rev. Allergy Immunol.* **2016**, *51*, 338–352. [CrossRef] [PubMed]
63. Jensen-Jarolim, E.; Bax, H.J.; Bianchini, R.; Crescioli, S.; Daniels-Wells, T.R.; Dombrowicz, D.; Fiebiger, E.; Gould, H.J.; Irshad, S.; Janda, J.; et al. AllergoOncology: Opposite outcomes of immune tolerance in allergy and cancer. *Allergy* **2017**, *73*, 328–340. [CrossRef] [PubMed]
64. Pellizzari, G.; Bax, H.J.; Josephs, D.H.; Gotovina, J.; Jensen-Jarolim, E.; Spicer, J.; Karagiannis, S.N. Harnessing Therapeutic IgE Antibodies to Re-educate Macrophages against Cancer. *Trends Mol. Med.* **2020**, *26*, 615–626. [CrossRef]

65. Ender, F.; Wiese, A.V.; Schmudde, I.; Sun, J.; Vollbrandt, T.; König, P.; Laumonnier, Y.; Köhl, J. Differential regulation of C5a receptor 1 in innate immune cells during the allergic asthma effector phase. *PLoS ONE* **2017**, *12*, e0172446. [CrossRef]
66. Rhoads, D.D.; Roufa, D.J. Emetine resistance of Chinese hamster cells: Structures of wild-type and mutant ribosomal protein S14 mRNAs. *Mol. Cell. Biol.* **1985**, *5*, 1655–1659. [CrossRef]

2

ER Stress is Involved in Epithelial-to-Mesenchymal Transition of Alveolar Epithelial Cells Exposed to a Hypoxic Microenvironment

Eva Delbrel [1], Yurdagül Uzunhan [1,2], Abdoulaye Soumare [1], Thomas Gille [1,2], Dominique Marchant [1], Carole Planès [1,2] and Emilie Boncoeur [1,*]

1 Université Paris 13, Sorbonne Paris Cité, Laboratoire 'Hypoxie & Poumon' (Inserm U1272), F-93017 Bobigny, France; eva.delbrel@univ-paris13.fr (E.D.); yurdagul.uzunhan@aphp.fr (Y.U.); abdoulaye.soumare@hotmail.com (A.S.); gille.tom@gmail.com (T.G.); dom.marchant@yahoo.fr (D.M.); carole.planes@aphp.fr (C.P.)

2 Assistance Publique Hôpitaux de Paris (APHP), Hôpital Avicenne, F-93017 Bobigny, France

* Correspondence: emilie.boncoeur@univ-paris13.fr

Abstract: Background: Idiopathic pulmonary fibrosis (IPF) is a chronic, progressive and fatal interstitial lung disease of unknown origin. Alveolar epithelial cells (AECs) play an important role in the fibrotic process as they undergo sustained endoplasmic reticulum (ER) stress, and may acquire a mesenchymal phenotype through epithelial-to-mesenchymal transition (EMT), two phenomena that could be induced by localized alveolar hypoxia. Here we investigated the potential links between hypoxia, ER stress and EMT in AECs. Methods: ER stress and EMT markers were assessed by immunohistochemistry, western blot and qPCR analysis, both in vivo in rat lungs exposed to normoxia or hypoxia (equivalent to 8% O_2) for 48 h, and in vitro in primary rat AECs exposed to normoxia or hypoxia (1.5% O_2) for 2–6 days. Results: Hypoxia induced expression of mesenchymal markers, pro-EMT transcription factors, and the activation of ER stress markers both in vivo in rat lungs, and in vitro in AECs. In vitro, pharmacological inhibition of ER stress by 4-PBA limited hypoxia-induced EMT. Calcium chelation or hypoxia-inducible factor (HIF) inhibition also prevented EMT induction under hypoxic condition. Conclusions: Hypoxia and intracellular calcium are both involved in EMT induction of AECs, mainly through the activation of ER stress and HIF signaling pathways.

Keywords: hypoxia; ER stress; alveolar epithelial cell; loss of phenotype

---

1. Introduction

Idiopathic pulmonary fibrosis (IPF) is a chronic, progressive and fatal interstitial lung disease of unknown origin. According to the prevailing hypothesis, IPF could be caused due to repetitive micro-injuries of the alveolar epithelium, followed by inefficient and/or aberrant epithelial repair and uncontrolled (myo)fibroblast proliferation, leading to excessive extracellular matrix deposition and destruction of distal lung architecture [1]. Indeed, in IPF lungs, some alveolar epithelial cells (AECs) become hyperplastic with abnormal activation and production of profibrotic factors such as TGF-β1, while other AECs undergo massive apoptosis. AECs may even acquire a mesenchymal phenotype through a process of epithelial-to-mesenchymal transition (EMT) [2–4]. In the last decade, chronic endoplasmic reticulum (ER) stress of AECs has been recognized as a key pathogenic event in lung fibrosis. ER stress is defined by the activation of the unfolded protein response (UPR) pathways to restore ER homeostasis [5,6].

This implies activation of the following transcription factors: activating transcription factor 4 (ATF4), ATF6N, and spliced X-box binding protein 1 (sXBP1), in order to inhibit protein translation, to increase chaperon synthesis, and to promote the ER activated degradation (ERAD) machinery. Altogether, ER stress and the UPR activation contribute to improve protein folding, and limit the formation of protein aggregates. First described in familial cases of lung fibrosis due to surfactant protein mutations, ER stress in AECs was also evidenced in sporadic cases of IPF [7,8]. We and others recently proposed that localized alveolar hypoxia could represent an important trigger for ER stress and subsequent UPR activation in AECs from sporadic IPF [9,10].

Localized alveolar hypoxia may likely occur in the course of IPF because of fibrotic lung remodeling and collapse of distal airspaces. Accordingly, the expression of the hypoxia-inducible factor 1α (HIF-1α) has been evidenced in AECs from IPF lungs as well as in AECs from mouse lungs treated with bleomycin, a drug known to induce pulmonary fibrosis [11,12]. We and others have reported in vitro, that hypoxic microenvironment induces phenotypic changes of primary AECs characterizing the EMT process. Indeed, HIF-1α can directly regulate EMT-inducing-genes through fixation on its hypoxia responsive element (HRE), but also promotes the pro-EMT transforming growth factor β (TGF-β) signaling pathways [13,14]. Furthermore, modulation of intracellular calcium has been reported in AECs exposed to hypoxia [15] and could be related to the induction of EMT features [16]. Hypoxic exposure may also lead to calcium depletion from the ER [15], thereby inducing ER stress. Although ER stress may promote EMT in some cell types [17], the potential involvement of chronic ER stress in hypoxia-induced EMT of AECs has never been studied. Here, we hypothesized that ER stress and activation of UPR pathways could contribute to EMT-associated phenotypic changes observed in AECs exposed to hypoxic stress, and that disturbance of intracellular calcium signaling could play a role in this process.

The objectives of the present study were therefore to examine the role of ER stress in the induction of EMT features in AECs exposed to hypoxia in vivo and in vitro, and to decipher the cellular mechanisms involved. We particularly studied the potential role of calcium, an important determinant of ER homeostasis. Our results provide evidence that ER stress and HIF-1 signaling pathways are both involved in the induction of EMT of AECs exposed to hypoxia, and suggest that any disturbance of intracellular calcium homeostasis plays a crucial role in this process.

2. Results

2.1. Acute Hypoxia Upregulates UPR Pathways and Induces Phenotypic Alterations of Alveolar Epithelial Cells in Rat Lungs

To evaluate the effect of hypoxia on UPR pathways in vivo, rats were exposed to a hypoxic atmosphere (equivalent to 8% FiO_2) for 16 to 72 h. Compared to normoxia, exposure to hypoxia induced the three pathways of UPR signaling in lung tissues, as shown by western blot experiments (Figure 1A–C). A significant increase in ATF4 expression was observed after 24 h exposure ($p < 0.05$) as compared to normoxia, with no significant decrease at 48 h exposure (Figure 1A). To study the activation of the ATF6α pathway, the cleaved form of ATF6N (50 kDa) was quantified and the ATF6N/ATF6 ratio was compared in normoxic and hypoxic conditions. When normalized to β-actin, the exposure of rats to 24 h hypoxia led to a 4.2-fold increase of the ATF6N protein level compared to normoxia (Figure 1B), as well as an increase in the ATF6N/ATF6 ratio (2.8 ± 1.1, $p < 0.05$). This ATF6N expression was maintained at 48 h of hypoxic exposure, and a more than two-fold increase of the ATF6N/ATF6 ratio was still observed (2.08 ± 0.9). To study the activation of the XBP1 pathway, the spliced form of XBP1 (sXBP1: 55 kDa) was quantified, and sXBP1/XBP1 ratio was compared in normoxic and hypoxic conditions. When normalized to β-actin, exposure of rats to 24 h hypoxia led to a 3.8-fold increase of the sXBP1 protein level compared to normoxia (Figure 1C). This expression was maintained at 48 h of hypoxic exposure. However, no change in the sXBP1/XBP1 ratio was observed.

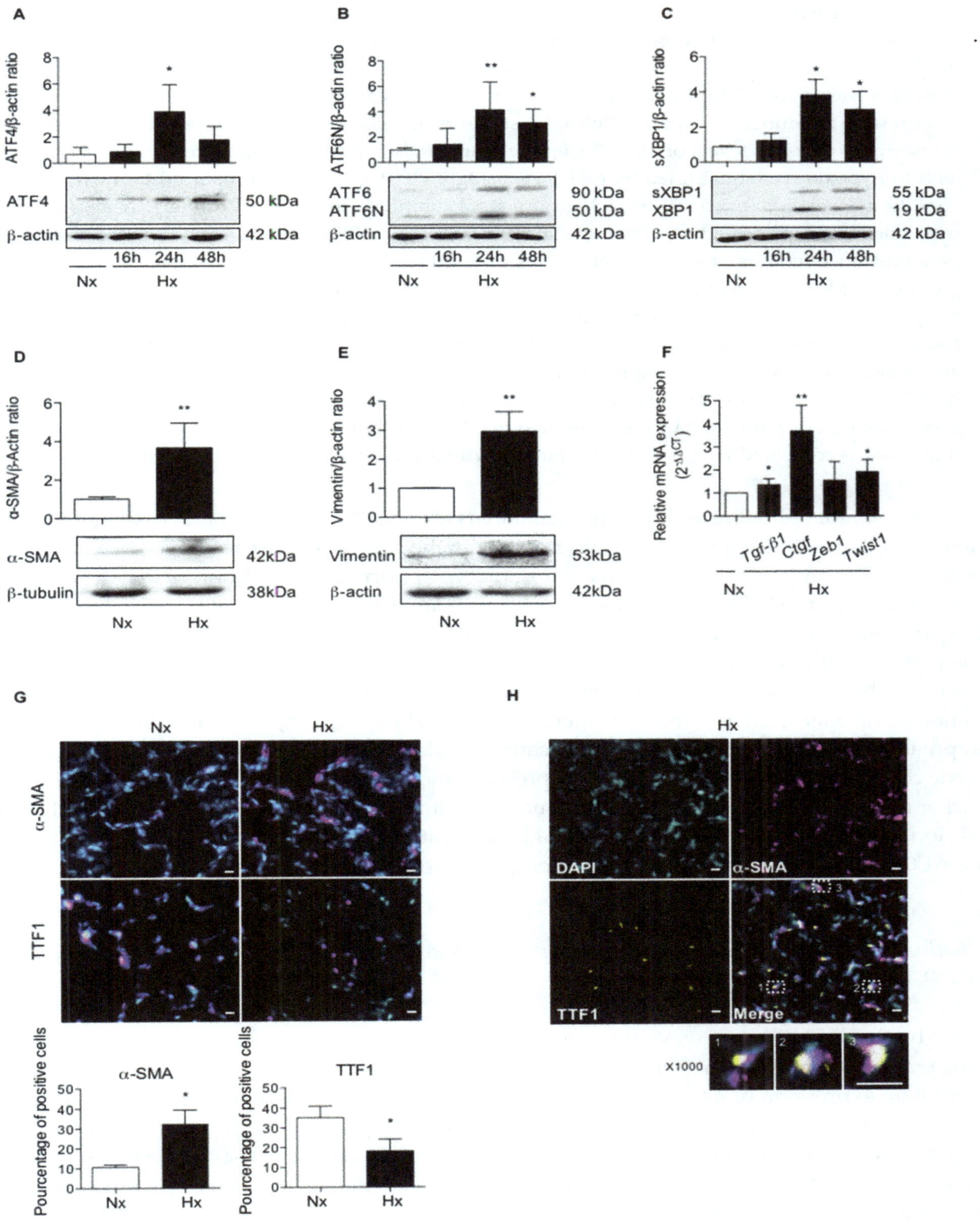

Figure 1. Hypoxia induces UPR pathways and modulates epithelial and mesenchymal markers expression in lungs of rats exposed to hypoxia. (**A**) Lungs of rats stabulated in normoxia (Nx) (21% O_2) or exposed to hypoxia (Hx) (equivalent to 8% FiO_2) during 16 h, 24 h, 48 h or 72 h were isolated and used for western blotting, immunohistochemistry and RT-qPCR analyses. Western blot of ATF4 protein, (**B**) ATF6N/ATF6 and (**C**) spliced XBP1 (sXBP1)/XBP1 were performed in lung homogenates. Representative blot of $n = 8$ experiments is shown. Quantification has been done and expression levels of ATF4, ATF6N or sXBP1 was reported to the β-actin expression level for each condition. Raw data were submitted to a Kruskal-Wallis one-way analysis of variance. * indicate a significant difference as

compared with normoxic condition ($p < 0.05$). (**D**) Western blot of α-SMA protein and (**E**) vimentin were performed in lung homogenates from rat exposed to a 72 h-hypoxia. Representative blot of $n = 5$ experiments is shown. Quantification has been done and the expression of α-SMA (**D**) and vimentin was reported to the β-actin expression for each condition. Raw data ($n = 5$ rats in each group) were submitted to a Mann-Whitney test and relative expression was represented. (**F**) mRNA transcript expression levels of *Tgf-β1, Ctgf, Zeb1* and *Twist1* in lungs homogenates of rats exposed 48 h to hypoxia were quantified by qRT-PCR using $2^{-\Delta\Delta CT}$ method and reported to the normoxic condition. Raw data ($n = 5$ rats in each group) were submitted to a Mann-Whitney test and relative expression was represented. (**G**) Immunostaining of α-SMA or TTF1 were performed on 5 μm slices of paraffin-embedded from the left lobe of rat lung exposed to 72 h normoxia or hypoxia. A representative picture of at least $n = 5$ independent experiments for each condition has been presented. Original magnification: × 200 and scale bars represent 20 μm. Raw data were submitted to a Mann-Whitney test and relative expression was represented. (**H**) Co-staining for α-SMA (magenta), TTF1 (yellow), and DAPI to localize nuclei (in cyan) is shown (original magnification: × 400 or × 1000). Percentage of α-SMA or TTF1 positive cells in the lung of rats exposed 72 h to hypoxia as compared to normoxia ($n = 5$ rats in each group). Raw data were submitted to a Mann-Whitney test * and ** indicate a significant difference as compared with normoxic condition with a $p < 0.05$ and $p < 0.01$, respectively.

Expression of epithelial and mesenchymal markers was studied in parallel in lung homogenates of rat exposed to a 72 h-hypoxia. A 3-fold increase in the protein expression of α-SMA and vimentin was observed in hypoxic condition, as compared with normoxic condition ($p < 0.01$ and $p < 0.01$, respectively) (Figure 1D,E). In a previous work, our team demonstrated that hypoxia induces in vitro the expression of *Tgf-β1, Ctgf, Zeb1* and *Twist1* mRNA in AECs, four well-known genes involved in the process of EMT [18]. The effect of exposure to 48 h hypoxia on mRNA transcript expression levels of all these markers was therefore studied in rat lung homogenates (Figure 1F). As compared with normoxic condition, a significant increase in *Tgf-β1* expression, *Ctgf*, and *Twist1* was observed in hypoxic lungs ($p < 0.05$), while no significant modulation of *Zeb1* expression was observed in the hypoxic condition (Figure 1F). Finally, the expression and the localization of α-SMA and TTF1 (used as a marker of alveolar epithelial cells), were studied by immunofluorescence (Figure 1G,H). In hypoxic condition, co-immunostaining studies strongly suggest that α-SMA and TTF1 were co-expressed in some AECs (Figure 1H), consistent with an ongoing process of EMT.

2.2. Activation of UPR Pathways is Involved in the Loss of Alveolar Epithelial Cell Phenotype Induced in Vitro by Hypoxic Exposure

Activation of UPR pathways was confirmed in vitro in primary rat AECs exposed for 6 h to hypoxia. As compared with normoxia, hypoxia led to a significant increase of ATF4 and ATF6N/ATF6 ratio protein expression ($p < 0.01$) (Figure 2A,B). Of note, we recently reported that the XBP1 spliced form was induced only after 16 h of hypoxic exposure [10]. In primary AECs transfected with plasmids coding for luciferase reporter activity of amino acid response element (ATF4-luc) or ER stress response element (ATF6N/sXBP1-luc), a significant induction of the luciferase activity was observed in response to hypoxia ($p < 0.01$) (Figure 2C,D). The ER stress inhibitor 4-phenylbutyrate (4-PBA), known as a chemical chaperone, limits UPR pathway activation. Indeed, treatment of AECs with 4-PBA fully prevented the increase in ATF4 protein expression and the ATF6N/ATF6 ratio ($p < 0.05$) (Figure 2A,B). Furthermore, treatment with 4-PBA also abolished the increase in ATF4 (Figure 2C) and ATF6N (Figure 2D) response element activities induced by hypoxia ($p < 0.05$).

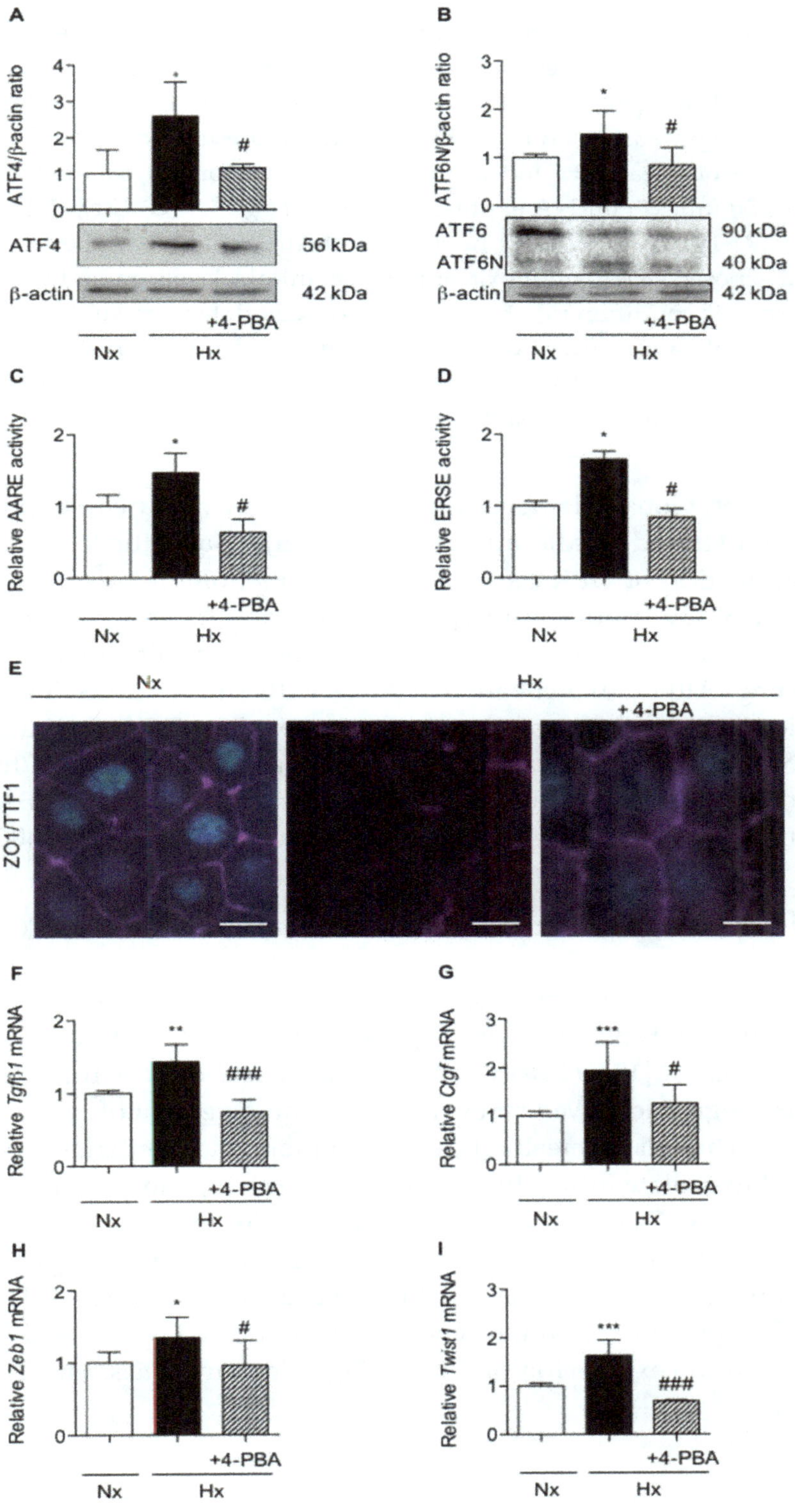

Figure 2. Inhibition of UPR pathways prevents loss of alveolar epithelial cells phenotype in primary rat alveolar epithelial cells exposed to hypoxia. Isolated primary rat AECs were cultured in normoxia (Nx) (21% O_2) or hypoxia (Hx) (1.5% O_2) during various periods in the presence or absence of 100 mM 4-phenylbutyrate (4-PBA). (**A**) Western blot of ATF4 protein and (**B**) ATF6N/ATF6 ratio were performed primary AECs exposed 6 h to hypoxia. Representative blot of $n = 5$ experiments is shown. Quantification has been done and the expression levels of ATF4 and ATF6 were reported to the β-actin expression for each condition. (**C**) Primary rat AECs transfected with plasmid coding for luciferase reporter activity

of amino acid response element (AARE: i.e., ATF4-luc) or (**D**) endoplasmic reticulum stress element (ERSE: i.e., ATF6N/sXBP1-luc), were treated or not with 100 mM 4-PBA and exposed 6 h in hypoxic condition. (**C**) Luciferase activity corresponding to the transcriptional capacity of ATF4 or (**D**) ATF6N was measured. (**E**) ZO-1 (magenta) and TTF1 (cyan) immunostaining were performed on rat AECs cultured on filter and exposed for 6-days to hypoxia in the presence or absence of 100 mM 4-PBA. A representative picture of at least $n = 5$ independent experiments for each condition has been presented. Scale bar represents 50 µm. (**F**) mRNA expression levels of *Tgf-β1*, (**G**) *Ctgf*, (H) *Zeb1* and (I) *Twist1* were quantified by qRT-PCR using $2^{-\Delta\Delta CT}$ method in rat AECs cultured in the presence or absence of 100 mM 4-PBA and exposed 48 h to normoxia or hypoxia. mRNA levels under hypoxic condition were reported to the normoxic condition ($n = 5$ experiments). Raw data were submitted a Kruskal-Wallis test. *, ** and *** indicate a significant difference as compared with normoxic value with $p < 0.05$, $p < 0.01$ and $p < 0.001$ respectively. # and ### indicate a significant difference as compared with value in untreated hypoxic cells with $p < 0.05$ and $p < 0.001$, respectively.

We and others have previously demonstrated that a 6 day-exposure to hypoxia led to a change of AECs morphology, as illustrated by alteration of ZO-1 staining and the loss of TTF1 expression [18]. To investigate the implication of UPR pathways in this phenomenon, AECs were incubated with 4-PBA and cultured for 6 days under the hypoxic condition. As shown in Figure 2E, exposure of AECs to hypoxia led to a decrease in TTF1 expression and to modifications in cell morphology as assessed by ZO-1 staining. Although incubation of AECs with 4-PBA limited TTF1 and ZO-1 decreases, no significant modification in cell morphology was observed by ZO-1 staining. Then, *Tgf-β1*, *Ctgf*, *Zeb1* and *Twist1* mRNA levels were measured in rat primary AECs exposed for 48 h to hypoxia in the presence or absence of 4-PBA (Figure 2F–I). Treatment of AECs with 4-PBA fully prevented the hypoxia-induced increase in *Tgf-β1*, *Ctgf*, *Zeb1* and *Twist1* mRNA levels ($p < 0.05$) (Figure 2F–I).

2.3. Calcium Chelation Limits Cell Alterations and UPR Pathways Activation in AECs Exposed to Hypoxia

A fine tuning of calcium concentration is essential for ER homeostasis [19]. In AECs, hypoxia may induce calcium influx through L-type calcium channels located at the plasma membrane [20], as well as calcium depletion of the ER [15]. However, little is known about the role of intracellular calcium modulation on ER stress regulation. We first evaluated the involvement of calcium in hypoxia-induced loss of AECs phenotype. The cell permeable 1,2-bis(o-aminophenoxy)ethane-N,N,N,N-tetraacetic acid (BAPTA-AM) was used to chelate intracellular calcium. No change in cell morphology or phenotype was observed in normoxic-AECs treated with BAPTA-AM. Pre-treatment of AECs with BAPTA-AM just before a 6-day hypoxic exposure prevented the changes in cell morphology induced by hypoxia as illustrated by ZO-1 staining and the decrease in TTF1 expression (Figure 3A). The key role of calcium in the change of the AECs phenotype under hypoxia was reinforced by the observation that treatment with BAPTA-AM blunted the expression of *Tgf-β1*, *Ctgf*, *Zeb1* and *Twist1* mRNAs in hypoxic AECs ($p < 0.05$) (Figure 3B–E).

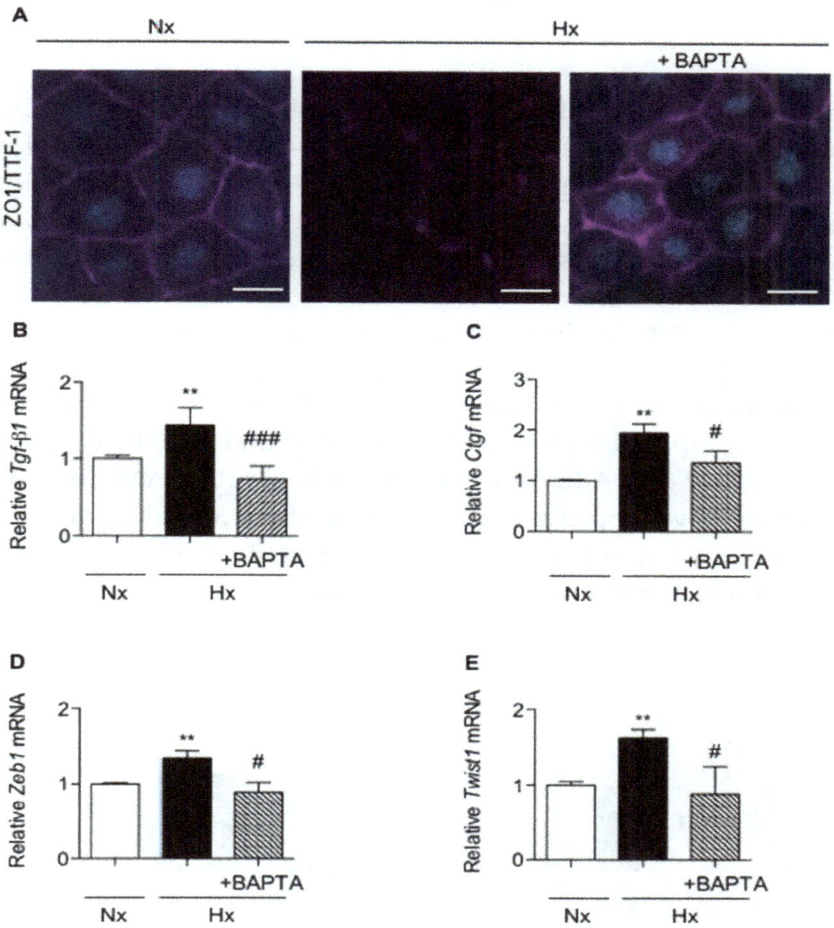

Figure 3. Calcium chelation prevents the loss of epithelial phenotype in primary rat alveolar epithelial cells exposed to hypoxia. Primary rat AECs were treated or not with 1 µM 1,2-bis(o-aminophenoxy)ethane-N,N,N,N-tetraacetic acid (BAPTA-AM) 90 min before exposure to normoxia (Nx) (21% O_2) or hypoxia (Hx) (1.5% O_2) for increasing times. (**A**) ZO-1 (magenta) and TTF1 (cyan) immunostainings were performed after a 6-day exposure. A representative picture of at least $n = 4$ independent experiments for each condition has been presented and scale bar represents 50 µm. (**B**) Expression levels of *Tgf-β1*, (**C**) *Ctgf*, (**D**) *Zeb1* and (**E**) *Twist1* mRNA transcripts were assessed after a 48 h exposure. mRNA levels were quantified by qRT-PCR using $2^{-\Delta\Delta CT}$ method and values in hypoxic cells were reported to values obtained in normoxic condition ($n = 4$ experiments). Raw data were submitted a Kruskal-Wallis test. ** indicate a significant difference as compared with normoxic condition with $p < 0.01$, respectively. # and ## indicate a significant difference as compared with value in untreated hypoxic cells with $p < 0.05$ and $p < 0.01$, respectively.

Furthermore, any expression and transcriptional activity of ATF4 and ATF6N/sXBP1 were fully prevented when AECs were pre-treated with BAPTA before exposure to hypoxia (Figure 4A–D, respectively, $p < 0.05$).

2.4. Pharmacological Inhibition of UPR Pathways and Chelation of Calcium Modulates HIF-1 Expression and Activity

Numerous studies reported that HIF transcription factor could be involved in loss of AECs phenotype [21]. In our model, we showed by immunochemistry that treatment of AECs with the HIF-1 inhibitor YC-1 partially blunted the hypoxic effects on ZO-1 and TTF1 expression (Figure 5A). YC-1 limited TTF1 decrease in response to hypoxia, but no effect on cell morphology as assessed by ZO-1 expression was observed. As ER stress inhibition or calcium chelation also prevented the effect of hypoxia on ZO-1 and TTF1 expression, we next investigated the impact of UPR pathways inhibition or calcium chelation on HIF-1α stabilization and HIF capacity to transactivate the hypoxia responsive elements (HRE) upstream the luciferase gene in response to hypoxia (Figure 5B,C). In AECs exposed for 7 h to hypoxia, HIF-1α protein expression (Figure 5B) and the HRE activity (Figure 5C) were significantly increased as compared with normoxia ($p < 0.05$ and $p < 0.01$ respectively). Interestingly, treatment of AECs with either 4-PBA (to limit ER stress), or BAPTA-AM (to chelate calcium) during hypoxic exposure, completely suppressed the accumulation of HIF-1α protein (Figure 5B) and significantly blunted HIF transcriptional activity (Figure 5C) ($p < 0.01$), suggesting a link between ER stress, intracellular calcium concentration and the HIF pathway.

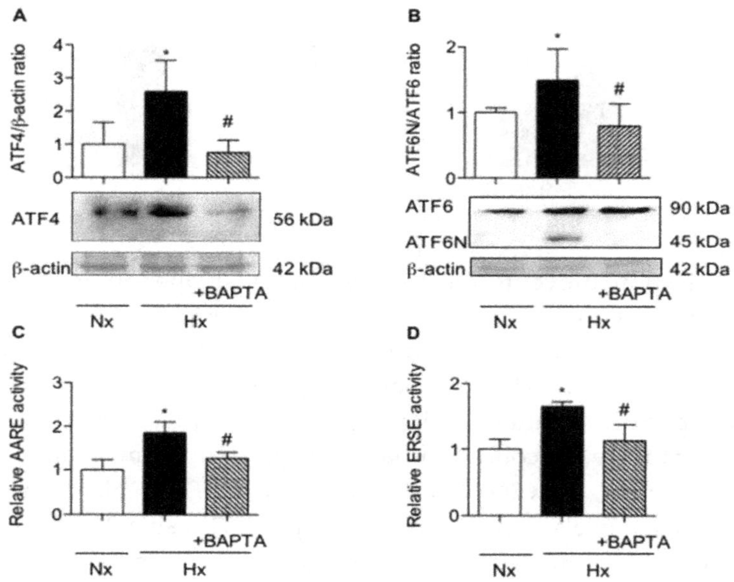

Figure 4. Calcium chelation prevents the induction of UPR pathways in primary rat alveolar epithelial cells exposed to hypoxia. Primary rat AECs were treated or not with 1 μM 1,2-bis(o-aminophenoxy)ethane-N,N,N,N-tetraacetic acid (BAPTA-AM) 90 min before a 6-h exposition to normoxia (Nx) (21% O_2) or hypoxia (Hx) (1.5% O_2). (**A**) Western blot of ATF4 and (**B**) ATF6N/ATF6 ratio were performed. Representative blot of $n = 5$ experiments is shown. Quantification of ATF4 and ATF6N protein expression was performed and was reported to the β-actin expression for each condition. (**C**) Primary rat AECs were transfected with plasmid coding for luciferase reporter activity of amino acid response element (AARE: i.e., ATF4-luc) or (**D**) endoplasmic reticulum stress element (ERSE: i.e., ATF6N/sXBP1-luc), and cultured as describe. (**C**) Luciferase activity corresponding to the transcriptional capacity of ATF4 or (**D**) ATF6N/sXBP1 was measured ($n = 4$ experiments). Raw data were submitted to a Kruskal-Wallis test. * indicates a significant difference against control or normoxic condition ($p < 0.05$). # indicates a significant difference as compared with value in untreated hypoxic cells ($p < 0.05$).

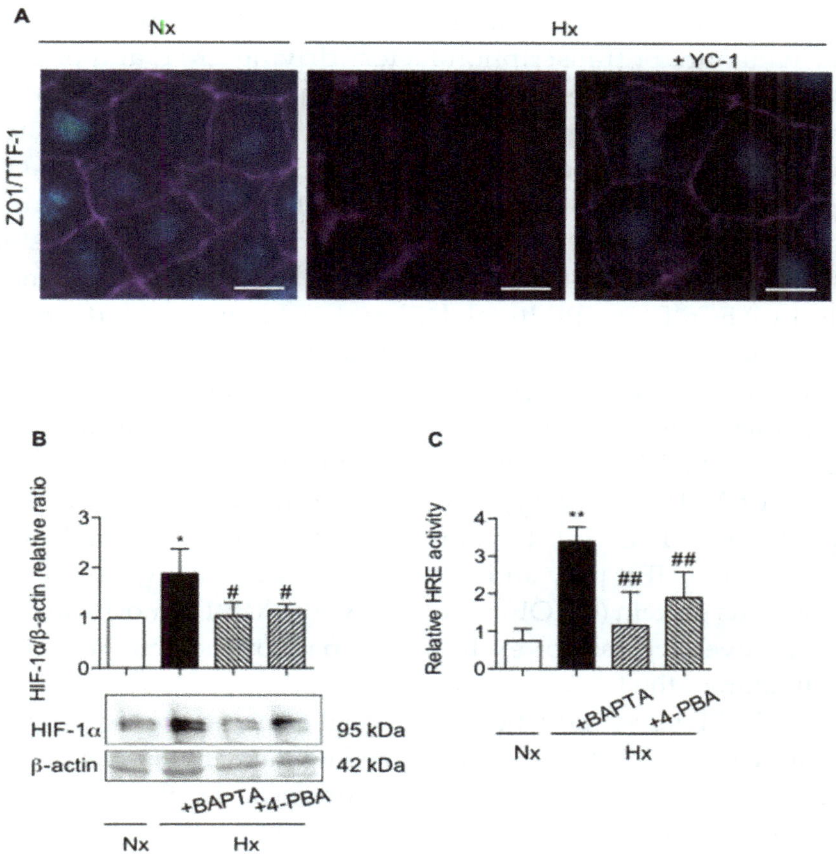

Figure 5. Involvement of HIF-1α in alveolar epithelial cell phenotypic changes induced by hypoxia. Primary rat AECs were cultured in normoxia (Nx) (21% O_2) or hypoxia (Hx) (1.5% O_2) during 6 days in presence or absence of 10 μM YC-1. (**A**) Immunostaining of ZO-1 (magenta) and TTF1 (cyan) were performed. $n = 4$ experiments were performed. Isolated primary rat AECs were cultured in normoxia (Nx) (21% O_2) or hypoxia (Hx) (1.5% O_2) during 6 h in the presence or absence of 100 mM 4-phenylbutyrate (4-PBA) or pre-treated or not with 1 μM BAPTA-AM 90 min before exposition to hypoxia. A representative picture of at least $n = 4$ independent experiments for each condition has been presented and scale bar represents 50 μm. (**B**) Western blot of HIF-1α protein levels was performed. Representative blot of $n = 5$ experiments is shown. Expression levels of HIF-1α were quantified and reported to β-actin expression for each condition. Primary rat AECs were transfected with plasmid coding for luciferase reporter activity of hypoxia responsive element (HRE: i.e., HIF-luc), and cultured as described. (**C**) Luciferase activity corresponding to the transcriptional capacity of HIF was reported ($n = 4$ experiments). Raw data were submitted a Kruskal-Wallis test. * and ** indicate a significant difference as compared with normoxic value with $p < 0.05$ and $p < 0.01$ respectively. # and ## indicate a significant difference as compared with value in untreated hypoxic cells with $p < 0.05$ and $p < 0.01$, respectively.

3. Discussion

Extracellular matrix remodeling and accumulation of fibroblasts and myofibroblasts is a hallmark of IPF. Epithelial-to-mesenchymal transition (EMT) of AECs has been increasingly documented in the fibrogenesis. EMT is mainly initiated by the presence of TGF-β, and we and others proposed that the hypoxic microenvironment of the cells could be an additive trigger for the EMT process in IPF [18,21]. In the present study, we provide evidence that hypoxic exposure and HIF induce EMT-like features in vivo and in vitro in AECs, and that ER stress and UPR-dependent signaling pathways are involved in this process.

Classically, loss of epithelial phenotype and acquisition of mesenchymal characteristics comprise upregulation of α-SMA and vimentin [4,21], modification of tight junction protein ZO-1 [4,17], and induction of transcription factors driving EMT such as *Zeb1* and *Twist1* [21]. In our study, prolonged exposure to hypoxia induced in vivo in rat lungs an overall increase in the expression of mesenchymal markers α-SMA and vimentin, of transcription factors driving EMT, and of pro-fibrotic mediators known to induce EMT. These in vivo results reinforce our previous in vitro work, demonstrating that prolonged exposure to hypoxia is a trigger for epithelial to mesenchymal modifications of AECs [21]. Furthermore, our results show increased expression of α-SMA in alveolar area in lung tissues from rats exposed to hypoxia. Co-immunostaining experiments suggest that the mesenchymal marker α-SMA and the epithelial marker TTF1 are co-expressed in some AECs, consistent with an ongoing process of EMT. Of note, co-expression of alveolar epithelial and mesenchymal markers has been observed previously in AECs from IPF lungs [17] and in bleomycin-induced lung fibrosis in the mouse [22]. Our observation favors the ambiguous role of AECs in the EMT phenomenon contributing to myofibroblasts accumulation in IPF, as previously described [2].

Our in vivo experiments also show that exposure to hypoxia induces the expression of ER stress signaling pathways, ATF4, ATF6N and sXBP1 with a specific time course in rat lung homogenates. Of note, the activation of XBP1 under hypoxia seems to be more delayed than the activation of ATF4 and ATF6α pathways. This result is consistent with previous studies suggesting that the ATF4/ATF6α branches of the UPR play an important role in early events such as apoptosis partly through C/EBP homologous protein (CHOP) induction, while XBP1 is mostly involved in the induction of EMT [10,23,24]. However we cannot exclude that part of the activation of XBP1 could be an implication in the induction of the late apoptosis [25].

Interestingly, in AECs, ER stress induction by thapsigargin or tunicamycin was shown to decrease epithelial markers E-cadherin and ZO-1, to increase the mesenchymal marker α-SMA, and to induce a fibroblast-like morphology consistent with EMT [17]. Furthermore, pharmacological inhibition of ER stress prevents TGF-β1-inducted EMT features [26]. Here, in line with *Mo* et al. [26] work, we observed that the incubation of primary rat AECs with the ER stress pharmacological inhibitor 4-PBA fully prevented the decrease in TTF1 expression induced by hypoxia, and the increase in EMT-like markers *Tgf-β1*, *Ctgf*, *Twist1* and *Zeb1*. However, no significant modification on cell morphology is observed through ZO-1 immunostaining. Interestingly, intracellular calcium chelation with BAPTA-AM had the same effect and prevented the loss of epithelial phenotype induced by hypoxic microenvironment. An important role of calcium as an intracellular messenger within this process has ever been proposed by others since inhibition of specific calcium channels or calcium chelation [16] in lung cancer cells limits TGF-β-induced EMT [27] though the limitation of N-cadherin and vimentin expression. Modulation of intracellular calcium level and ER homeostasis is largely documented. ER senses and integrates changes in calcium concentrations in and outside of the ER, and maintains cellular homeostasis through specific calcium dependent ER-associated proteins and the activation of the UPR pathways [28]. In our work, calcium chelation is able to limit hypoxia-induced ER stress and as a consequence to limit the EMT-like process. This observation is consistent with previous findings highlighting the impact of hypoxia on calcium homeostasis of AECs. Indeed, hypoxic exposure lead to an induction of calcium influx in cultured AECs, mostly through L-type calcium channels [20].

Next, we demonstrate the critical role of HIF-1α in the EMT process. Inhibition of HIF-1α stabilization by YC-1 prevented the loss of TTF1 expression. This observation is in line with studies conducted by Zhou et al. showing EMT features after HIF-1α stabilization in AECs exposed to hypoxia [21]. Interestingly, inhibition of HIF-1α was observed in hypoxic AECs treated either with the calcium chelator BAPTA, or with the ER stress inhibitor 4-PBA. These intriguing results may suggest that induction of EMT in AECs exposed to hypoxia results in a crosstalk between HIF-1α and ER stress signaling pathways. Interestingly, the induction of HIF-1 activity by ER stress has been previously reported in cardiomyocytes during myocardial ischemia-reperfusion [29]. Induction of HIF-1 could also be the result of an unbalance between pro-oxidative and anti-oxidative cellular responses. Interestingly, we previously demonstrated in vitro that hypoxic exposure increases reactive oxygen species (ROS) within AECs, and that this could be related to the activation of HIF-1 [30]. Here, we confirmed in vivo that exposure of rats to hypoxia increases ROS in the lungs (see Supplemental Figure S1A,B). As oxidizing environment is required for disulfide bonds formation within the ER, we tested the impact of antioxidant treatment of AECs with N-acetylcysteine (NAC) on the expression endoplasmic reticulum oxidoreductase 1 (ERO-1) involved in the disulfide bonds formation (Supplemental Figure S1C,D).

We demonstrated ERO-1 induction in response to hypoxia, and showed that treatment of AECs with NAC limited this induction. However, the treatment with NAC did modify neither UPR activation (through the activation of ATF4 or ATF6N/sXBP1 responsive element) nor EMT induction (through the expression of ZO-1 and TTF1) in hypoxic cells (Supplemental Figure S1E,F and Figure 1G,H respectively). These findings suggest that the production of ROS does not play a prominent role in hypoxia-induced ER stress and related EMT.

In conclusion, the present study shows that hypoxia and the microenvironment of injured AECs can trigger epithelial cell dysfunction through induction of EMT features. Our study identifies the ER stress and the calcium present in the environment of the ER as critical elements governing the fate of injured cells. We provide evidence that inhibition of HIF-1α stabilization or pharmacological molecules that relieve ER stress can prevent hypoxia-induced alterations of AECs phenotype, at least in vitro (Figure 6). Taken together, and in accordance with recently published data from Burman et al. [9], our study strengthens the hypothesis that the hypoxic milieu of injured AECs could trigger lung fibrosis. Hypoxic-dependent ER stress signaling pathways could represent an attractive therapeutic approach to ameliorate epithelial abnormalities IPF.

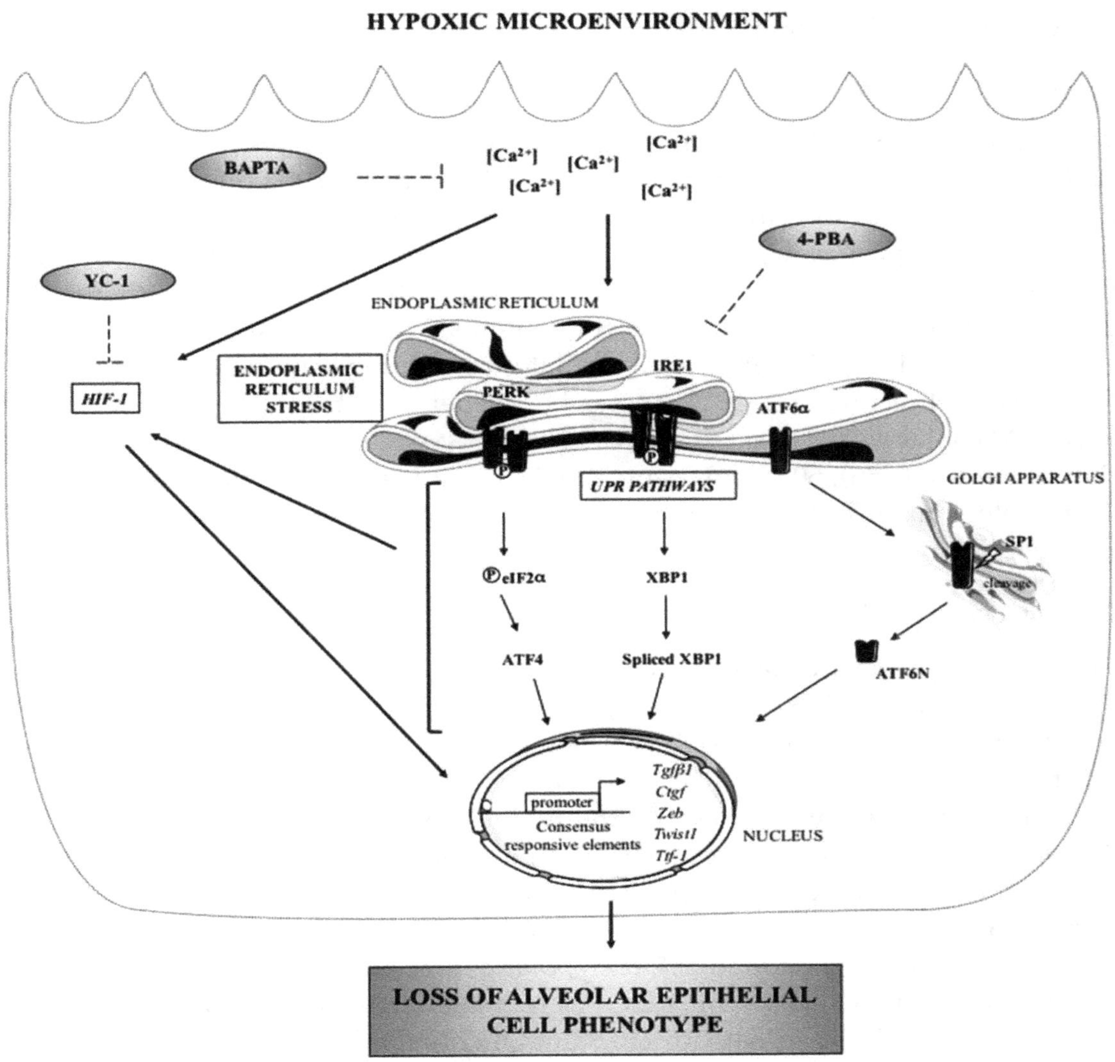

Figure 6. ER stress: a major regulator of the loss of epithelial cell phenotype in hypoxic environment. Loss of alveolar phenotype is a consequence of a long term exposure of the cells to a hypoxic

microenvironment. Hypoxia leads to the activation of the PERK/ATF4 and ATF6α/ATF6N branches of the UPR, to the upregulation of *Tgfβ1*, *Ctgf*, *Zeb1* and *Twist1* gene expression, to a decrease in TTF1 expression, and finally to a disruption of ZO-1 expression (black arrows). In vitro, pharmacological inhibitors (dotted arrow) revealed that this effect is partly mediated by the stabilization of HIF-1α. Calcium chelation induced by BAPTA-AM prevents the loss of epithelial phenotype observed under hypoxia, by blunting the induction of the UPR and HIF-1 transcriptional activity.

4. Materials and Methods

4.1. Rat Model of Acute Hypoxic Exposure

Experiments have been approved by the local ethical committee (Charles Darwin, CE5) in accordance with the European Communities Council for animal care (C2EA-06, authorization APAFIS #7846, approved on September 2017, the 1st). 21-days old male Sprague-Dawley rats (Janvier Labs, St Berthevin, France) were housed four per cage and cared for a 12/12 light/dark cycle in a free food and water environment. Rats were placed for 16 h, 24 h, 48 h or 72 h (n = 6–8 rats per group) in a hypobaric chamber maintained at a pressure of 337 mmHg by a vacuum source at flow rates sufficient to prevent CO2 buildup to simulate an 8% FiO_2. Control rats were kept outside of the hypobaric chamber in the same room. At the end of exposure, animals were anesthetized by intraperitoneal pentobarbital injection (60 mg/kg) and sacrificed by abdominal artery section. The left lobe of the lung was fixed by intratracheal instillation of fresh 4% paraformaldehyde (at 25 cm H_2O transpulmonary pressure). The right lobe of the lung was snap frozen in liquid nitrogen.

4.2. Alveolar Epithelial Cells Isolation

Primary AECs were isolated from four weeks male Sprague-Dawley rats, as describe previously [21] according to a procedure approved by the local ethical committee (Charles Darwin, CE5) (C2EA-06, authorisation C9300801, authorization APAFIS #8150, approved on august 2017, the 8th). Briefly, perfused lungs were digested with 60 U elastase (Worthington, Serlabo, Entraigues-sur-la-Sorgue, France) and AECs were purified by a differential adherence technique on plastic plates (Greiner dishes, Fisher Scientific, Rungis, France). AECs were seeded at 4.5×10^6 cells in 6-well plates or 1×10^6 cells in 24-well plates containing polycarbonate membrane inserts with a pore size of 0.4 µm (Corning™ Transwell™, Fisher Scientific, Rungis, France). Cells were cultured in DMEM containing 25 mM D-glucose, 10 mM Hepes, 23.8 mM NaHCO3, 2 mM L-glutamine, 10% fetal bovine serum (FBS), 50 U/mL penicillin, 50 µg/mL streptomycin, 10 µg/mL gentamycin, 10 µg/mL amphotericin B (Thermo Fisher, Illkirch cedex, France) and placed at 37 °C with 5% CO_2 in a humidified incubator.

4.3. Alveolar Epithelial Cells Treatments

On day 1 after isolation, primary rat AECs were placed in a humidified airtight incubator with inflow and outflow valves and exposed to a hypoxic gas mixture containing 1.5% O_2-5% CO_2-94.5% N_2 (oxygen tension in culture media: 45 mmHg), and kept at 37 °C for six days. Control normoxic cells were maintained in a 21% O_2-5% CO_2-74% N_2 humidified incubator during the same time (oxygen tension in culture media: 140 mmHg). For shorter hypoxic exposure experiments, primary rats AECs were used at day 3 after isolation. Calcium chelation was performed by a 90 min pre-treatment with 1 µM of the cell permeable 1,2-bis(o-aminophenoxy)ethane-N,N,N,N-tetraacetic acid (BAPTA-AM) (Sigma Aldrich, Saint Quentin Fallavier, France). Culture medium was removed, cells were washed with PBS and fresh medium was added before hypoxic exposure.

To inhibit UPR pathways activation, AECs were treated with 100 mM of the ER stress inhibitor 4-phenylbutyric acid (4-PBA) (Sigma Aldrich, Saint Quentin Fallavier, France) and exposed for 6 h or 6-days hypoxia. To inhibit HIF-1α stabilization, AECs were treated with 10 µM 5′-hydroxymethyl-2′-furyl)-1-benzyl indazole (YC-1) and exposed for 6 h or 6-days hypoxia.

4.4. In Vivo and In Vitro Immunofluorescence Stainings

In vivo, after exposure for 72 h to hypoxia, fixed rat lungs were dehydrated, paraffin embedded, and sections of 5 μM were collected on classical Superfrost™ Plus microscope slides (Fisher Scientific, Rungis, France). Tissue sections were submitted to a pH 6 antigen retrieval, kept in a 2% BSA-5% goat serum blocking solution for 1 h at room temperature and incubated overnight at 4 °C with 1:500 anti-mouse alpha-smooth muscle actin (α-SMA) (A2547, Sigma Aldrich, Saint Quentin Fallavier, France) and 1:500 anti-rabbit thyroid transcription factor-1 (TTF1) solution antibodies (WRAB-1231, Seven hills, Cincinnati, OH, USA). Tissue sections were rinsed with PBS and incubated in 1:200 Alexa 568 Fluor® conjugated secondary antibody solution (Invitrogen, Thermo Fisher, Illkirch cedex, France) and protected from light. In vitro, zonula occludens-1 (ZO-1) and TTF1 immunostaining were realized on AECs cultured 6 days in hypoxic condition as previously described [18]. Briefly, after 4% paraformaldehyde fixation and permeabilization with 0.1% Triton X100, AECs were incubated in 2% BSA blocking solution for 30 min and then 1 h with 1:200 anti-rabbit ZO-1 (AB2272, Sigma Aldrich, Saint Quentin Fallavier, France) and 1:50 anti-mouse TTF1 (180221, Invitrogen, Thermo Fisher, Illkirch cedex, France) antibodies solution. AECs were then washed with PBS and incubated in 1:200 Alexa 488 and 568 Fluor® conjugated secondary antibodies solution (Invitrogen, Thermo Fisher, Illkirch cedex, France). For in vivo and in vitro immunofluorescence studies, nuclear labeling was performed by a DAPI (300 nM) staining during 8 min and washed with PBS. Slides were mounted with Immun-Mount solution (Thermo Fisher, Illkirch cedex, France) and imaged with a Retiga 2000R CCD camera with Image-proexpress 6.0 (QImaging, Briscous, France) connected to an Axio Observer D1 inverted epifluorescence microscope (Zeiss, Paris, France).

4.5. Transient Transfection of AECs and Luciferase Activity Assay

AECs were transiently transfected with the NEON™ transfection system (Life Technologies, Thermo Fisher, Illkirch cedex, France) allowing a 25–30% transfection efficiency as previously described [31]. ATF4 transcriptional activity was evaluated with the amino acid response element (AARE) cloned upstream of the firefly luciferase reporter gene (6.1 kb pGL3-2xAARE) [32]. ATF6N/sXBP1 transcriptional activity were evaluated with the endoplasmic reticulum response element (ERSE) also cloned upstream of the firefly luciferase reporter gene (pGL4.39 Promega, Charbonnières-les-Bains, France). Finally, HIF transactivation capacity was evaluated with a plasmid containing hypoxia response element (HRE) cloned upstream the luciferase reporter gene (pGL4.42 Promega, Charbonnières-les-Bains, France). The plasmid pRL-SV40 expressing renilla reniformis luciferase (RL) reporter gene (Promega, Charbonnières-les-Bains, France) was used for normalization of the luciferase response.

Freshly isolated AECs were plated at 1.5×10^7 cells in 100 mm dishes. On day 1 after isolation, AECs were washed with PBS, dissociated with trypsin, centrifuged at 800 rpm during 8 min and resuspended in the resuspension buffer R (NEON, Invitrogen, Thermo Fisher, Illkirch cedex, France). In each tip, 4×10^5 cells were mixed with 1 μg of the plasmid of interest (AARE-luc, ERSE-luc, HRE-luc) and with 0.4 μg of pRL-SV40. After electroporation, cells were seeded in 24-well plates without antibiotics in supplemented DMEM. On day 3, AECs were exposed to several treatments. At the end of exposition, AECs were lysed and Firefly and Renilla Luciferase assays were undertaken with the Dual-Luciferase Reporter Assay System, as specified by the manufacturer (Promega, Charbonnières-les-Bains, France). AARE, ERSE and HRE activities were assessed by quantifying the relative light units (RLU) ratio of firefly to RL measured with the Clarity™ luminescence microplate reader (BioTek, Colmar, France).

4.6. Western Blot Analyses

For in vivo study, 30 mg of snap-frozen rat lung biopsies exposed several times (16–48 h) to hypobaric hypoxia or normoxia were washed twice in PBS and then subjected to an Ultra-Turrax®

homogenizer (IKA, Staufen, Germany) in protein lysis buffer containing 20 mM Tris base, 150 mM NaCl, 1% Triton X100, 1% SDS, 0.5% deoxycholate and 0.01% cocktail protease inhibitors (Fisher Scientific, Rungis, France).

For in vitro study, AECs exposed to normoxia or hypoxia were washed twice in ice-cold PBS and extracted in lysis buffer containing H_2O, 62.5 mM Tris-HCl (pH 6.8), 10% Glycerol, 2% SDS and 0.01% cocktail protease inhibitors. Cells were submitted to three repeated cycles of sonication and speed freezing in azote. Cell lysates were then centrifuged at 13,000 rpm for 30 min at 4 °C to eliminate debris. Total protein content in lung homogenates or in AECs was determined by BCA assay (Thermo Fisher, Illkirch cedex, France). Samples (30 μg protein per sample in Laemmli buffer containing 5% β-mercapto-ethanol) were then resolved through 7.5% or 12% acrylamide gels, electrically transferred to nitrocellulose membrane, and incubated overnight at 4 °C with 1:2000 anti-mouse ATF4 (sc-200, Santa Cruz Biotechnology, Cliniscience, Nanterre, France) anti-mouse α-SMA (A2547, Sigma Aldrich, Saint Quentin Fallavier, France), anti-mouse vimentin (V6630, Sigma Aldrich, Saint Quentin Fallavier, France) or with 1:500 anti-rabbit ATF6α (sc-22799, Santa Cruz Biotechnology, Cliniscience, Nanterre, France), anti-mouse XBP1 (sc-7160, Santa Cruz Biotechnology, Nanterre, France), anti-rabbit HIF-1α (NB100-479, Novus, Biotechne, Lille, France) antibody solution. Next day, the membrane was incubated with appropriate anti-rabbit or mouse HRP-conjugated secondary antibody (Dako, P0448 and P0447 respectively, DAKO, Agilent technologies, Les Ulis Cedex, France). The signals revealed after membrane incubation in SuperSignal™ chemiluminescent HRP substrates (Thermo Fisher, Illkirch cedex, France) were quantified by densitometric analysis using Image Lab™ software (BioRad, Marnes-la-Coquette, France), normalized using quantification of the β-actin or β-tubulin in each lane and expressed in arbitrary units.

4.7. RNA Extraction and Reverse Transcription-Quantitative Polymerase Chain Reaction

AECs freshly isolated were seeded at 3.5×10^6 cells on 12-well plates. After normoxia or hypoxia and treatments exposition, cells were washed twice with PBS, extracted in ice-cold PBS and centrifuged 5 min at 1500 rpm. For in vivo study, 30 mg of snap-frozen rat lung biopsies exposed 48 h to hypobaric hypoxia or normoxia were washed twice in PBS. TRIzol™ Reagent (Qiagen, Courtaboeuf, France) was added and lung tissue was homogenized with an Ultra-Turrax® system. AECs pellet was also incubated with TRIzol™ Reagent. After vigorous mixing cell and lung homogenates, chloroform was added and centrifuged 15 min at 12,000 g. After transferring aqueous phase, nucleic acids were precipitated by isopropanol and then by 75% ethanol. Extracted ARN were resuspended in 20 μL H_2O and quantified using a BioSpec-Nano spectrophotometer (Life Science, Shimadzu, Marne-la-Vallée, France) at 260 nm. Single-strand cDNAs were synthesized from 0.5 age of total RNA using maxima first strand cDNA synthesis kit composed by a mixture of oligo (dT) and random hexamer primers according to the manufacturer's instructions (Thermo Fisher, Illkirch cedex, France). Resulting cDNA samples were amplified by quantitative polymerase chain reaction (PCR) with Absolute qPCR SybrGreen Rox mix (Thermo Fisher, Illkirch cedex, France) on StepOne Plus Real-Time PCR system (Applied Biosystem, Life technology, Thermo Fisher, Illkirch cedex, France). Loss of epithelial phenotype was evaluated by measurement of *Tgf-β1*, *Ctgf*, *Twist1* and *Zeb1* transcripts levels. Length and sequence of primers used for quantitative real-time PCR are described in Table 1. All samples were performed in duplicate. Cycle threshold values were normalized to the amplification of the endogenous reference gene β-actin for each transcript. The expression levels were calculated using the $2^{-\Delta\Delta CT}$ method and fold increase expression were reported to normoxia condition.

Table 1. Primers used for Real-Time Polymerase Chain Reaction.

GENE	Forward Primer	Reverse Primer
Twist1 (108 bp)	5′-CTACGCCTTCTCCGTCTGGA-3′	5′-CAATGACATCTAGGTCTCCGGC-3′
Ctgf (100 bp)	5′-CCTAGCTGCCTACCGACTGG-3′	5′-CTTAGAACAGGCGCTCCACT-3′
Tgf-β1 (146 bp)	5′-TGAGTGGCTGTCTTTTGACG-3′	5′-TGGGACTGATCCCATTGATT-3′
Zeb1 (90 bp)	5′-CCGTAAGTTCAAGTGCACCG-3′	5′-GTGGGACTGCCACTGTGGAT-3′
β-actin (74 bp)	5′-ACCGTGAAAAGATGACCCAGA-3′	5′-CACAGCCTGGATGGCTACGT-3′

4.8. Statistical Analyses

Results were presented as means ± SD. To evaluate differences between groups, all raw data were submitted to a Mann-Whitney and Kruskal-Wallis one-way analysis of variance followed by a Dunn's multiple comparison tests and graphics were performed by PRISM software (version 6, GraphPad, San Diego, CA, USA). A p value < 0.05 was considered a significant difference between conditions.

Author Contributions: Conceptualization, E.B., E.D., Y.U., and C.P.; methodology and validation: E.B., E.D., A.S., D.M. and T.G.; writing—review and editing, E.B., E.D., Y.U. and C.P.; supervision, E.B. and C.P.; funding acquisition, E.B. and C.P.

Acknowledgments: We thank Rabab Label, Geoffrey Tremblais for their excellent technical assistance and Pierre Fafournoux for generous gift of pGL3-2xAARE plasmid.

Abbreviations

4-PBA	4-phenylbutyrate
AARE	Amino-acid responsive element
AEC	Alveolar epithelial cell
ATF	Activating transcription factor
BAPTA	1,2-bis(o-aminophenoxy)ethane-N,N,N,N-tetraacetic acid
ER	Endoplasmic reticulum
ERSE	ER stress element
HIF	Hypoxia inducible factor
HRE	Hypoxia responsive element
IPF	Idiopathic pulmonary fibrosis
IRE-1	Inositol-requiring endonuclaease-1
mRNA	messenger RNA
PERK	PKR-ER like kinase
RL	Renilla reniformis luciferase
TTF1	Thyroid transcription factor 1
UPR	Unfolded protein response
YC-1	5′-hydroxymethyl-2′-furyl)-1-benzyl indazole
ZO-1	Zonula occludens 1

References

1. Selman, M.; King, T.E.; Pardo, A.; American Thoracic Society; European Respiratory Society; American College of Chest Physicians. Idiopathic Pulmonary Fibrosis: Prevailing and Evolving Hypotheses about Its Pathogenesis and Implications for Therapy. *Ann. Intern. Med.* **2001**, *134*, 136–151. [CrossRef]
2. Goldmann, T.; Zissel, G.; Watz, H.; Drömann, D.; Reck, M.; Kugler, C.; Rabe, K.F.; Marwitz, S. Human Alveolar Epithelial Cells Type II Are Capable of TGFβ-Dependent Epithelial-Mesenchymal-Transition and Collagen-Synthesis. *Respir. Res.* **2018**, *19*, 138. [CrossRef]

3. Kugler, K.; Matthias, C.; Wolters, P.J.; Robillard, L.; Galvez, M.G.; Brumwell, A.N.; Sheppard, D.; Chapman, H.A. Alveolar Epithelial Cell Mesenchymal Transition Develops in Vivo during Pulmonary Fibrosis and Is Regulated by the Extracellular Matrix. *Proc. Natl. Acad. Sci. USA* **2006**, *103*, 13180–13185. [CrossRef]
4. Willis, B.C.; Liebler, J.M.; Luby-Phelps, K.; Nicholson, A.G.; Crandall, E.D.; du Bois, R.M.; Borok, Z. Induction of Epithelial-Mesenchymal Transition in Alveolar Epithelial Cells by Transforming Growth Factor-Beta1: Potential Role in Idiopathic Pulmonary Fibrosis. *Am. J. Pathol.* **2005**, *166*, 1321–1332. [CrossRef]
5. Gora, S.; Maouche, S.; Atout, R.; Wanherdrick, K.; Lambeau, G.; Cambien, F.; Ninio, E.; Karabina, S.-A. Phospholipolyzed LDL Induces an Inflammatory Response in Endothelial Cells through Endoplasmic Reticulum Stress Signaling. *FASEB J.* **2010**, *24*, 3284–3297. [CrossRef]
6. Guleria, A.; Singh, V.; Chandna, S. An Attenuated Calcium Signaling and Pre-Emptive Activation of UPR Pathway Together Contribute to ER and Calcium Stress Resilience of Lepidopteran Insect Cells. *Biochim. Biophys. Acta (BBA) Gen. Subj.* **2017**, *1861*, 504–521. [CrossRef]
7. Korfei, M.; Ruppert, C.; Mahavadi, P.; Henneke, I.; Markart, P.; Koch, M.; Lang, G.; Fink, L.; Bohle, R.-M.; Seeger, W.; et al. Epithelial Endoplasmic Reticulum Stress and Apoptosis in Sporadic Idiopathic Pulmonary Fibrosis. *Am. J. Respir. Crit. Care Med.* **2008**, *178*, 838–846. [CrossRef]
8. Lawson, W.E.; Crossno, P.F.; Polosukhin, V.V.; Roldan, J.; Cheng, D.-S.; Lane, K.B.; Blackwell, T.R.; Xu, C.; Markin, C.; Ware, L.B.; et al. Endoplasmic Reticulum Stress in Alveolar Epithelial Cells Is Prominent in IPF: Association with Altered Surfactant Protein Processing and Herpesvirus Infection. *Am. J. Physiol. Lung Cell. Mol. Physiol.* **2008**, *294*, L1119–L1126. [CrossRef]
9. Burman, A.; Kropski, J.A.; Calvi, C.L.; Serezani, A.P.; Pascoalino, B.D.; Han, W.; Sherrill, T.; Gleaves, L.; Lawson, W.E.; Young, L.R.; et al. Localized Hypoxia Links ER Stress to Lung Fibrosis through Induction of C/EBP Homologous Protein. *JCI Insight* **2018**, *3*. [CrossRef]
10. Delbrel, E.; Soumare, A.; Naguez, A.; Label, R.; Bernard, O.; Bruhat, A.; Fafournoux, P.; Tremblais, G.; Marchant, D.; Gille, T.; et al. HIF-1α Triggers ER Stress and CHOP-Mediated Apoptosis in Alveolar Epithelial Cells, a Key Event in Pulmonary Fibrosis. *Sci. Rep.* **2018**, *8*. [CrossRef]
11. Guo, L.; Xu, J.; Liu, L.; Liu, S.; Zhu, R. Hypoxia-Induced Epithelial-Mesenchymal Transition Is Involved in Bleomycin-Induced Lung Fibrosis. *BioMed Res. Int.* **2015**, *2015*, 1–10. [CrossRef]
12. Tzouvelekis, A.; Harokopos, V.; Paparountas, T.; Oikonomou, N.; Chatziioannou, A.; Vilaras, G.; Tsiambas, E.; Karameris, A.; Bouros, D.; Aidinis, V. Comparative Expression Profiling in Pulmonary Fibrosis Suggests a Role of Hypoxia-Inducible Factor-1α in Disease Pathogenesis. *Am. J. Respir. Crit. Care Med.* **2007**, *176*, 1108–1119. [CrossRef]
13. Zhang, W.; Shi, X.; Peng, Y.; Wu, M.; Zhang, P.; Xie, R.; Wu, Y.; Yan, Q.; Liu, S.; Wang, J. HIF-1α Promotes Epithelial-Mesenchymal Transition and Metastasis through Direct Regulation of ZEB1 in Colorectal Cancer. *PLoS ONE* **2015**, *10*, e0129603. [CrossRef]
14. Mingyuan, X.; Qianqian, P.; Shengquan, X.; Chenyi, Y.; Rui, L.; Yichen, S.; Jinghong, X. Hypoxia-Inducible Factor-1α Activates Transforming Growth Factor-B1/Smad Signaling and Increases Collagen Deposition in Dermal Fibroblasts. *Oncotarget* **2017**, *9*, 3188–3197. [CrossRef]
15. Gusarova, G.A.; Trejo, H.E.; Dada, L.A.; Briva, A.; Welch, L.C.; Hamanaka, R.B.; Mutlu, G.M.; Chandel, N.S.; Prakriya, M.; Sznajder, J.I. Hypoxia Leads to Na,K-ATPase Downregulation via Ca2+ Release-Activated Ca2+ Channels and AMPK Activation. *Mol. Cell. Biol.* **2011**, *31*, 3546–3556. [CrossRef]
16. Davis, F.M.; Azimi, I.; Faville, R.A.; Peters, A.A.; Jalink, K.; Putney, J.W.; Goodhill, G.J.; Thompson, E.W.; Roberts-Thomson, S.J.; Monteith, G.R. Induction of Epithelial–Mesenchymal Transition (EMT) in Breast Cancer Cells Is Calcium Signal Dependent. *Oncogene* **2014**, *33*, 2307–2316. [CrossRef]
17. Zhong, Q.; Zhou, B.; Ann, D.K.; Minoo, P.; Liu, Y.; Banfalvi, A.; Krishnaveni, M.S.; Dubourd, M.; Demaio, L.; Willis, B.C.; et al. Role of Endoplasmic Reticulum Stress in Epithelial–Mesenchymal Transition of Alveolar Epithelial Cells: Effects of Misfolded Surfactant Protein. *Am. J. Respir. Cell Mol. Biol.* **2011**, *45*, 498–509. [CrossRef]
18. Uzunhan, Y.; Bernard, O.; Marchant, D.; Dard, N.; Vanneaux, V.; Larghero, J.; Gille, T.; Clerici, C.; Valeyre, D.; Nunes, H.; et al. Mesenchymal Stem Cells Protect from Hypoxia-Induced Alveolar Epithelial-Mesenchymal Transition. *Am. J. Physiol. Lung Cell. Mol. Physiol.* **2016**, *310*, L439–L451. [CrossRef]
19. Williams, J.A.; Hou, Y.; Ni, H.-M.; Ding, W.-X. Role of Intracellular Calcium in Proteasome Inhibitor-Induced Endoplasmic Reticulum Stress, Autophagy and Cell Death. *Pharm. Res.* **2013**, *30*, 2279–2289. [CrossRef]

20. Planes, C.; Friedlander, G.; Loiseau, A.; Amiel, C.; Clerici, C. Inhibition of Na-K-ATPase Activity after Prolonged Hypoxia in an Alveolar Epithelial Cell Line. *Am. J. Physiol. Lung Cell. Mol. Physiol.* **1996**, *271*, L70–L78. [CrossRef]
21. Zhou, G.; Dada, L.A.; Wu, M.; Kelly, A.; Trejo, H.; Zhou, Q.; Varga, J.; Sznajder, J.I. Hypoxia-Induced Alveolar Epithelial-Mesenchymal Transition Requires Mitochondrial ROS and Hypoxia-Inducible Factor 1. *Am. J. Physiol. Lung Cell. Mol. Physiol.* **2009**, *297*, L1120–L1130. [CrossRef]
22. Tanjore, H.; Xu, X.C.; Polosukhin, V.V.; Degryse, A.L.; Li, B.; Han, W.; Sherrill, T.P.; Plieth, D.; Neilson, E.G.; Blackwell, T.S.; et al. Contribution of Epithelial-Derived Fibroblasts to Bleomycin-Induced Lung Fibrosis. *Am. J. Respir. Crit. Care Med.* **2009**, *180*, 657–665. [CrossRef]
23. Chen, X.; Iliopoulos, D.; Zhang, Q.; Tang, Q.; Greenblatt, M.B.; Hatziapostolou, M.; Lim, E.; Tam, W.L.; Ni, M.; Chen, Y.; et al. XBP1 Promotes Triple-Negative Breast Cancer by Controlling the HIF1α Pathway. *Nature* **2014**, *508*, 103–107. [CrossRef]
24. Li, H.; Chen, X.; Gao, Y.; Wu, J.; Zeng, F.; Song, F. XBP1 Induces Snail Expression to Promote Epithelial-to-Mesenchymal Transition and Invasion of Breast Cancer Cells. *Cell. Signal.* **2015**, *27*, 82–89. [CrossRef]
25. Banerjee, A.; Ahmed, H.; Yang, P.; Czinn, S.J.; Blanchard, T.G. Endoplasmic Reticulum Stress and IRE-1 Signaling Cause Apoptosis in Colon Cancer Cells in Response to Andrographolide Treatment. *Oncotarget* **2016**, *7*. [CrossRef]
26. Mo, X.-T.; Zhou, W.-C.; Cui, W.-H.; Li, D.-L.; Li, L.-C.; Xu, L.; Zhao, P.; Gao, J. Inositol-Requiring Protein 1 —X-Box-Binding Protein 1 Pathway Promotes Epithelial–Mesenchymal Transition via Mediating Snail Expression in Pulmonary Fibrosis. *Int. J. Biochem. Cell Biol.* **2015**, *65*, 230–238. [CrossRef] [PubMed]
27. Bhattacharya, A.; Kumar, J.; Hermanson, K.; Sun, Y.; Qureshi, H.; Perley, D.; Scheidegger, A.; Singh, B.B.; Dhasarathy, A. The Calcium Channel Proteins ORAI3 and STIM1 Mediate TGF-& β2; Induced *Snai1* Expression. *Oncotarget* **2018**, *9*. [CrossRef]
28. Krebs, J.; Agellon, L.B.; Michalak, M. Ca2+ Homeostasis and Endoplasmic Reticulum (ER) Stress: An Integrated View of Calcium Signaling. *Biochem. Biophys. Res. Commun.* **2015**, *460*, 114–121. [CrossRef]
29. Belaidi, E.; Thomas, A.; Bourdier, G.; Moulin, S.; Lemarié, E.; Levy, P.; Pépin, J.-L.; Korichneva, I.; Godin-Ribuot, D.; Arnaud, C. Endoplasmic Reticulum Stress as a Novel Inducer of Hypoxia Inducible Factor-1 Activity: Its Role in the Susceptibility to Myocardial Ischemia-Reperfusion Induced by Chronic Intermittent Hypoxia. *Int. J. Cardiol.* **2016**, *210*, 45–53. [CrossRef]
30. Bernard, O.; Jeny, F.; Uzunhan, Y.; Dondi, E.; Terfous, R.; Label, R.; Sutton, A.; Larghero, J.; Vanneaux, V.; Nunes, H.; et al. Mesenchymal Stem Cells Reduce Hypoxia-Induced Apoptosis in Alveolar Epithelial Cells by Modulating HIF and ROS Hypoxic Signaling. *Am. J. Physiol. Lung Cell. Mol. Physiol.* **2018**, *314*, L360–L371. [CrossRef]
31. Migneault, F.; Boncoeur, É.; Morneau, F.; Pascariu, M.; Dagenais, A.; Berthiaume, Y. Cycloheximide and Lipopolysaccharide Downregulate AENaC MRNA via Different Mechanisms in Alveolar Epithelial Cells. *Am. J. Physiol. Lung Cell. Mol. Physiol.* **2013**, *305*, L747–L755. [CrossRef]
32. Chaveroux, C.; Sarcinelli, C.; Barbet, V.; Belfeki, S.; Barthelaix, A.; Ferraro-Peyret, C.; Lebecque, S.; Renno, T.; Bruhat, A.; Fafournoux, P.; et al. Nutrient Shortage Triggers the Hexosamine Biosynthetic Pathway via the GCN2-ATF4 Signalling Pathway. *Sci. Rep.* **2016**, *6*. [CrossRef]

3

Voluntary Activity Modulates Sugar-Induced Elastic Fiber Remodeling in the Alveolar Region of the Mouse Lung

Julia Hollenbach [1], Elena Lopez-Rodriguez [1,2], Christian Mühlfeld [1,2,3] and Julia Schipke [1,2,3,*]

[1] Institute of Functional and Applied Anatomy, Hannover Medical School, 30625 Hannover, Germany; Julia.Hollenbach@tiho-hannover.de (J.H.); Lopez-Rodriguez.Elena@mh-hannover.de (E.L.-R.); Muehlfeld.Christian@mh-hannover.de (C.M.)

[2] Biomedical Research in Endstage and Obstructive Lung Disease Hannover (BREATH), Member of the German Center for Lung Research (DZL), 30625 Hannover, Germany

[3] Cluster of Excellence REBIRTH (From Regenerative Biology to Reconstructive Therapy), 30625 Hannover, Germany

* Correspondence: schipke.julia@mh-hannover.de

Abstract: Diabetes and respiratory diseases are frequently comorbid conditions. However, the mechanistic links between hyperglycemia and lung dysfunction are not entirely understood. This study examined the effects of high sucrose intake on lung mechanics and alveolar septal composition and tested voluntary activity as an intervention strategy. C57BL/6N mice were fed a control diet (CD, 7% sucrose) or a high sucrose diet (HSD, 35% sucrose). Some animals had access to running wheels (voluntary active; CD-A, HSD-A). After 30 weeks, lung mechanics were assessed, left lungs were used for stereological analysis and right lungs for protein expression measurement. HSD resulted in hyperglycemia and higher static compliance compared to CD. Lung and septal volumes were increased and the septal ratio of elastic-to-collagen fibers was decreased despite normal alveolar epithelial volumes. Elastic fibers appeared more loosely arranged accompanied by an increase in elastin protein expression. Voluntary activity prevented hyperglycemia in HSD-fed mice. The parenchymal airspace volume, but not the septal volume, was increased. The septal extracellular matrix (ECM) composition together with the protein expression of ECM components was similar to control levels in the HSD-A-group. In conclusion, HSD was associated with elastic fiber remodeling and reduced pulmonary elasticity. Voluntary activity alleviated HSD-induced ECM alterations, possibly by preventing hyperglycemia.

Keywords: dietary sugar; hyperglycemia; lung mechanics; alveolar septal composition; physical activity; extracellular matrix remodeling

1. Introduction

Over the last decades sugar consumption has risen dramatically and in most parts of the world sucrose—a disaccharide composed of glucose and fructose—is the most common sweetener [1]. Glucose is metabolized in every cell of the body and its metabolism is tightly regulated by insulin, whereas fructose is primarily metabolized in the liver promoting de novo lipogenesis [2]. High sucrose and/or high fructose consumption leads to persistent blood hyperglycemia and systemic disorders like metabolic syndrome (MetS) and diabetes type 2 [3].

There is evidence that the lung is a target organ for glucotoxicity-induced complications. MetS defined by hyperglycemia, hypertriglyceridemia, and hypertension among others is a risk factor for diabetes type 2, but also for lung function impairment and lung diseases like chronic obstructive pulmonary disease (COPD) and asthma [4]. In diabetic patients, a poor glycemic control leads to a progressive decline of lung function [5], and respiratory conditions including COPD and obstructive sleep apnea are frequent comorbidities of diabetes [6,7]. Moreover, high blood glucose levels were shown to affect fetal and postnatal lung development by generalized slowing of alveolar septal growth [8]. The underlying mechanistic links between hyperglycemia and lung dysfunction are not entirely understood. A better insight could help to develop novel therapeutic approaches and might identify hyperglycemia as an early risk factor for lung diseases.

Physical exercise was shown to be effective against a number of diseases including MetS and type 1 and type 2 diabetes, and to reduce blood glucose levels, triglycerides, blood pressure, or waist circumference [9,10]. Moreover, it also exerts beneficial effects on lung function [11]. Generally, exercise has an anti-inflammatory effect by induction of anti-inflammatory mediators such as IL-6, IL-1ra, TNF-R, and IL-10 [12]. In mice which were exposed to cigarette smoke for several weeks, physical exercise reduced oxidative stress in the lung and was therefore able to protect against emphysema development [13].

The present study tested the hypotheses, that: (i) prolonged excess dietary sucrose intake affects lung mechanics and structure in mice and that (ii) voluntary activity alleviates these sucrose-induced changes.

2. Results

2.1. Body Weight and Blood Glucose Concentrations

As already published by Schipke et al. [14], high sucrose diet (HSD)-fed mice had higher body weights (control diet (CD): 40.5 ± 3.6 g, HSD: 45.6 ± 2.0 g, $p = 0.001$) and elevated fasting blood glucose concentrations (CD: 8.4 ± 0.5 mmol/L, HSD: 9.8 ± 1.2 mmol/L, $p < 0.001$) in comparison to CD-fed mice after 30 weeks. Voluntary activity had no impact on the HSD-related body weight increase (CD-active (A): 39.2 ± 4.1 g, HSD-A: 43.4 ± 2.8 g, $p = 0.045$; HSD vs. HSD-A $p = 0.176$), but prevented hyperglycemia in the active HSD-group (CD-A: 8.0 ± 0.5 mmol/L, HSD-A: 8.3 ± 0.3 mmol/L, $p = 0.373$; HSD vs. HSD-A $p < 0.001$).

2.2. Lung Mechanics

HSD resulted in lower Elastance H ($p = 0.015$; Figure 1A) and higher static lung compliance ($p = 0.012$; Figure 1B) and inspiratory capacity ($p = 0.043$; Figure 1C) compared to CD. Voluntary activity did not influence the HSD-induced changes in lung mechanics; however, H was reduced in active CD-fed mice compared to non-active CD-fed mice ($p = 0.03$; Figure 1A).

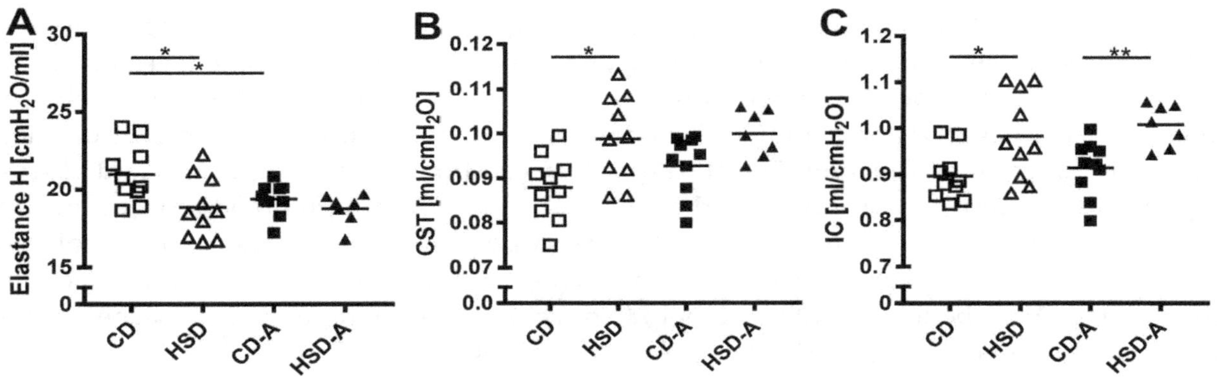

Figure 1. Effects of high sucrose intake and voluntary activity on lung mechanics. Mice were fed a control diet (CD) or a high sucrose diet (HSD) and were left untreated or had access to running wheels (CD-A, HSD-A). Lung mechanics measurements were performed after 30 weeks. (**A**) Elastance H, (**B**) Static lung compliance, (**C**) Inspiratory capacity. Values are individual data points, with means indicated by horizontal lines. Data were compared by 2-Way ANOVA followed by Tukey test; p-values < 0.05 are indicated: * $p < 0.05$, ** $p < 0.01$.

2.3. Lung Structure

Left lung volumes were higher in the HSD- as well as in the HSD-A-group compared to their respective controls (CD vs. HSD $p = 0.039$, CD-A vs. HSD-A $p = 0.002$, Figure 2A). This was due to an increase in the parenchyma volume (HSD vs. CD $p = 0.043$, HSD-A vs. CD-A $p < 0.001$, Figure 2B), whereas the non-parenchyma volume was not significantly altered (Figure 2C).

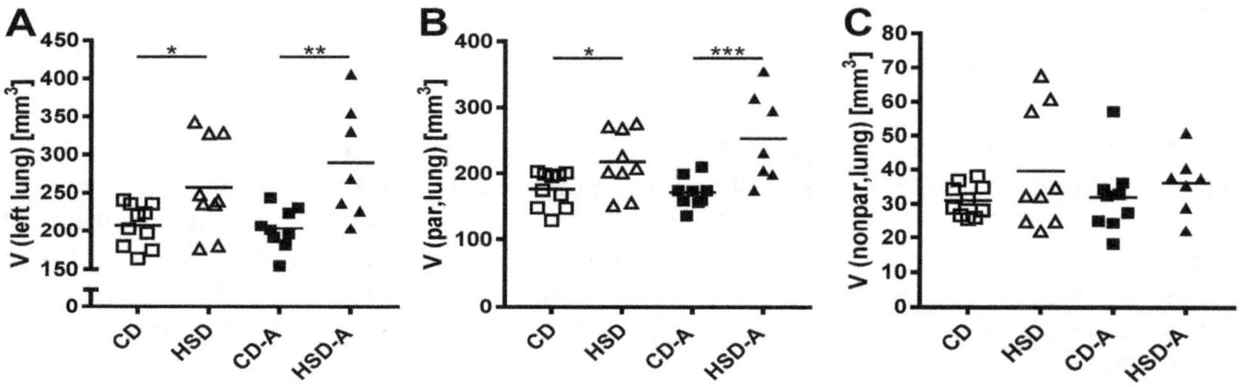

Figure 2. Effects of high sucrose intake and voluntary activity on lung and parenchyma volumes. Mice were fed a control diet (CD) or a high sucrose diet (HSD) and were left untreated or had access to running wheels (CD-A, HSD-A) for 30 weeks. (**A**) Volume of the left lung; (**B**) Volume of left lung parenchyma, (**C**) Volume of left lung non-parenchyma. Values are individual data points, with means indicated by horizontal lines. Data were compared by 2-Way ANOVA followed by Tukey test; p-values < 0.05 are indicated: * $p < 0.05$, ** $p < 0.01$, *** $p < 0.001$.

2.4. Parenchyma Composition

The parenchymal composition differed between inactive and active HSD-groups (Figure 3A,E). HSD alone induced a higher septal volume (CD vs. HSD $p = 0.001$, Figure 3B) and surface area (CD vs. HSD $p < 0.001$, Figure 3C) compared to controls. In contrast, the combination of activity and HSD resulted in a higher airspace volume (CD-A vs. HSD-A $p < 0.001$, Figure 3F), which was due to increases in both ductal (CD-A vs. HSD-A $p = 0.001$; Figure 3G) and alveolar (CD-A vs. HSD-A $p = 0.002$, Figure 3H) airspace, accompanied by a higher septal surface area (CD-A vs. HSD-A $p < 0.001$, Figure 3C). The thickness of alveolar septa did not differ significantly among the groups (Figure 3D).

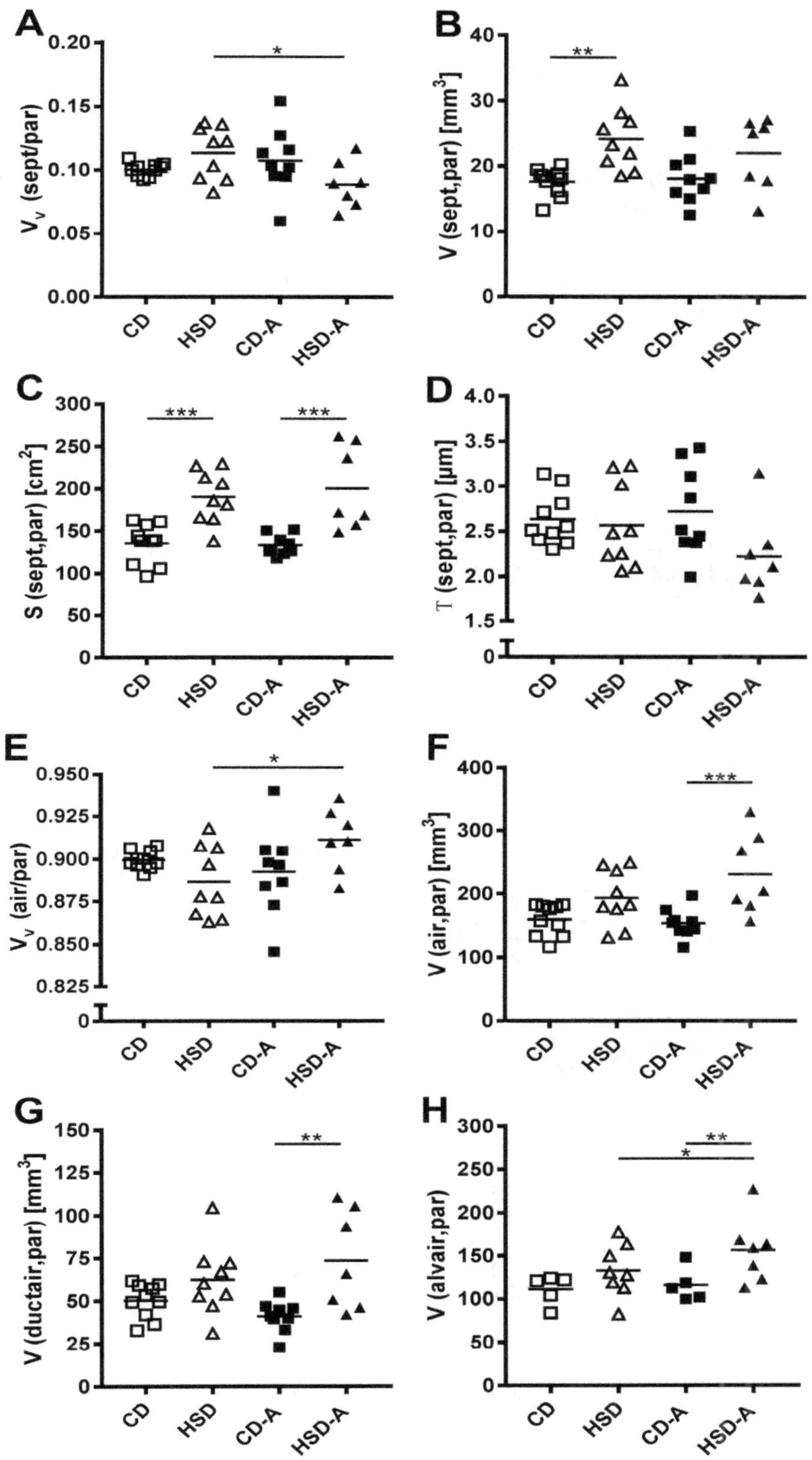

Figure 3. Effects of high sucrose intake and voluntary activity on parenchyma composition. Mice were fed a control diet (CD) or a high sucrose diet (HSD) and were left untreated or had access to running wheels (CD-A, HSD-A) for 30 weeks. (**A**) Septal volume density, (**B**) Septal volume, (**C**) Septal surface area; (**D**) Septal thickness; (**E**) Airspace volume density; (**F**) Airspace volume; (**G**) Ductal airspace volume; (**H**) Alveolar airspace volume. Values are individual data points, with means indicated by horizontal lines. Data were compared by 2-Way ANOVA followed by Tukey test; p-values < 0.05 are indicated: * $p < 0.05$, ** $p < 0.01$, *** $p < 0.001$.

2.5. Septal Composition

The increased septal volume in HSD-fed animals was accompanied by volume increases of endothelial cells (CD vs. HSD $p < 0.001$, Figure 4A) and the capillary lumen (CD vs. HSD $p = 0.003$, Figure 4B) compared to CD. Similarly, the absolute volume of interstitial cells (mainly fibroblasts) showed a strong tendency to higher levels (CD vs. HSD $p = 0.053$, Figure 4C). In contrast, the epithelial cell volume was not significantly changed in response to HSD (Figure 4D). Voluntary activity in combination with HSD resulted in elevated absolute volumes of interstitial cells compared to CD-A ($p = 0.005$, Figure 4C). The volume of lipid droplets within interstitial cells was not significantly affected by diet or activity (Figure 4 E).

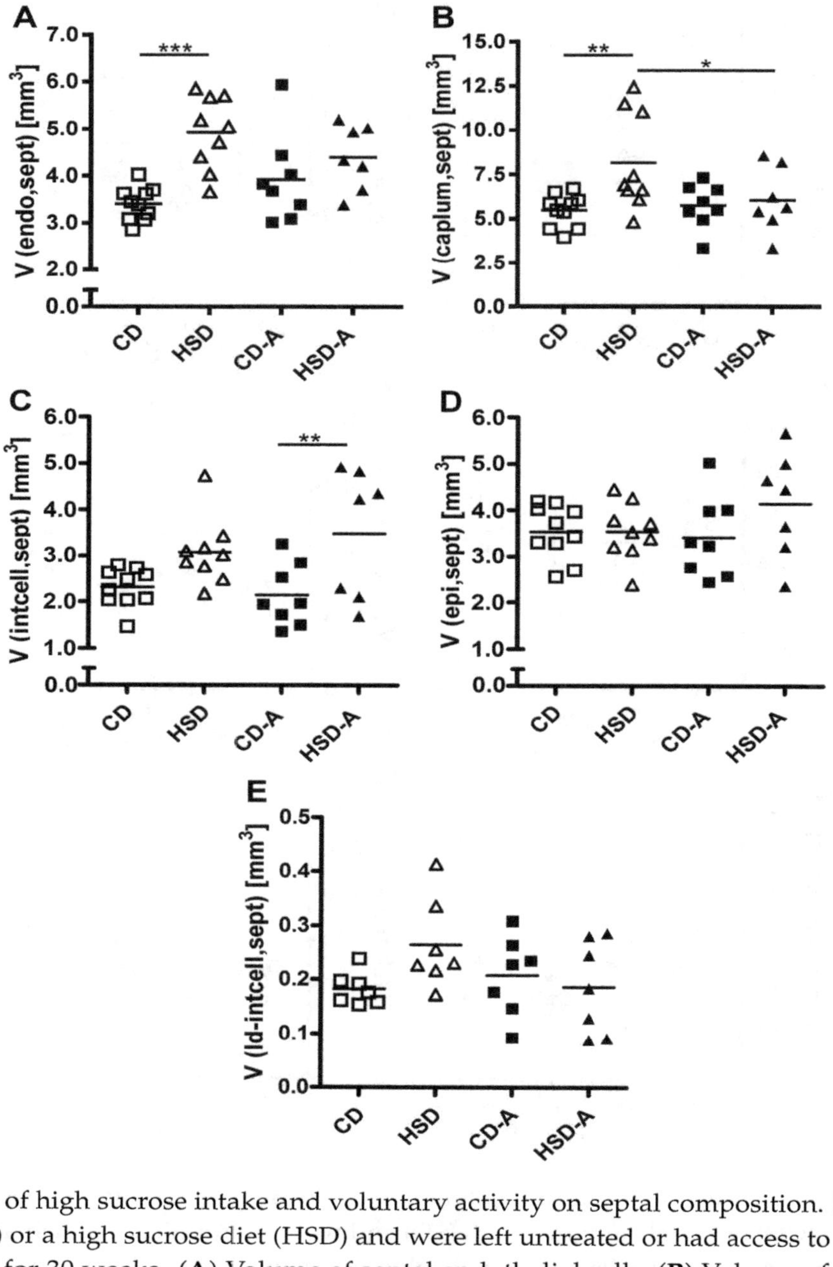

Figure 4. Effects of high sucrose intake and voluntary activity on septal composition. Mice were fed a control diet (CD) or a high sucrose diet (HSD) and were left untreated or had access to running wheels (CD-A, HSD-A) for 30 weeks. (**A**) Volume of septal endothelial cells; (**B**) Volume of septal capillary lumen; (**C**) Volume of septal interstitial cells; (**D**) Volume of septal epithelial cells; (**E**) Volume of lipid droplets within septal interstitial cells. Values are individual data points, with means indicated by horizontal lines. Data were compared by 2-Way ANOVA followed by Tukey test; p-values < 0.05 are indicated: * $p < 0.05$, ** $p < 0.01$, *** $p < 0.001$.

2.6. Extracellular Matrix Composition

Compared to CD, the absolute volumes of the extracellular matrix (ECM) (defined as all non-cellular spaces of the septum which includes proteoglycans, collagen fibers and elastic fibers among others; CD vs. HSD $p = 0.001$, Figure 5A) and of collagen fibers within the ECM (CD vs. HSD $p = 0.009$, Figure 5B) were significantly increased in HSD-fed animals. This was consistent with the higher septal volume in these animals. In contrast, the volume of elastic fibers was unchanged in the HSD-group (Figure 5C) and the ratio of elastic-to-collagen fiber volumes was reduced in HSD compared to CD ($p = 0.003$, Figure 5D).

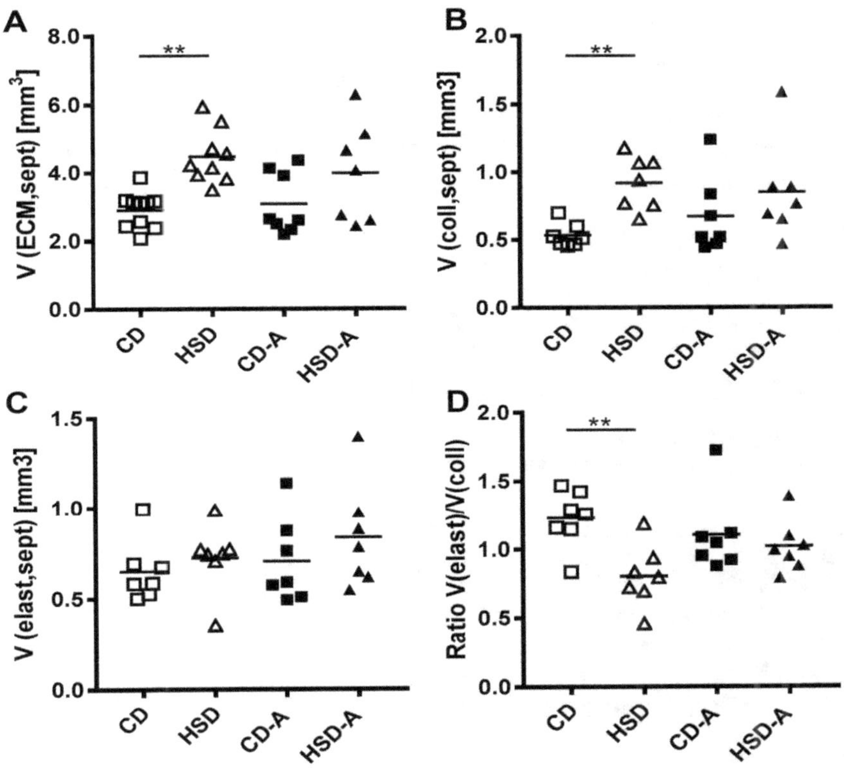

Figure 5. Effects of high sucrose intake and voluntary activity on extracellular matrix composition. Mice were fed a control diet (CD) or a high sucrose diet (HSD) and were left untreated or had access to running wheels (CD-A, HSD-A) for 30 weeks. (**A**) Volume of septal extracellular matrix; (**B**) Volume of septal collagen fibers; (**C**) Volume of septal elastic fibers; (**D**) Ratio of the elastic fiber volume to the collagen fiber volume. Values are individual data points, with means indicated by horizontal lines. Data were compared by 2-Way ANOVA followed by Tukey test; p-values < 0.05 are indicated: ** $p < 0.01$.

The structural appearance of septal elastic fibers differed between animals. They appeared either loosely arranged, densely packed, or showed an intermediate phenotype (Figure 6A). Scoring revealed that elastic fibers of HSD-fed animals resembled the loose phenotype in contrast to the more densely packed elastic fibers in control mice (Figure 6B). Voluntary activity partly changed this categorization. Regarding collagen fibers, there was no morphological difference between the groups.

Next, the parenchymal protein expression of elastin and fibrillin as main components of elastic fibers, and of collagen I and collagen III as most common collagen types within the lung parenchyma (4) was assessed. The elastin expression was markedly increased to about 500% of control levels in response to HSD (CD vs. HSD $p < 0.001$, Figure 6C). Fibrillin protein expression was increased to 200% of control levels (CD vs. HSD $p < 0.001$, Figure 6D), whereas collagen I and III levels were similar to CD (Figure 6E,F). Voluntary activity significantly alleviated the HSD-induced changes in elastin (HSD vs. HSD-A $p = 0.006$, Figure 6C) and fibrillin (HSD vs. HSD-A $p = 0.014$, Figure 6D) expression.

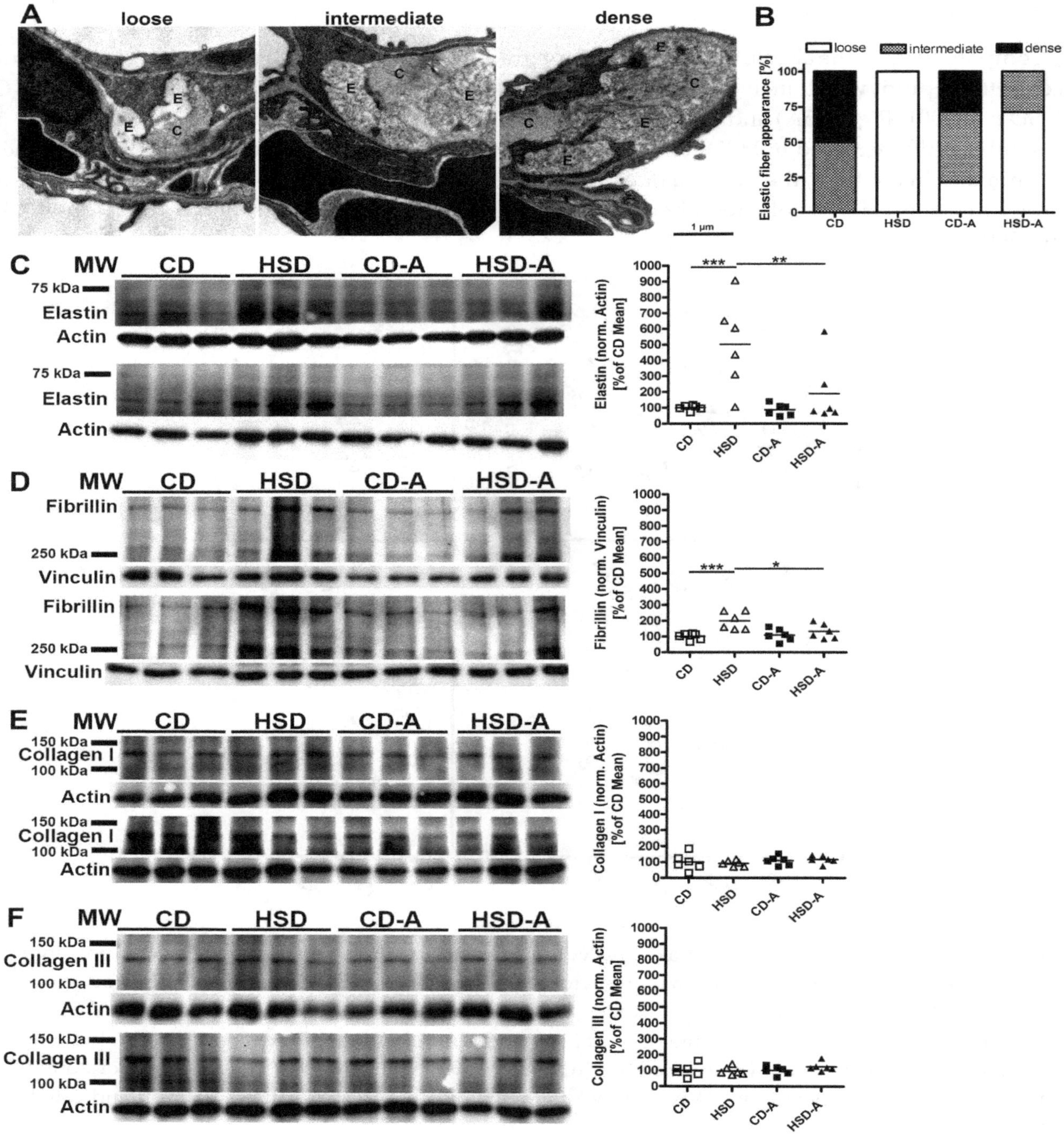

Figure 6. Effects of high sucrose intake and voluntary activity on composition of elastic fibers and collagen fibers. Mice were fed a control diet (CD) or a high sucrose diet (HSD) and were left untreated or had access to running wheels (CD-A, HSD-A) for 30 weeks. (**A**) Representative electron microscopical images showing loose, intermediate or dense structural composition of elastic fibers. E, elastic fibers; C, collagen fibers. (**B**) Scoring of elastic fiber appearance. (**C**) Elastin protein expression; (**D**) Fibrillin-1 protein expression; (**E**) Collagen I protein expression; (**F**) Collagen III protein expression. (**C–F**) left: PVDF membranes with protein bands used for quantification, molecular marker bands are indicated; right: protein band intensity signals normalized to the respective loading control and expressed as percentage of the CD mean value of the respective membrane; values are individual data points, with means indicated by horizontal lines. Data were compared by 2-Way ANOVA followed by Tukey test; p-values < 0.05 are indicated: * $p < 0.05$, ** $p < 0.01$, *** $p < 0.001$.

3. Discussion

Excess dietary sucrose intake for 30 weeks resulted in hyperglycemia and lung mechanics alterations indicating reduced elasticity, higher septal volumes, and elastic fiber remodeling. Voluntary activity prevented hyperglycemia and alleviated ECM alterations in HSD-fed mice. Moreover, the parenchymal airspace volume, but not the septal volume, was increased in the HSD-A-group.

Within the lung, the ECM significantly influences the elastic properties [15]. The ECM is mainly composed of elastic fibers, collagen fibers, and proteoglycans. The molecular components are synthesized by interstitial fibroblasts and released into the interstitium, where they assemble into their fibrillar structure. Collagen and elastic fibers cooperate to create a stable, but also elastic septal architecture [15]. In HSD-fed mice, the collagen fiber volume was higher in accordance with the septal volume increase. Moreover, the protein amount of collagen I and III (as the main collagen types of the lung) within 20 μg total parenchymal protein was similar to control levels. This indicates that the amount and the composition of septal collagen fibers in HSD-fed mice are comparable to control conditions. In contrast, the volume of elastic fibers was similar between HSD- and CD-fed mice despite the higher septal volume in the HSD-group, and the ratio of elastic-to-collagen fiber volumes was reduced. Additionally, the structural appearance of the elastic fibers was different in HSD-fed mice. They appeared loosely arranged with more amorphous material and less electron dense structures in contrast to the more densely packed elastic fibers in the control group. Analysis of the parenchymal protein composition revealed that in response to HSD, the amount of elastin was markedly increased to on average 500% of control levels. Also, the fibrillin amount was higher in HSD-fed mice, although this reached only about 200% of control levels. Thus, the prolonged high dietary sucrose intake influenced the expression of the main elastic fiber components elastin and fibrillin. The altered elastin-to-fibrillin ratio might have caused a divergent composition and thus altered structural appearance of the elastic fibers. Since elastic fibers are mainly responsible for the pulmonary elastic recoil during expiration, this finding could at least contribute to the lower lung elasticity we observed upon HSD feeding.

Elastic fibers are complex structures and the largest ECM component of the lung. Their extracellular assembly is directed by the fibroblast and requires the coordinated expression of tropoelastin and microfibril components as well as enzymes essential for elastin cross-linking [16]. In other organs like the heart, hyperglycemia-induced effects on fibroblasts are well studied with upregulation of collagen expression as one main effect [17–20]. In contrast, little is known about glucotoxic effects on pulmonary fibroblasts. Glucose-stimulation of fetal rat lung explants results in greater lipid inclusions within fibroblasts [21], contradicting the unchanged lipid droplet volumes in fibroblasts of HSD-fed mice found in this study. This might be due to differences in age (fetal vs. adult) and/or experimental design (lung explant vs. living organism). In cultured human lung fibroblasts, insulin stimulates collagen synthesis [22], however, direct glucose-related effects on lung fibroblasts are not well studied. Also endothelial cells influence pulmonary ECM composition, either via nitric oxide production or by endothelial-mesenchymal transition, and may therefore contribute to the sucrose-induced changes observed in this study [23].

A functional correlation between hyperglycemia and elastic fiber remodeling could add important insight into the complex and not well understood association between diabetes and pulmonary dysfunction. Abnormal elastic fiber assembly and integrity as a result of genetic mutations is associated with an increased susceptibility for lung diseases [24] and changes in content and composition of ECM components significantly contribute to pathogenesis and progression of asthma, COPD, idiopathic pulmonary fibrosis, pulmonary arterial hypertension, and lung cancer [15,25]. On the other hand, type 1 diabetes mellitus leads to a decrease of lung elasticity [26,27]. Moreover, a poor glycemic control indicated by high HbA1c concentrations in diabetic patients results in a progressive decline in lung function [5] and diabetic individuals are at higher risk of COPD, asthma, pulmonary fibrosis, and pneumonia [28]. While diabetic microangiopathy in the lung is one explanation for these alterations, also structural changes are considered to play a major role [29,30]. In diabetic rats, the relative amounts of collagen, elastin, and basal laminae in the septum are increased [31] and diabetes induction by streptozotocin, in 3 week old rats, results in increased collagen and elastin [32]. Another study examining normally fed and undernourished diabetic rats concludes that experimental diabetes affects lung connective tissue metabolism and breakdown and thereby leads to increases in lung collagen and elastin [33]. In humans, fasting plasma glucose concentrations of 6.1–6.9 mmol/L without or with impaired glucose clearance indicate a prediabetic state, whereas a fasting plasma glucose concentration equal to or higher than 7 mmol/L is defined as diabetes [34]. This is not directly transferable to mice, as plasma glucose concentrations of 5–8 mmol/L are reported for mice under control conditions [14,35]. Severe diabetes upon streptozotocin injection is reflected by blood glucose concentrations greater than 14 mmol/L [35]. The HSD-fed mice examined here had blood glucose concentrations around 10 mmol/L, which was significantly higher than CD-fed mice (8.5 mmol/L), but below the severe diabetes conditions of other studies [35]. Moreover, glucose tolerance measured by an oral glucose tolerance test was unimpaired in the HSD-group [14], pointing to a prediabetic or early diabetic state. Thus, elastic fiber remodeling seems to be an early hyperglycemia-induced pulmonary alteration that might prime the lung for injury or disease. Moreover, the mouse model used in this study is suitable to monitor for early hyperglycemia-induced pulmonary alterations and to test therapeutic options against disease progression.

One intervention strategy already known to be effective against many metabolic disorders is physical exercise [9]. Here, voluntary activity prevented hyperglycemia in HSD-fed mice [14] in line with others showing improved blood sugar control due to physical exercise in prediabetic or diabetic individuals [36,37]. In active, HSD-fed mice the parenchymal airspace volume, but not the septal volume, was increased and the absolute volume of interstitial cells was higher compared to CD-A. Moreover, the septal amount of elastic fibers, the elastic-to-collagen fiber ratio and the protein expression of elastic fiber components was similar to control levels. This indicates that voluntary activity alleviated the HSD-induced septal remodeling processes, possibly by prevention of hyperglycemia. Although this did not result in normalization of lung mechanics, the increase in airspace volume instead of septal volume in HSD-A may point to a beneficial effect for elasticity. It was shown before that physical activity affects expression and activity of matrix metalloprotease- 2 (MMP-2) and MMP-9 and their inhibitors TIMP-1 and TIMP-2 in human muscle and tendon tissue [38,39] which are involved in degradation and stabilization of ECM components. In line with that, physical exercise has a positive effect on ECM remodeling in patients with diabetes type 2 by influencing expression of MMP-2 and its tissue inhibitor TIMP-2 [40].

4. Materials and Methods

4.1. Animals and Study Design

All animal experiments were approved by the Local Institutional Animal Care and Research Advisory committee and permitted by the Lower Saxony State Office for Consumer Protection and Food Safety (Reference number 33.14-42502-04-13/1244, approval date 11.09.2013). Male C57BL/6N mice were purchased from Charles River (Sulzfeld, Germany) at the age of five weeks. After one week of acclimatization in the local housing facility, animals were randomly assigned to four groups. Animals were housed separately under 12 h light and 12 h dark cycle and were fed ad libitum either a CD with a carbohydrate:protein:fat ratio of 70:20:10 kcal% containing 7% sucrose (D12450J, Research diets, New Brunswick, NJ, USA) [14] or a HSD with a carbohydrate:protein:fat ratio of 70:20:10 kcal% containing 35% sucrose (D12450B, Research diets) [14]. Some animals had free access to running wheels for voluntary activity resulting in four experimental groups: (1) CD (n = 10), (2) CD-A (n = 9), (3) HSD (n = 9) and (4) HSD-A (n = 7).

For all animals used in this study, basic data (body weight, energy intake, running distance, circulating plasma lipid levels and glucose homeostasis) were recently published in another context and compared with additional experimental groups by 3-Way ANOVA [14]. Therefore, body weights and fasting blood glucose concentrations of the mice in this study were subjected to the statistical analysis used here (2-Way ANOVA and Tukey post-hoc test) and means and p-values are reported in the results section of this paper.

4.2. Lung Mechanics

After 30 weeks, mice were anesthetized with Ketamine (100 mg/kg body weight; Dr. Graeub AG, Bern, Switzerland) and Xylazin (5 mg/kg body weight; Rompun®, Bayer, Leverkusen, Germany) via intraperitoneal injection. Afterwards mice were tracheostomized and mechanically ventilated using the Flexivent small animal ventilator (SCIREQ, Montreal, QC, Canada) with a frequency of 150/min and a tidal volume of 10 mL/kg body weight. To prevent spontaneous breathing, 0.8 mg/kg body weight pancuronium bromide (Actavis®, Inresa Arztneimittel GmbH, Freiburg, Germany) was injected intraperitoneally. Three different mechanical parameters were assessed: the tissue elastance (H), the static lung compliance (CST) and the inspiratory capacity (IC) as described elsewhere [41,42]. In brief, elastance H was assessed using the broadband forced oscillation technique at a positive end-expiratory pressure (PEEP) of 3 cm H_2O. Quasi-static pressure volume loops were measured to calculate CST according to the Salazar-Knowls equation and IC was determined by deep inflation of the lung at a pressure of 30 cm H_2O.

4.3. Lung Fixation, Sampling, and Processing

Right lung lobes were ligated and the left lung was fixed via tracheal instillation at a hydrostatic pressure of 20 cm H_2O using 1.5% paraformaldehyde (Sigma-Aldrich, St. Louis, MO, USA) and 1.5% glutaraldehyde (Merck, Darmstadt, Germany) in 0.15 M HEPES buffer (Sigma-Aldrich). Right lung lobes were snap frozen and stored at −80 °C. The left lung was kept in fixative for at least 24 h. The left lung volume was determined by fluid displacement (Principle of Archimedes) [43]. Afterwards, systematic uniform random sampling (SURS) was performed [44] and tissue slices were randomly allocated to light microscopy (LM) or transmission electron microscopy (TEM) analysis.

Slices for LM analysis were embedded in Technovit 7100 (Heraeus Kulzer, Wehrheim, Germany) as described previously [45]. In brief, tissue slices were osmicated for 2 h followed by an overnight incubation in a half saturated aqueous solution of uranyl acetate. After dehydration with ascending acetone concentrations, samples were embedded in Technovit 7100, 1.5 μm thick sections were cut and stained with toluidine blue.

Slices for TEM analysis were randomly subsampled into 1 mm^3 tissue blocks and embedded in epoxy resin (Epon®, Serva, Heidelberg, Germany) as described previously [45]. In brief, tissue blocks were post-fixed with osmium tetroxide followed by an overnight en bloc incubation with uranyl acetate. After dehydration with ascending acetone concentrations, samples were embedded in epoxy resin and 60 nm ultrathin sections were cut for analysis.

4.4. Stereological Analysis—Light Microscopy

The following parameters were determined by design-based stereology at the LM level: Volume densities and total volumes of the parenchyma and non-parenchyma, the alveolar septa and the alveolar and ductal airspace as well as the surface density and the total surface area of the alveolar septa. Three to four tissue slices per animal were digitized using a slide scanner (Axio Scan.Z1, ZEISS, Oberkochen, Germany) and analyzed using the newCast software (Visiopharm, Hørsholm, Denmark). The analyst was blinded for experimental groups throughout the analysis.

Volumes were determined by point counting [44]. For estimating the parenchyma (V(par,lung)) and non-parenchyma volume (V(nonpar,lung)), random fields of view were provided by the Visiopharm software at a sampling fraction of 50% and an objective lens magnification of 5 x. The test grid consisted of 24 points and points hitting the structure of interest (parenchyma and non-parenchyma) as well as points hitting the reference space (lung tissue) were counted. Volume densities (V_V) were calculated by dividing the sum of the points hitting the structure of interest by the sum of the points hitting the reference space (Equation (1)) and total volumes (V) were calculated by multiplying the volume density by the total volume of the reference space (Equation (2)):

$$V_V(\text{struct/ref}) = \sum P(\text{struct})/\sum P(\text{ref}) \tag{1}$$

$$V(\text{struct,ref}) = V_V\ (\text{struct/ref}) \times V(\text{lung}) \tag{2}$$

For estimating the septal volume (V(sept,par)) and the airspace volume (V(air,par)) within the parenchyma, fields of view obtained with a sampling fraction of 5% and an objective lens magnification of 20 x were analyzed using the same test grid as above. Volumes were calculated as shown in Equations (1) and (2) with septum or airspace representing the structure of interest and the parenchyma representing the reference space.

For estimating the alveolar (V(alvair,par)) and ductal (V(ductair,par)) airspace volumes within the parenchyma, random images were obtained at a sampling fraction of 5–10% and an objective lens magnification of 10 x using the same test system as above. Volumes were calculated as shown in Equations (1) and (2) with the alveolar or ductal airspace representing the structure of interest and the parenchyma representing the reference space.

For estimating the septal surface area within the parenchyma (S(sept,par)), random images obtained at a sampling fraction of 5% and an objective lens magnification of 20 x were analyzed. The test grid consisted of two lines and four points with a known length per point (l/p = 34.14 μm). All intersections of the test lines with the septal surface and all points hitting the parenchyma were counted [43] and the surface area was calculated as shown in Equations (3) and (4):

$$S_V(\text{sept/par}) = 2 \times \sum I(\text{sept})/(l/p \times \sum P(\text{par})), \tag{3}$$

$$S(\text{sept,par}) = S_V\ (\text{sept/par}) \times V(\text{par,lung}). \tag{4}$$

The septal thickness (τ(sept)) was calculated as shown in Equation (5) [44].

$$\tau(\text{sept}) = 2 \times V_V(\text{sept/par})/S_V(\text{sept/par}) \tag{5}$$

4.5. Stereological Analysis—Transmission Electron Microscopy

The following parameters were estimated by design-based stereology at the TEM level: volume densities and total volumes of epithelial cells, endothelial cells, interstitial cells, the capillary lumen and the extracellular matrix (ECM; defined as all non-cellular spaces of the septum which includes proteoglycans, water, collagen and elastic fibers among others). Moreover, volume densities and total volumes of collagen fibers and elastic fibers within the septal ECM and of lipid droplets within interstitial cells were quantified in a separate analysis. Three tissue blocks per animal were analyzed. At least 90 random images per animal were taken according to SURS standards with a Morgagni 268 microscope (FEI, Eindhoven, Netherlands) at a primary magnification of 14,000 x. Images were analyzed using the STEPanizer stereology online tool [46] by an analyst blinded for experimental groups.

Volume densities were estimated by point counting as described above. For estimation of epithelium, endothelium, capillary lumen, interstitial cells and ECM, the test grid consisted of 16 points and for estimation of collagen fibers, elastic fibers and lipid droplets within interstitial cells the test grid consisted of 400 points. Points hitting epithelial cells (P(epi)), endothelial cells (P(endo)), capillary lumen (P(caplum)), interstitial cells (P(intcell)), ECM (P(ECM)), elastic fibers (P(elast)), collagen fibers (P(coll)) and lipid droplets (P(LD-intcell)) and points hitting the reference space (septum; P(sept)) were counted. Volume densities and total volumes were calculated as described in Equations (1) and (2).

4.6. *Scoring of Structural Elastic Fiber Appearance*

The structural appearance of elastic fibers was assessed by an analyst who was blinded for experimental groups. At least 90 random images at a primary magnification of 14,000 x per animal were analyzed and elastic fibers were assigned to one of three groups: (i) loosely arranged, more amorphous components, (ii) intermediate, (iii) densely packed, more electron dense, fibrillar structures (Figure 6A).

4.7. *Protein Islolation And Western Blot*

Lung samples were homogenized with a tissue lyser (Qiagen, Hilden, Germany), proteins were isolated using the NucleoSpin®RNA/Protein Kit (Macherey-Nagel, Düren, Germany) and protein concentration was measured with a protein quantification assay (Macherey-Nagel).

20 μg proteins per lane were loaded, fractionated by SDS-PAGE (polyacrylamide gel concentrations in Table 1) and transferred to PVDF membranes (Bio-Rad, Hercules, CA, USA). Membranes were blocked (blocking conditions in Table 1), incubated with the primary antibody, washed, incubated with the secondary antibody (antibody details in Table 1), washed and developed using the Clarity Max™ Western ECL Blotting Substrate (Bio-Rad) and the ChemiDocTM Touch Imager (Bio-Rad). Protein bands intensities were assessed with the Image LabTM Software (Bio-Rad), normalized according to the loading control and expressed as percentage of the CD mean of the respective membrane.

Table 1. Gel concentrations, blocking conditions, and antibodies used for Western Blot analysis.

Protein	Gel Concentration	Blocking Conditions	Primary Antibody, Dilution, Incubation Conditions	Secondary Antibody, Dilution, Incubation Conditions
		Target Proteins		
Fibrillin-1	5%	drying and equilibration in 3% BSA for 10 min	Anti-Fibrillin 1 antibody (ab231094; Abcam, Cambridge, Great Britain) 1:1000 overnight, 4 °C	Peroxidase-AffiniPure F(ab')2 Fragment Goat Anti-Rabbit IgG (111-036-045, Dianova, Hamburg, Germany) 1:20,000 1 h, room temperature
Elastin	10%	drying and equilibration in 3% BSA for 10 min	Anti-Elastin antibody (ab217356, Abcam) 1:2000 overnight, 4 °C	Peroxidase-AffiniPure F(ab')2 Fragment Goat Anti-Rabbit IgG (111-036-045, Dianova) 1:20,000 1 h, room temperature
Collagen I	10%	1 h 3% BSA/TBS	COL1A1 (3G3) (sc-293182, Santa Cruz Biotechnology, Dallas, TX, USA) 1:500 overnight, 4 °C	m-IgGκ BP-HRP (sc-516102, Santa Cruz Biotechnology) 1:20,000 1 h, room temperature
Collagen III	8%	1 h 3% BSA/TBS	COL3A1 (B-10) (sc-271249, Santa Cruz Biotechnology) 1:500 overnight, 4 °C	m-IgGκ BP-HRP (sc-516102, Santa Cruz Biotechnology) 1:20,000 1 h, room temperature
		Loading Controls		
α-Actin			α-Actin Antibody (G-12) (sc-130619, Santa Cruz Biotechnology) 1:2000 1 h, room temperature	Peroxidase-AffiniPure F(ab')2 Fragment Goat Anti-Rabbit IgG (111-036-045, Dianova) 1:20,000 1 h, room temperature
Vinculin			Vinculin antibody (7F9) (sc-73614, Santa Cruz Biotechnology) 1:2000 1 h, room temperature	m-IgGκ BP-HRP (sc-516102, Santa Cruz Biotechnology) 1:20,000 1 h, room temperature

4.8. Statistical Analysis

Data were analyzed with Sigma Plot (SYSTAT Software Inc., Erkrath, Germany) by two-way analysis of variance (2-Way ANOVA) followed by Tukey test for pairwise multiple comparisons. p-values < 0.05 were considered significant, p-values between 0.05 and 0.1 ($0.05 < p < 0.1$) were considered to show a tendency towards significance [47]. Data are expressed as means ± SD or means and individual data points for each mouse. Graphs were created using GraphPad Prism (version 4, GraphPad Software, San Diego, CA, USA) and figures were constructed with Photoshop CS6 (Adobe, San José, CA, USA).

5. Conclusions

In conclusion, high sucrose intake induced hyperglycemia and elastic fiber remodeling that resulted in reduced pulmonary elasticity. In contrast, the alveolar epithelium did not show alterations. This might contribute to the hyperglycemia-related decline in lung function observed in patients and could prime the lung for injury and disease. Future studies are needed to shed further light on this correlation between high blood sugar and ECM remodeling. Voluntary activity prevented hyperglycemia and significantly alleviated elastic fiber alterations in HSD-fed mice, indicating that physical exercise is a potent intervention strategy against sugar-induced pulmonary changes.

Author Contributions: Conceptualization, C.M. and J.S.; Data curation, J.H.; Formal analysis, J.H. and J.S.; Investigation, J.H., E.L.-R., and J.S.; Methodology, E.L.-R. and J.S.; Project administration, C.M.; Supervision, C.M. and J.S.; Writing – original draft, J.H. and J.S.; Writing – review & editing, E.L.-R. and C.M.

Acknowledgments: We thank Melanie Bornemann, Susanne Kuhlmann, and Rita Lichatz (Institute of Functional and Applied Anatomy, MHH) for excellent technical support. We thank Sheila Fryk for the linguistic revision of the manuscript.

Abbreviations

CD	Control diet
HSD	High sucrose diet
ECM	Extracellular matrix
MetS	Metabolic syndrome
COPD	Chronic obstructive pulmonary disease
CST	Static lung compliance
IC	Inspiratory capacity

References

1. Lustig, R.H.; Schmidt, L.A.; Brindis, C.D. The toxic truth about sugar. *Nature* **2012**, *482*, 27. [CrossRef] [PubMed]
2. Lustig, R.H. Fructose: Metabolic, Hedonic, and Societal Parallels with Ethanol. *J. Am. Diet. Assoc.* **2010**, *110*, 1307–1321. [CrossRef]
3. Malik, V.S.; Popkin, B.M.; Bray, G.A.; Després, J.-P.; Willett, W.C.; Hu, F.B. Sugar-Sweetened Beverages and Risk of Metabolic Syndrome and Type 2 Diabetes: A meta-analysis. *Diabetes Care* **2010**, *33*, 2477–2483. [CrossRef]
4. Baffi, C.W.; Wood, L.; Winnica, D.; Strollo, P.J., Jr.; Gladwin, M.T.; Que, L.G.; Holguin, F. Metabolic Syndrome and the Lung. *Chest* **2016**, *149*, 1525–1534. [CrossRef] [PubMed]
5. Davis, W.A.; Knuiman, M.; Kendall, P.; Grange, V.; Davis, T.M.E. Glycemic Exposure Is Associated with Reduced Pulmonary Function in Type 2 Diabetes: The Fremantle Diabetes Study. *Diabetes Care* **2004**, *27*, 752–757. [CrossRef] [PubMed]

6. Punjabi, N.M.; Beamer, B.A. Alterations in Glucose Disposal in Sleep-disordered Breathing. *Am. J. Respir. Crit. Care Med.* **2009**, *179*, 235–240. [CrossRef] [PubMed]
7. Cazzola, M.; Rogliani, P.; Calzetta, L.; Lauro, D.; Page, C.; Matera, M.G. Targeting Mechanisms Linking COPD to Type 2 Diabetes Mellitus. *Trends Pharmacol. Sci.* **2017**, *38*, 940–951. [CrossRef] [PubMed]
8. Grant, M.M.; Cutts, N.R.; Brody, J.S. Influence of maternal diabetes on basement membranes, type 2 cells, and capillaries in the developing rat lung. *Dev. Biol.* **1984**, *104*, 469–476. [CrossRef]
9. Pedersen, B.K.; Saltin, B. Exercise as medicine—Evidence for prescribing exercise as therapy in 26 different chronic diseases. *Scand. J. Med. Sci. Sports* **2015**, *25*, 1–72 doi 101111/sms12581. [CrossRef]
10. Lemes, Í.R.; Turi-Lynch, B.C.; Cavero-Redondo, I.; Linares, S.N.; Monteiro, H.L. Aerobic training reduces blood pressure and waist circumference and increases HDL-c in metabolic syndrome: A systematic review and meta-analysis of randomized controlled trials. *J. Am. Soc. Hypertens.* **2018**, *12*, 580–588. [CrossRef]
11. Salcedo, P.A.; Lindheimer, J.B.; Klein-Adams, J.C.; Sotolongo, A.M.; Falvo, M.J. Effects of Exercise Training on Pulmonary Function in Adults with Chronic Lung Disease: A Meta-Analysis of Randomized Controlled Trials. *Arch. Phys. Med. Rehabil.* **2018**, *99*, 2561.e7–2569.e7. [CrossRef] [PubMed]
12. Petersen, A.M.W.; Pedersen, B.K. The anti-inflammatory effect of exercise. *J. Appl. Physiol.* **2005**, *98*, 1154–1162. [CrossRef] [PubMed]
13. Toledo, A.C.; Magalhaes, R.M.; Hizume, D.C.; Vieira, R.P.; Biselli, P.J.C.; Moriya, H.T.; Mauad, T.; Lopes, F.D.T.Q.S.; Martins, M.A. Aerobic exercise attenuates pulmonary injury induced by exposure to cigarette smoke. *Eur. Respir. J.* **2012**, *39*, 254–264. [CrossRef]
14. Schipke, J.; Vital, M.; Schnapper-Isl, A.; Pieper, D.H.; Mühlfeld, C. Spermidine and Voluntary Activity Exert Differential Effects on Sucrose- Compared with Fat-Induced Systemic Changes in Male Mice. *J. Nutr.* **2019**, *149*, 451–462. [CrossRef]
15. Burgstaller, G.; Oehrle, B.; Gerckens, M.; White, E.S.; Schiller, H.B.; Eickelberg, O. The instructive extracellular matrix of the lung: Basic composition and alterations in chronic lung disease. *Eur. Respir. J.* **2017**, 50. [CrossRef]
16. Kielty, C.M.; Sherratt, M.J.; Shuttleworth, C.A. Elastic fibres. *J. Cell Sci.* **2002**, *115*, 2817–2828.
17. Shamhart, P.E.; Luther, D.J.; Adapala, R.K.; Bryant, J.E.; Petersen, K.A.; Meszaros, J.G.; Thodeti, C.K. Hyperglycemia enhances function and differentiation of adult rat cardiac fibroblasts. *Can. J. Physiol. Pharmacol.* **2014**, *92*, 598–604. [CrossRef] [PubMed]
18. Aguilar, H.; Fricovsky, E.; Ihm, S.; Schimke, M.; Maya-Ramos, L.; Aroonsakool, N.; Ceballos, G.; Dillmann, W.; Villarreal, F.; Ramirez-Sanchez, I. Role for high-glucose-induced protein O-GlcNAcylation in stimulating cardiac fibroblast collagen synthesis. *Am. J. Physiol. Cell Physiol.* **2014**, *306*, C794–C804. [CrossRef]
19. Sedgwick, B.; Riches, K.; Bageghni, S.A.; O'Regan, D.J.; Porter, K.E.; Turner, N.A. Investigating inherent functional differences between human cardiac fibroblasts cultured from nondiabetic and Type 2 diabetic donors. *Cardiovasc. Pathol.* **2014**, *23*, 204–210. [CrossRef]
20. Hutchinson, K.R.; Lord, C.K.; West, T.A.; Stewart, J.A., Jr. Cardiac fibroblast-dependent extracellular matrix accumulation is associated with diastolic stiffness in type 2 diabetes. *PLoS ONE* **2013**, *8*, e72080. [CrossRef]
21. Gewolb, I.; Torday, J. High glucose inhibits maturation of the fetal lung in vitro. Morphometric analysis of lamellar bodies and fibroblast lipid inclusions. *Lab. Investig.* **1995**, *73*, 59–63. [PubMed]
22. Goldstein, R.; Poliks, C.F.; Pilch, P.F.; Smith, B.D.; Fine, A. Stimulation of Collagen Formation by Insulin and Insulin-Like Growth Factor I in Cultures of Human Lung Fibroblasts. *Endocrinology* **1989**, *124*, 964–970. [CrossRef] [PubMed]
23. Kato, S.; Inui, N.; Hakamata, A.; Suzuki, Y.; Enomoto, N.; Fujisawa, T.; Nakamura, Y.; Watanabe, H.; Suda, T. Changes in pulmonary endothelial cell properties during bleomycin-induced pulmonary fibrosis. *Respir. Res.* **2018**, *26*, 127. [CrossRef] [PubMed]
24. Shifren, A.; Mecham, R.P. The stumbling block in lung repair of emphysema: Elastic fiber assembly. *Proc. Am. Thorac. Soc.* **2006**, *3*, 428–433. [CrossRef]
25. Burgess, J.K.; Mauad, T.; Tjin, G.; Karlsson, J.C.; Westergren-Thorsson, G. The extracellular matrix—The under-recognized element in lung disease? *J. Pathol.* **2016**, *240*, 397–409. [CrossRef] [PubMed]
26. Schuyler, M.R.; Niewoehner, D.E.; Inkley, S.R.; Kohn, R. Abnormal Lung Elasticity in Juvenile Diabetes Mellitus. *Am. Rev. Respir. Dis.* **1976** *113*, 37–41. [CrossRef]

27. Sandler, M.; Bunn, A.E.; Stewart, R.I. Cross-Section Study of Pulmonary Function in Patients with Insulin-dependent Diabetes Mellitus. *Am. Rev. Respir. Dis.* **1987**, *135*, 223–229. [CrossRef]
28. Ehrlich, S.F.; Quesenberry, C.P., Jr.; Van Den Eeden, S.K.; Shan, J.; Ferrara, A. Patients diagnosed with diabetes are at increased risk for asthma, chronic obstructive pulmonary disease, pulmonary fibrosis, and pneumonia but not lung cancer. *Diabetes Care* **2010**, *33*, 55–60. [CrossRef]
29. Pitocco, D.; Fuso, L.; Conte, E.G.; Zaccardi, F.; Condoluci, C.; Scavone, G.; Incalzi, R.A.; Ghirlanda, G. Thediabetic lung-a new target organ? *Rev. Diabet. Stud.* **2012**, *9*, 23–35. [CrossRef]
30. Zheng, H.; Wu, J.; Jin, Z.; Yan, L.-J. Potential Biochemical Mechanisms of Lung Injury in Diabetes. *Aging Dis.* **2017**, *8*, 7–16. [CrossRef] [PubMed]
31. Kida, K.; Utsuyama, M.; Takizawa, T.; Thurlbeck, W.M. Changes in Lung Morphologic Features and Elasticity Caused by Streptozotocin-induced Diabetes Mellitus in Growing Rats. *Am. Rev. Respir. Dis.* **1983**, *128*, 125–131. [CrossRef]
32. Ofulue, A.F.; Kida, K.; Thurlbeck, W.M. Experimental Diabetes and the Lung: I. Changes in Growth, Morphometry, and Biochemistry. *Am. Rev. Respir. Dis.* **1988**, *137*, 162–166. [CrossRef]
33. Ofulue, A.F.; Thurlbeck, W.M. Experimental Diabetes and the Lung: II. In Vivo Connective Tissue Metabolism. *Am. Rev. Respir. Dis.* **1988**, *138*, 284–289. [CrossRef]
34. World Health Organization. Fact Sheet: Diabetes. 2018. Available online: https://www.who.int/news-room/fact-sheets/detail/diabetes (accessed on 12 May 2019).
35. Lee, Y.-S.; Eun, H.S.; Kim, S.Y.; Jeong, J.-M.; Seo, W.; Byun, J.-S.; Jeong, W.-I.; Yi, H.-S. Hepatic immunophenotyping for streptozotocin-induced hyperglycemia in mice. *Sci. Rep.* **2016**, *6*, 30656. [CrossRef] [PubMed]
36. Colberg, S.R.; Sigal, R.J.; Fernhall, B.; Regensteiner, J.G.; Blissmer, B.J.; Rubin, R.R.; Chasan-Taber, L.; Albright, A.L.; Braun, B.; Medicine, A.C.; et al. Exercise and type 2 diabetes: The American College of Sports Medicine and the American Diabetes Association: Joint position statement. *Diabetes Care* **2010**, *33*, e147–e167. [CrossRef] [PubMed]
37. Jelleyman, C.; Yates, T.; O'Donovan, G.; Gray, L.J.; King, J.A.; Khunti, K.; Davies, M.J. The effects of high-intensity interval training on glucose regulation and insulin resistance: A meta-analysis. *Obes. Rev.* **2015**, *16*, 942–961. [CrossRef] [PubMed]
38. Rullman, E.; Norrbom, J.; Strömberg, A.; Wågsäter, D.; Rundqvist, H.; Haas, T.; Gustafsson, T. Endurance exercise activates matrix metalloproteinases in human skeletal muscle. *J. Appl. Physiol.* **2009**, *106*, 804–812. [CrossRef]
39. Koskinen, S.O.A.; Heinemeier, K.M.; Olesen, J.L.; Langberg, H.; Kjaer, M. Physical exercise can influence local levels of matrix metalloproteinases and their inhibitors in tendon-related connective tissue. *J. Appl. Physiol.* **2004**, *96*, 861–864. [CrossRef] [PubMed]
40. Kadoglou, N.P.E.; Vrabas, I.S.; Sailer, N.; Kapelouzou, A.; Fotiadis, G.; Noussios, G.; Karayannacos, P.E.; Angelopoulou, N. Exercise ameliorates serum MMP-9 and TIMP-2 levels in patients with type 2 diabetes. *Diabetes Metab.* **2010**, *36*, 144–151. [CrossRef]
41. Lopez-Rodriguez, E.; Boden, C.; Echaide, M.; Perez-Gil, J.; Kolb, M.; Gauldie, J.; Maus, U.A.; Ochs, M.; Knudsen, L. Surfactant dysfunction during overexpression of TGF-β1 precedes profibrotic lung remodeling in vivo. *Am. J. Physiol. Lung Cell. Mol. Physiol.* **2016**, *310*, L1260–L1271. [CrossRef] [PubMed]
42. Knudsen, L.; Atochina-Vasserman, E.N.; Massa, C.B.; Birkelbach, B.; Guo, C.-J.; Scott, P.; Haenni, B.; Beers, M.F.; Ochs, M.; Gow, A.J. The role of inducible nitric oxide synthase for interstitial remodeling of alveolar septa in surfactant protein D-deficient mice. *Am. J. Physiol. Lung Cell. Mol. Physiol.* **2015**, *309*, L959–L969. [CrossRef] [PubMed]
43. Scherle, W. A simple method for volumetry of organs in quantitative stereology. *Mikroskopie* **1970**, *26*, 57–60.
44. Ochs, M.; Mühlfeld, C. Quantitative microscopy of the lung: A problem-based approach. Part 1: Basic principles of lung stereology. *Am. J. Physiol. Lung Cell. Mol. Physiol.* **2013**, *305*, L15–L22. [CrossRef]
45. Schneider, J.P.; Ochs, M. Alterations of mouse lung tissue dimensions during processing for morphometry: A comparison of methods. *Am. J. Physiol. Lung Cell. Mol. Physiol.* **2013**, *306*, L341–L350. [CrossRef] [PubMed]
46. Tschanz, S.A.; Burri, P.H.; Weibel, E.R. A simple tool for stereological assessment of digital images: The STEPanizer. *J. Microsc.* **2011**, *243*, 47–59. [CrossRef] [PubMed]
47. Curran-Everett, D.; Benos, D.J. Guidelines for reporting statistics in journals published by the American Physiological Society. *Am. J. Physiol. Metab.* **2004**, *287*, E189–E191. [CrossRef]

4

Hypercapnia Impairs Na,K-ATPase Function by Inducing Endoplasmic Reticulum Retention of the β-Subunit of the Enzyme in Alveolar Epithelial Cells

Vitalii Kryvenko [1,2], Miriam Wessendorf [1], Rory E. Morty [1,2,3], Susanne Herold [1,2], Werner Seeger [1,2,3], Olga Vagin [4,5], Laura A. Dada [6], Jacob I. Sznajder [6] and István Vadász [1,2,*]

1 Department of Internal Medicine, Justus Liebig University, Universities of Giessen and Marburg Lung Center (UGMLC), Member of the German Center for Lung Research (DZL), 35392 Giessen, Germany
2 The Cardio-Pulmonary Institute (CPI), 35392 Giessen, Germany
3 Department of Lung Development and Remodeling, Max Planck Institute for Heart and Lung Research, 61231 Bad Nauheim, Germany
4 Department of Physiology, David Geffen School of Medicine, University of California at Los Angeles, Los Angeles, CA 90095, USA
5 Veterans Administration Greater Los Angeles Healthcare System, Los Angeles, CA 90073, USA
6 Division of Pulmonary and Critical Care Medicine, Feinberg School of Medicine, Northwestern University, Chicago, IL 60611, USA
* Correspondence: Istvan.Vadasz@innere.med.uni-giessen.de

Abstract: Alveolar edema, impaired alveolar fluid clearance, and elevated CO_2 levels (hypercapnia) are hallmarks of the acute respiratory distress syndrome (ARDS). This study investigated how hypercapnia affects maturation of the Na,K-ATPase (NKA), a key membrane transporter, and a cell adhesion molecule involved in the resolution of alveolar edema in the endoplasmic reticulum (ER). Exposure of human alveolar epithelial cells to elevated CO_2 concentrations caused a significant retention of NKA-β in the ER and, thus, decreased levels of the transporter in the Golgi apparatus. These effects were associated with a marked reduction of the plasma membrane (PM) abundance of the NKA-α/β complex as well as a decreased total and ouabain-sensitive ATPase activity. Furthermore, our study revealed that the ER-retained NKA-β subunits were only partially assembled with NKA α-subunits, which suggests that hypercapnia modifies the ER folding environment. Moreover, we observed that elevated CO_2 levels decreased intracellular ATP production and increased ER protein and, particularly, NKA-β oxidation. Treatment with α-ketoglutaric acid (α-KG), which is a metabolite that has been shown to increase ATP levels and rescue mitochondrial function in hypercapnia-exposed cells, attenuated the deleterious effects of elevated CO_2 concentrations and restored NKA PM abundance and function. Taken together, our findings provide new insights into the regulation of NKA in alveolar epithelial cells by elevated CO_2 levels, which may lead to the development of new therapeutic approaches for patients with ARDS and hypercapnia.

Keywords: carbon dioxide; hypercapnia; Na,K-ATPase; endoplasmic reticulum; sodium transport; protein oxidation; alveolar epithelium

---

1. Introduction

Na,K-ATPase (NKA) is a heterodimeric enzyme and a member of the P-type ATPase family. NKA is located at the basolateral plasma membrane (PM) of polarized cells, where the primary function of the enzyme is to extrude three sodium ions while taking up two potassium ions per pump cycle in an ATP-dependent manner [1,2]. A functional NKA requires a catalytic α-subunit and a regulatory β-subunit [2]. Additionally, a γ-subunit has also been identified, which represents a family of single-span transmembrane proteins containing the FXYD motif that is not an integral part of the transporter but rather regulates the activity and membrane abundance of the enzyme [3,4]. In the alveolar epithelium of the lung, the activity of NKA creates an Na^+ gradient that drives reabsorption of fluid from the alveolar space, which keeps the alveoli relatively "dry," which is essential for an effective gas exchange. The catalytic α-subunit of the transporter contains the binding sites for Na^+, K^+, and ATP [2]. The NKA β-subunit, which is a type II membrane glycoprotein, has a pivotal role in delivery and appropriate insertion of the NKA-α subunit in the PM [1]. Remarkably, mice deficient in the NKA-β subunit in alveolar epithelial cells have reduced alveolar fluid clearance, which results in aggravation of acute lung injury (ALI) and further underlies the pivotal role of NKA-β in the overall transporter function [5]. Additionally, numerous reports have shown that the function of NKA-β is not limited to regulation of NKA-α, but is centrally involved in establishing epithelial cell polarity, formation of adherens junctions, and regulation of paracellular permeability, which are key for maintaining a functional epithelial barrier [6–10].

Carbon dioxide (CO_2) is a byproduct of mitochondrial respiration and cellular metabolism. Excess of CO_2, in mammals, is eliminated by the lungs under physiological conditions [11,12]. Thus, any condition that leads to alveolar hypoventilation or impairs diffusion of CO_2 across the alveolar-capillary barrier results in retention of CO_2 in the blood, which is termed hypercapnia. During ALI and in patients with acute respiratory distress syndrome (ARDS), disruption of the alveolar-capillary barrier, and, thus, accumulation of edema fluid in the interstitial and alveolar spaces, may result in hypercapnia. Moreover, hypercapnia is often further potentiated or even directly caused by protective ventilation strategies with low tidal volumes to limit further lung damage [12,13]. Remarkably, hypercapnia was found to decrease alveolar fluid clearance and resolution of alveolar edema by decreasing the PM abundance of the Na,K-ATPase [14–16]. Since ALI is often associated with hypercapnia and is characterized by alveolar edema and disruption of epithelial junctions [17], further understanding of the mechanisms impairing the NKA function and of the potential rescue mechanisms might be of critical importance promoting the resolution of epithelial injury, alveolar repair processes, and edema resolution.

About one-third of all cellular proteins interact with the endoplasmic reticulum (ER) during folding and maturation processes [18]. Of note, in the ER, the NKA-β undergoes various post-translational modifications, including glycosylation and assembly with NKA-α, before leaving the ER and, subsequently, being transferred to the PM [19,20]. Whether hypercapnia affects ER protein folding of NKA has not been previously investigated. In the current study, we explored how elevated CO_2 levels influence the ER environment and expression, PM abundance, and function of the NKA-β subunit. Understanding the molecular mechanisms underlying the effects of hypercapnia on the folding and maturation of the NKA-β in the alveolar epithelium might provide new therapeutic strategies for the treatment of patients with ARDS and hypercapnia.

2. Results

2.1. *Hypercapnia Increases the Endoplasmic Reticulum Fraction of the Na,K-ATPase β-Subunit*

The NKA-β subunit is a glycoprotein that undergoes posttranslational maturation processing in the ER and Golgi prior to delivery to the plasma membrane. After the initial step of ER folding, the addition of an oligosaccharide core results in the formation of a specific high mannose N-glycan type NKA-β, which resides exclusively in the ER [19]. To investigate whether hypercapnia affects cellular levels of NKA-β, we exposed alveolar epithelial cells (AEC) for up to 72 h to physiological or increased levels of CO_2 and analyzed the protein expression pattern of NKA-β and NKA-α (Figure 1A).

We observed a transient and time-dependent increase in the abundance of ER-resident NKA-β, which reached a maximum at 12 h and lasted for at least 24 h upon hypercapnic exposure. Our subsequent experiments were performed after a 12-h hypercapnia exposure, where the highest ER-resident NKA-β abundance was observed. To demonstrate whether this effect was directly driven by CO_2 or the elevated CO_2-associated acidosis, AEC were treated with increasing CO_2 concentrations (up to 120 mmHg) with normal (pH = 7.4) or acidic (pH = 7.2) extracellular pH (Figure 1B). Of note, we observed that the acidic environment per se did not affect the levels of the ER-resident NKA-β. In addition, we did not find significant differences in the total protein levels of NKA-α and NKA-β subunits upon hypercapnic exposure for up to 12 h (Figure 1C,D).

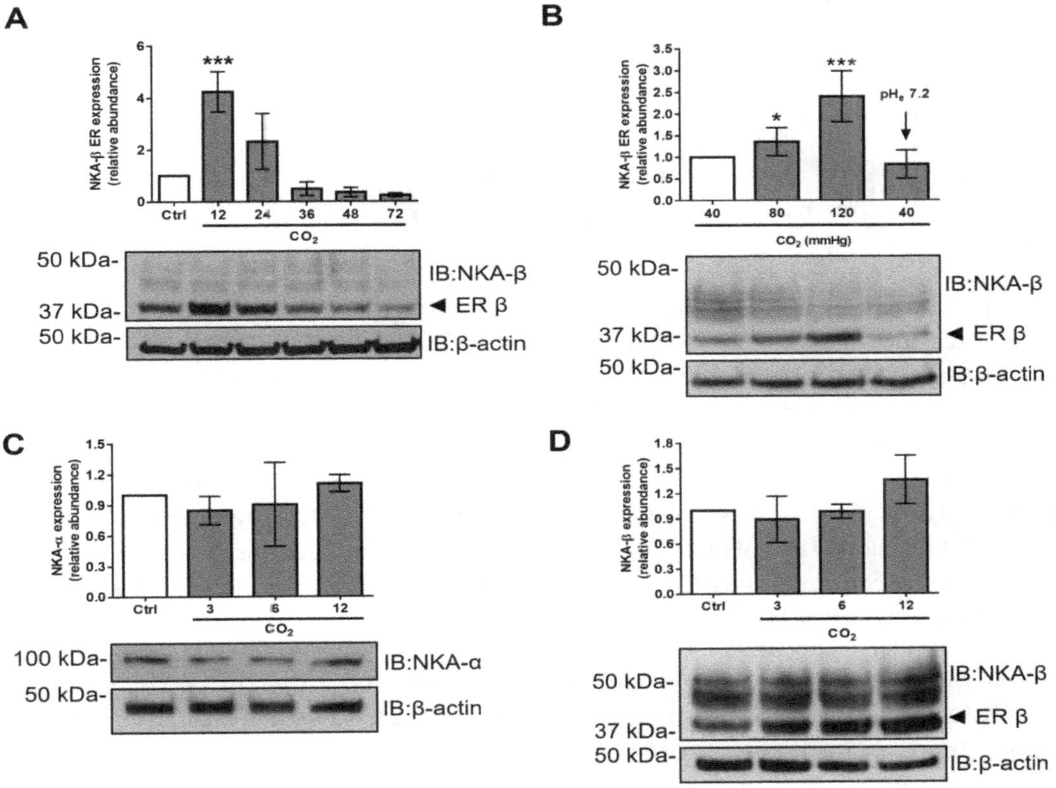

Figure 1. Hypercapnia increases Na,K-ATPase (NKA)-β abundance in the endoplasmic reticulum (ER). (**A**) A549 cells were exposed to 40 (Ctrl) or 120 mmHg CO_2 (CO_2) with an extracellular pH = 7.4 for the different time-points up to 72 h. Total cellular level of NKA-β was measured by immunoblotting. Representative immunoblots of NKA-β are shown. Bars represent ER-resident NKA-β/β-actin ratio. Values are expressed as mean ± SD (n = 3, *** $p < 0.001$). (**B**) A549 cells were treated with 40, 60, 80, and 120 mmHg of CO_2 with an extracellular pH = 7.4 or to 40 mmHg CO_2 with a pH = 7.2 for 12 h. NKA-β levels were measured by immunoblotting. Representative immunoblots of NKA-β are shown. Bars represent total NKA-β/β-actin ratio. Values are expressed as mean ± SD (n = 3, * $p < 0.05$, *** $p < 0.001$). (**C**) A549 cells were exposed to 40 (Ctrl) or 120 mmHg CO_2 (CO_2) with an extracellular pH = 7.4 for different time-points. Total cellular levels of NKA-α were measured by immunoblotting. Representative immunoblots of NKA-α are shown. Bars represent total NKA-α/β-actin ratio. Values are expressed as mean ± SD (n = 3). (**D**) A549 cells were exposed to 40 (Ctrl) or 120 mmHg CO_2 (CO_2) for different time-points. Total cellular levels of NKA-β were measured by immunoblotting. Representative immunoblots of NKA-β are shown. Bars represent total NKA-β/β-actin ratio. Values are expressed as mean ± SD (n = 3).

2.2. *Elevated CO_2 Levels Decrease Na,K-ATPase Plasma Membrane Abundance and Function*

It has been previously demonstrated that NKA-α cannot leave the ER before being assembled with the regulatory NKA-β subunit and that only a functional NKA α:β complex exported from the ER can reach the cellular surface [19,20]. Thus, to determine whether the hypercapnia-induced increase in the amount of ER-resident NKA-β influenced PM expression of the NKA, we performed a cell-surface protein biotinylation and the streptavidin pull-down assay (Figure 2A).

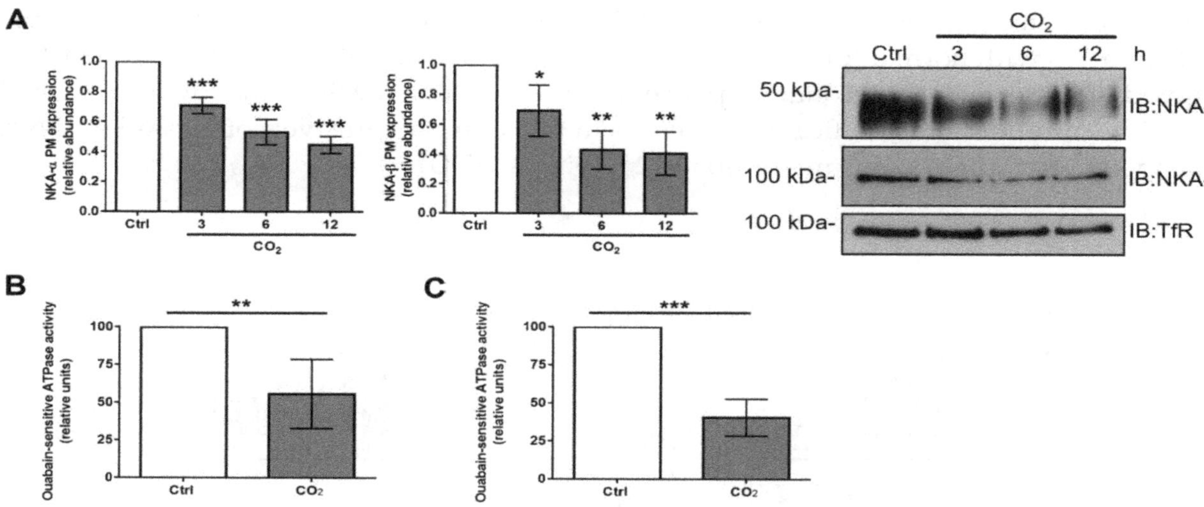

Figure 2. Exposure to elevated CO_2 levels for up to 12 h decreases Na,K-ATPase plasma membrane abundance and function. (**A**) A549 cells were exposed to 40 (Ctrl) or 120 mmHg CO_2 (CO_2) for different time-points. Plasma membrane (PM) abundance of NKA-α and NKA-β was determined by biotin-streptavidin pull-down and immunoblotting. Representative immunoblots of NKA-α, NKA-β, and transferrin receptor (TfR) at the PM are shown. Bars represent the NKA-α or NKA-β/TfR ratio. Values are expressed as mean ± SD ($n = 3$, * $p < 0.05$, ** $p < 0.01$, *** $p < 0.001$). (**B**) Primary rat ATII and (**C**) human A549 cells were exposed to 40 (Ctrl) or 120 mmHg CO_2 (CO_2) with extracellular pH = 7.4 for 12 h. The PM fraction was isolated by ultracentrifugation and ouabain-sensitive NKA activity was measured by using a colorimetric ATP bioluminescence assay kit. Values are expressed as mean ± SD ($n = 5$, ** $p < 0.01$, *** $p < 0.001$).

Exposure of AEC to elevated CO_2 concentrations decreased the cell surface abundance of the NKA-α and NKA-β subunits in a time-dependent manner. These findings correlated with the above-mentioned increase in the levels of ER-resident NKA-β (Figure 1D), which suggests that the ER retention of NKA-β contributed to the decreased cell-surface expression of the enzyme. Next, NKA function was assessed by measuring ouabain-sensitive ATPase activity in isolated PM fractions from primary rat alveolar epithelial type II (ATII) and human A549 cells (Figure 2B,C). Consistent with the results of our biotinylation assays, in both cellular cultures, elevated CO_2 levels markedly decreased ouabain-sensitive ATPase activity, which indicates reduced NKA function.

2.3. *Hypercapnia Induces Endoplasmic Reticulum Retention of the Na,K-ATPase β-Subunit*

The increased abundance of ER-resident NKA-β (that was not efficiently delivered to the plasma membrane) might be explained by retention of NKA-β in the ER [20]. To test this hypothesis, we performed isolation of ER and Golgi subcellular fractions from total cellular lysates and determined the amount of high mannose and complex N-glycan type NKA-β (Figure 3A). We observed increased amounts of NKA-β in the ER upon hypercapnia, which was associated with decreased Golgi-resident complex forms of the enzyme. These results suggested that newly synthesized forms of NKA were not processed to further maturation steps but were retained in the ER, which leads to decreased cell-surface abundance of the transporter.

Recent reports showed that the ER chaperones, binding immunoglobulin protein (BiP), and calnexin are required for the folding and retention of the NKA-β subunit upon normal and stress conditions [20]. To further assess if those chaperones were involved in the hypercapnia-induced ER retention of the NKA-β, AEC were exposed to normal or elevated CO_2 levels and localization of NKA-β, calnexin, and BiP were detected by immunofluorescent microscopy (Figure 3B,C). Enhanced co-localization of NKA-β with calnexin and BiP was observed upon hypercapnia, which indicates that both chaperons might be involved in the process of ER retention.

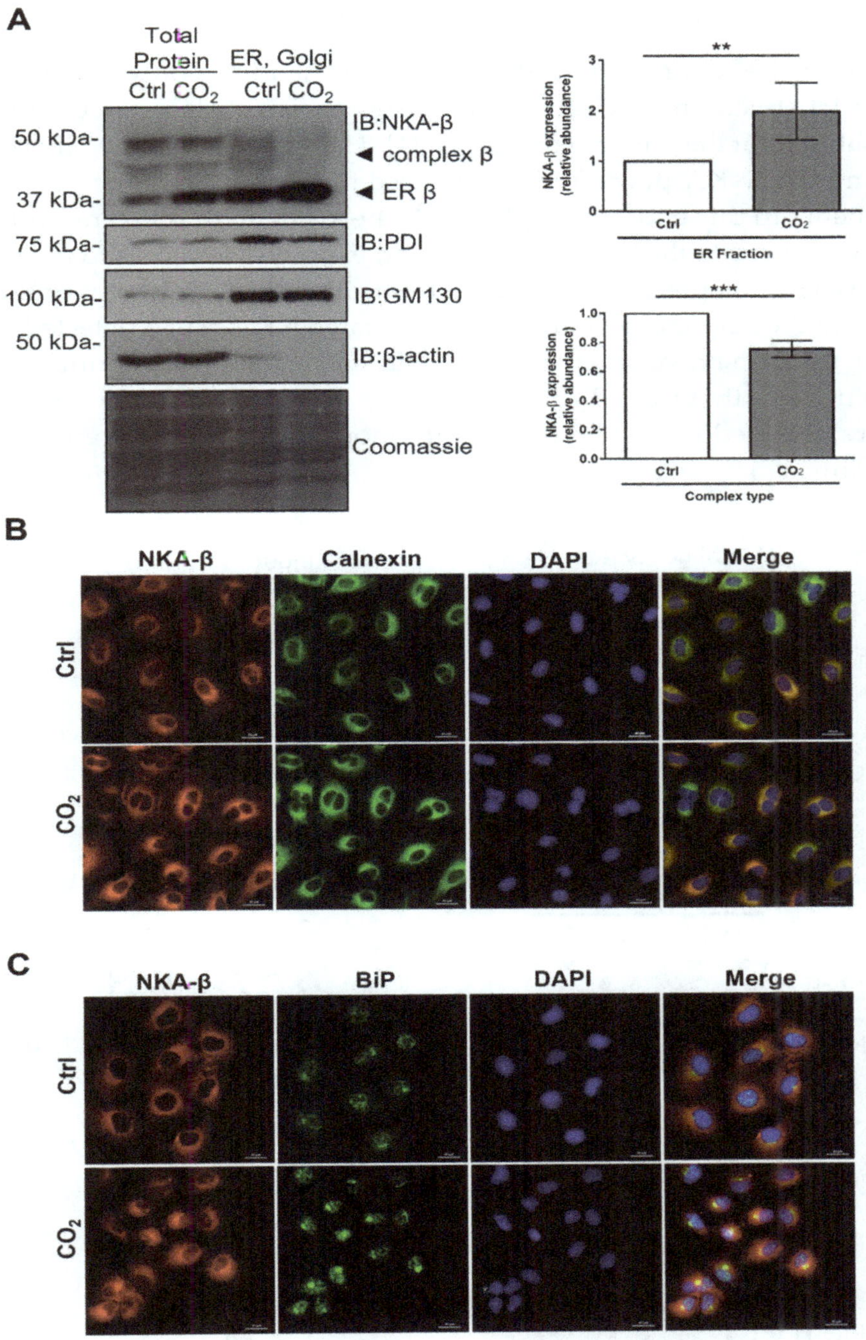

Figure 3. Elevated CO_2 levels promote endoplasmic reticulum (ER) retention of Na,K-ATPase-β. (**A**) A549 cells were exposed to 40 (Ctrl) or 120 mmHg CO_2 (CO_2) with an extracellular pH = 7.4 for 12 h. Subcellular fractions were isolated by ultracentrifugation and protein levels of the NKA-β, protein disulfide isomerase (PDI; an ER marker), and Golgin subfamily A member 2 (GM130;a Golgi marker) were analyzed by immunoblotting. Representative Western blots are shown. Bars represent ER NKA-β/Coomassie ratio or complex type NKA-β/Coomassie ratio. Values are expressed as mean ± SD ($n = 4$, ** $p < 0.01$, *** $p < 0.001$). (**B**) A549 cells were exposed to 40 (Ctrl) or 120 mmHg CO_2 (CO_2) with an extracellular pH = 7.4 for 12 h. Cellular localization of NKA-β and calnexin were determined by immunofluorescence. Immunofluorescence staining of NKA-β (red), calnexin (green), and nuclei (blue) are shown. Scale bar—20 μM. (**C**) A549 cells were exposed to 40 (Ctrl) or 120 mmHg CO_2 (CO_2) with an extracellular pH = 7.4 for 12 h. Cellular localization of NKA-β and BiP were determined by immunofluorescence. Representative immunofluorescence staining of NKA-β (red), BiP (green), and nuclei (blue) are shown. Scale bar—20 μM.

2.4. Hypercapnia Attenuates Na,K-ATPase α:β Complex Formation

Previous studies have reported that ER quality control allows only export of assembled NKA α:β complexes at a 1:1 stoichiometric ratio to the Golgi, which sustains an equimolar ratio of NKA α-subunits and β-subunits at the cellular surface [19,21]. Having demonstrated that elevated CO_2 levels caused ER retention of the NKA-β, we further analyzed the formation of the NKA α:β complex upon hypercapnia treatment. To this end, we employed A549-α_1-green fluorescent protein (A549-α_1-GFP) cells in which GFP was fused to the NKA-α subunit and exposed those cells to normal or elevated CO_2 levels. Afterward, we immunoprecipitated NKA-β from either total cell lysates or ER fractions by using specific antibodies and the amount of co-immunoprecipitated NKA-α was detected by immunoblotting (Figure 4A,B). Our results showed that hypercapnia decreased the amount of precipitated NKA α-subunit, which suggests that the ER-retained NKA-β was only partially assembled with NKA-α. Similar results were obtained when reverse co-immunoprecipitation with an antibody against GFP was performed (Figure 4C).

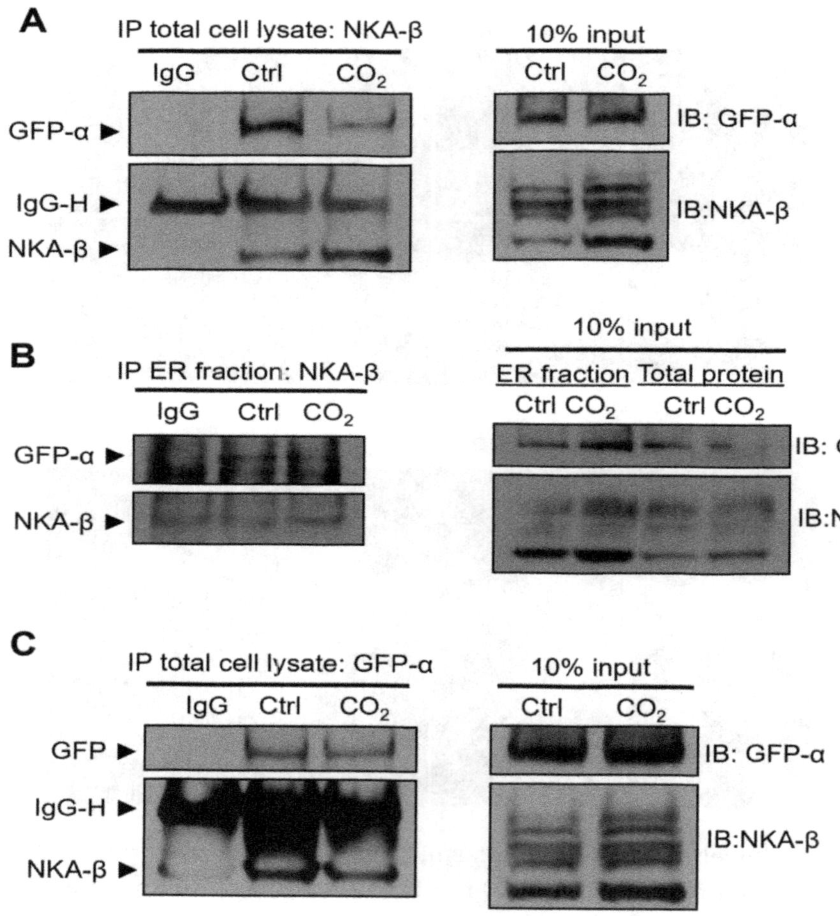

Figure 4. Elevated CO_2 levels decrease formation of the Na,K-ATPase-α:β complex. (**A**) A549-α_1-GFP expressing cells were exposed to 40 (Ctrl) or 120 mmHg CO_2 (CO_2) with an extracellular pH = 7.4 for 12 h. NKA-β was immunoprecipitated from the whole cell lysate by using an NKA-β-specific antibody and levels of co-immunoprecipitated NKA-α were analyzed by immunoblotting. Representative Western blots are shown (n = 4). (**B**) A549-α_1-GFP expressing cells were exposed to 40 (Ctrl) or 120 mmHg CO_2 (CO_2) with an extracellular pH = 7.4 for 12 h. The ER fraction was isolated and NKA-β was immunoprecipitated and the levels of co-immunoprecipitated NKA-α were analyzed by immunoblotting. Representative Western blots are shown (n = 3). (**C**) A549-α_1-GFP expressing cells were exposed to 40 (Ctrl) or 120 mmHg CO_2 (CO_2) with an extracellular pH = 7.4 for 12 h. NKA-α_1-GFP (GFP-α) was immunoprecipitated from the whole cell lysate by using a GFP-specific antibody and the levels of co-immunoprecipitated NKA-β were analyzed by immunoblotting. Representative Western blots are shown (n = 4).

2.5. *Elevated CO_2 Levels Alter the Oxidizing Environment of the Endoplasmic Reticulum and Promote Oxidation of the Na,K-ATPase β-Subunit*

It is well documented that a fully functional ER is dependent on physiological levels of Ca^{2+} and ATP and requires an oxidizing environment [22,23]. However, it has been shown that sustained hypercapnia and hypercapnic acidosis may decrease ATP production and perturb mitochondrial function [24,25]. Thus, we speculated that elevated CO_2 levels may prevent NKA-β maturation in the ER by altering the metabolic status of the cell. In line with this notion, we observed a significant decrease in intracellular ATP levels in hypercapnia-exposed AEC (Figure 5A). Of note, cell viability was not affected by elevated CO_2 levels even when AEC were exposed to hypercapnia for up to 72 h (Figure 5B).

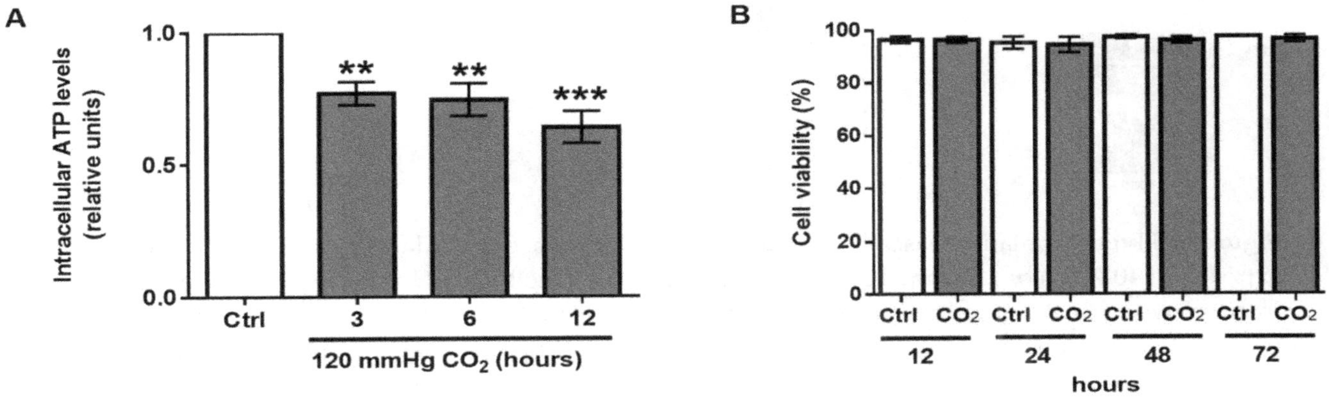

Figure 5. Hypercapnia decreases intracellular ATP production but does not affect cell viability. (**A**) A549 were treated with normal (Ctrl, 40 mmHg, pHe = 7.4) or elevated CO_2 levels (CO_2, 120 mmHg, pHe = 7.4) for different time-points. Intracellular ATP levels were measured by using an ATP bioluminescence assay kit. Bars represent total ATP/total protein ratio. Values are expressed as mean ± SD ($n = 3$, ** $p < 0.01$, *** $p < 0.001$). (**B**) A549 cells were exposed to normal (Ctrl, 40 mmHg, pHe = 7.4) or elevated CO_2 levels (CO_2, 120 mmHg, pHe = 7.4) for different time-points. Cell viability was measured by assessing the plasma membrane integrity. Graph bars represent the percentage of viable cells. Values are expressed as mean ± SD ($n = 3$).

It has been previously reported that decreased cellular ATP levels can promote protein oxidation by activating redox reactions [26,27]. Therefore, we next hypothesized that hypercapnia may alter the oxidizing environment of cells. To determine whether increased CO_2 levels affect protein oxidation in hypercapnia-treated AEC, we isolated total, cytosolic, and ER fractions from whole-cell homogenates by ultracentrifugation and, subsequently, assessed protein oxidation in these fractions. Importantly, in contrast to the total protein and cytosolic fractions (Figure 6A,B), hypercapnia treatment augmented the levels of protein oxidation in the ER (Figure 6C).

In addition, to determine whether NKA was a substrate of protein oxidation, AEC were exposed to normal or elevated CO_2 concentrations and the levels of protein oxidation in immunoprecipitated NKA-β were detected by immunoblotting (Figure 6C). Of note, we detected that the levels of NKA-β oxidation were increased when exposed to elevated CO_2 levels, which suggests that hypercapnia dysregulated the oxidizing status of the ER environment. Therefore, it induces the oxidation of NKA-β and potentially disrupts normal maturation of the enzyme.

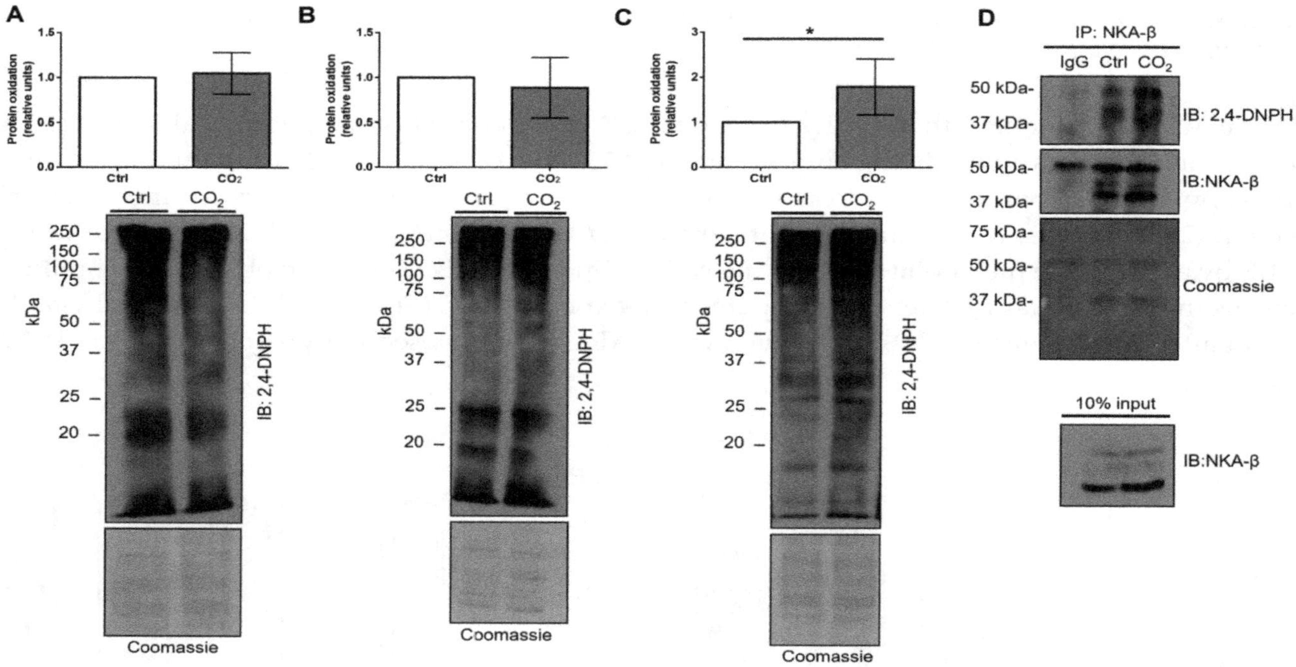

Figure 6. Hypercapnia increases ER protein and Na,K-ATPase-β oxidation levels. A549 cells were exposed to 40 (Ctrl) or 120 mmHg CO_2 (CO_2) with an extracellular pH = 7.4 for 12 h. Next, cellular fractions were isolated by ultracentrifugation and protein oxidation, which was determined in (**A**) total protein, (**B**) cytosolic, and (**C**) ER fraction by immunoblotting against 2,4-dinitrophenylhydrazone (2,4-DNPH). Bars represent a 2,4-DNPH/Coomassie ratio. Values are expressed as mean ± SD ($n = 5$, * $p < 0.05$). (**D**) A549 cells were exposed to normal (Ctrl, 40 mmHg, pHe = 7.4) or elevated CO_2 levels (CO_2, 120 mmHg, pHe = 7.4) for 12 h. NKA-β was then immunoprecipitated and protein oxidation was determined as described above. Representative Western blots are shown.

2.6. Treatment with α-Ketoglutaric Acid Ameliorates Hypercapnia-Induced ER Dysfunction and Restores Na,K-ATPase Function

Up to this point, our studies have suggested that hypercapnia enhances retention of ER-resident NKA-β due to increased protein oxidation in the ER. In a recent publication, it has been shown that elevated CO_2 levels inhibit expression of isocitrate dehydrogenase 2 (IDH2), which is a key enzyme in the tricarboxylic acid (TCA) cycle. Thereby, it causes mitochondrial dysfunction and ATP depletion [24]. Furthermore, treatment with α-ketoglutaric acid (α-KG) compensated the loss of IDH2 and raised ATP levels in hypercapnia-exposed cells [24]. Thus, we hypothesized that the increased ER oxidation by elevated CO_2 levels was due to mitochondrial dysfunction that might be rescued by administration of α-KG. Treatment of AEC with α-KG prevented the hypercapnia-induced increase in protein oxidation in the ER (Figure 7A).

Next, we determined the effects of α-KG treatment on ER-resident and PM-located NKA-β upon hypercapnia. AEC were exposed to normal or elevated levels of CO_2 for 12 h in the presence or absence of α-KG and, subsequently, the ER faction and cell surface abundance of NKA-β were measured (Figure 7B,C). Our results revealed that α-KG treatment rescues the effects of hypercapnia on the levels of NKA-β in the ER, which was associated with an increased expression of NKA-β at the PM. Moreover, to determine whether an increased cell surface abundance of the NKA-β resulted in an elevation of NKA activity, we measured ouabain-sensitive ATPase activity in primary and cultured AEC (Figure 7D,E) and observed that treatment with α-KG partially restored NKA function upon hypercapnia. Lastly, treatment with α-KG partially restored the hypercapnia-induced reduction in total intracellular ATP levels (Figure 7F). Taken together, these studies suggest that rescuing mitochondrial function and administration of α-KG restore the hypercapnia-induced ER retention of NKA-β, which increases PM abundance and activity of NKA.

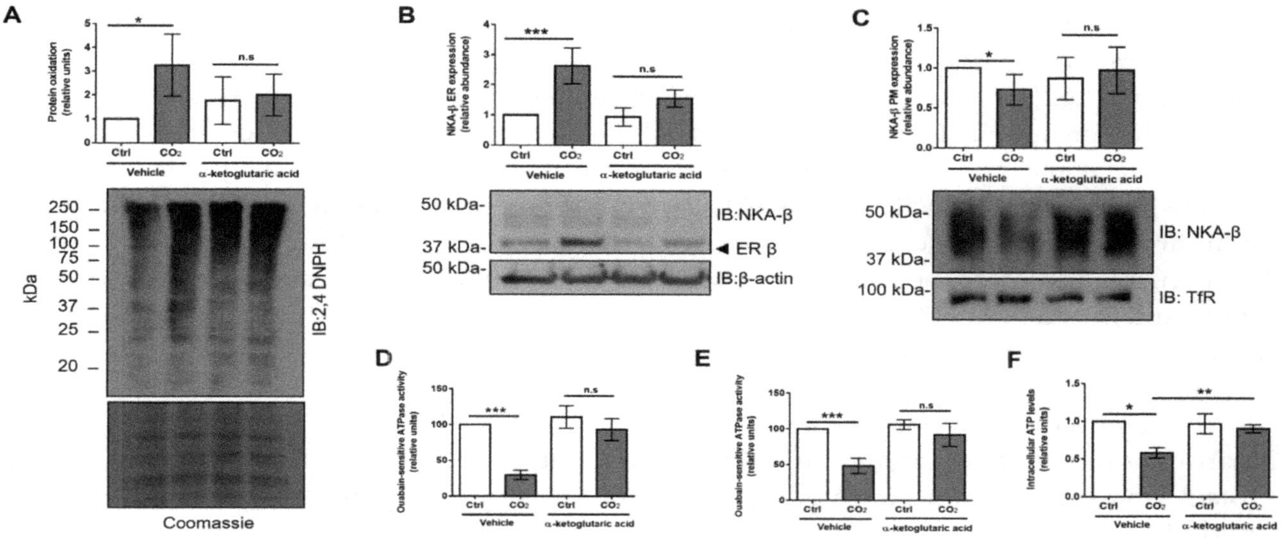

Figure 7. Treatment with α-KG reverses hypercapnia-induced protein oxidation and decreases ER-retained forms of Na,K-ATPase. (**A**) A549 cells were exposed to 40 (Ctrl) or 120 mmHg CO_2 (CO_2) with an extracellular pH = 7.4 for 12 h in the presence or absence of α-KG (10 mM) or vehicle. The ER fraction was isolated by ultracentrifugation and the level of protein oxidation was assessed as described above. Bars represent 2,4-DNPH/Coomassie ratio. Values are expressed as mean ± SD ($n = 3$, * $p < 0.05$, n.s—non-significant). (**B**) A549 cells were exposed to 40 (Ctrl) or 120 mmHg CO_2 (CO_2) with an extracellular pH = 7.4 for 12 h in the presence or absence of α-KG or vehicle. NKA-β levels were measured by immunoblotting. Representative immunoblots are shown. Bars represent the ER-resident NKA-β/β-actin ratio. Values are expressed as mean ± SD ($n = 5$, *** $p < 0.001$, n.s. – non-significant). (**C**) A549 cells were exposed to 40 (Ctrl) or 120 mmHg CO_2 (CO_2) for 12 h in the presence or absence of α-KG or vehicle. NKA-β PM abundance was determined by biotin-streptavidin pull-down and immunoblotting. Representative immunoblots of NKA-α, NKA-β, and TfR at the PM are shown. Bars represent the NKA-β/TfR ratio. Values are expressed as mean ± SD ($n = 5$, * $p < 0.05$, n.s—non-significant). (**D**) Primary rat ATII and (**E**) A549 cells were exposed to 40 (Ctrl) or 120 mmHg CO_2 (CO_2) with extracellular pH = 7.4 for 12 h in the presence or absence of α-KG or vehicle. The PM fraction was isolated by ultracentrifugation and ouabain-sensitive Na,K-ATPase activity was measured by using a colorimetric ATP bioluminescence assay kit. Values are expressed as mean ± SD ($n = 5$, *** $p < 0.001$, n.s. – non-significant). (**F**) A549 cells were exposed to 40 (Ctrl) or 120 mmHg CO_2 (CO_2) with an extracellular pH = 7.4 for 12 h in the presence or absence of α-KG or vehicle. Intracellular ATP levels were measured by using an ATP bioluminescence assay kit. Bars represent total ATP/total protein ratio. Values are expressed as mean ± SD ($n = 3$, * $p < 0.05$, ** $p < 0.01$).

3. Discussion

In the present study, we show that, in alveolar epithelial cells, hypercapnia downregulates NKA function by promoting oxidation of NKA-β, which, thereby, impairs its interaction with NKA-α and retains the misfolded NKA-β in the ER. This decreases PM abundance and activity of the transporter. In addition, we demonstrate that treatment with α-KG, which is an active metabolite, that has been previously shown to rescue the impaired TCA cycle and ATP production in hypercapnia-exposed cells, attenuates the elevated CO_2–induced NKA-β oxidation in the ER, which increases the abundance of the enzyme at the PM.

Effective alveolar gas exchange requires relatively "dry" airspaces achieved by an active vectorial Na^+ transport process across the alveolar epithelium [28], driven by the basolaterally-located NKA and the apical epithelial sodium channel, ENaC, which promotes alveolar fluid clearance [17,29,30]. It is well documented that impaired function/expression of these transporters have a deleterious impact on the resolution of lung edema in models of ALI [31,32]. In patients with ARDS, disruption of the alveolar-capillary barrier causes pulmonary edema that severely alters gas exchange and leads to hypoxia and hypercapnia. Since patients with ARDS require ventilation with low tidal volumes to limit ventilator-induced lung injury, hypercapnia is often further aggravated in this patient group [11,12], which has been tolerated in the last two decades. This is a concept termed "permissive hypercapnia." Hypercapnia is a double-edged sword and the associated acidosis may exhibit advantageous anti-inflammatory effects [33]. However, recent reports suggest that, in patients with severe hypercapnia, elevated levels of CO_2 are associated with higher complication rates, more organ failure, worse outcome, and increased risk of intensive care unit mortality [34]. A possible explanation, in addition to the recently established negative effects of elevated CO_2 levels on innate immunity and host defense [35–37], might be the hypercapnia-driven impairment of alveolar edema resolution due to the high CO_2-driven downregulation of PM abundance and function of NKA and ENaC [14,38].

We have previously reported that hypercapnia rapidly (within minutes) decreases NKA PM abundance by inducing phosphorylation of the α-subunit of the transporter at the Ser18 residue by protein kinase C- ζ that is activated by a CO_2-specific signaling pathway including subsequent phosphorylation of extracellular signal-regulated kinase and AMP-activated protein kinase, whereas the c-Jun N terminal kinase drives NKA retrieval from the cell surface [14–16,38]. In contrast, potential effects of elevated CO_2 levels on the regulatory β-subunit of NKA have not been previously reported. In the current study, we describe a novel mechanism by which sustained hypercapnia leads to misfolding of NKA-β in the ER. The NKA-β is a glycoprotein with a molecular mass depending on its glycosylation profile of ~35–55 kDa. Once being synthetized by the ribosomes, the nascent NKA-β protein is co-translationally transported to the ER, where high mannose N-glycan subunit forms are generated. In the ER, the NKA-β undergoes folding, posttranslational modifications, and assembling with the NKA-α. Subsequent maturation and further glycosylation of NKA-β results in the formation of complex-type N-glycan forms, which are located in the Golgi and at the PM [20]. The ER maturation steps play a pivotal role in the NKA-β glycosylation processing [19,21] as well as in the formation of the α:β complexes, which underline the pivotal role of NKA-β in trafficking and the correct membrane insertion of the NKA α-subunit [19,39].

We first investigated whether hypercapnia affects protein levels of NKA-β focusing on the above-mentioned glycosylation states in AEC. We observed a marked time-dependent and dose-dependent increase in the ER-resident high mannose glycosylation forms of NKA-β peaking at 12 h upon exposure to elevated CO_2 levels. Of note, these effects were independent of extracellular acidosis, which suggests that the observed effects were directly mediated by CO_2. This increase in ER-resident NKA-β forms was paralleled by a decreased PM abundance and activity of NKA-α:β. Moreover, while the levels of NKA-β were markedly increased in the ER where there was an enhanced interaction of NKA-β with the ER-resident chaperons, calnexin and BiP was evident and we observed a significant decrease in Golgi-resident forms of NKA. This is in line with previous reports that show that mutations in the NKA-α:β interaction regions [19], lipid peroxidation, and activation of oxidative stress by cadmium [20], removal of NKA-β glycosylation sites [20], and overexpression of unassembled NKA β-subunits [40] result in ER retention and increased binding of NKA-β to ER-resident chaperones [20,40]. Since the catalytic NKA-α-subunit cannot leave the ER (and, thus, reach the cellular surface) without being assembled with the regulatory NKA-β-subunit at a 1:1 stoichiometric ratio [19,20] and hypercapnia disturbs normal folding of NKA-β in the ER, which prevents its subsequent further maturation, collectively, our data suggest that elevated CO_2 levels disrupt the formation of the NKA-α:β complex in the ER, which impairs its delivery to the PM.

Changes in the ER environment or modifications of the protein structure may result in misfolding and protein retention in the ER [41]. It has been shown that high Ca^{2+} and sufficient ATP levels as well as a tightly regulated oxidizing environment are pivotal determinants of proper ER protein folding, glycosylating, and interaction with chaperones [42,43]. Thus, we hypothesized that the ER retention of NKA-β was due to changes in the ER environment. Of note, we establish, in this case, that elevated CO_2 alters the oxidizing environment of the ER and leads to protein carbonylation. Irreversible attachment of carbonyl groups to proteins is characteristic for a variety of oxidative pathways [44,45] that may promote protein misfolding and lead to various disease states [46,47]. The NKA-β contains a specific cysteine residue (Cys46) in its transmembrane domain that has been described to be highly susceptible to oxidative stress induced by glutathionylation [48], which possibly explains our findings regarding the enhanced ER retention of NKA-β. In addition, carbonylation of ER-resident chaperons may disrupt normal protein folding [46,49]. Whether hypercapnia leads to carbonylation of NKA-β at Cys46 and/or drives carbonylation of the above-mentioned ER-resident chaperons will need to be further investigated in future research. Furthermore, a common cellular response to transcriptional or translation errors is activation of protein carbonylation that "tags" peptides and, thereby, promotes their degradation [50]. Whether hypercapnia induces degradation of carbonylated proteins and NKA-β is currently being investigated in our laboratory.

In line with our previous findings in a different setting showing that elevated CO_2 reduces ATP production by inhibiting IDH2 in the TCA cycle and leads to mitochondrial dysfunction [24], our current study shows that sustained hypercapnia markedly decreases intracellular ATP levels. As mentioned above, normal mitochondrial function and sufficient ATP supply of the ER are essential for normal protein folding [23]. We next aimed to study the potential connection between NKA-β oxidation and ER retention upon hypercapnia and the metabolic status of the cell. To overcome the elevated CO_2-induced suppression of the TCA cycle, we treated AEC with α-KG (a TCA intermediate metabolite) that we have previously shown to rescue ATP production and cellular proliferation in CO_2 exposed cells [24]. We observed that hypercapnia-induced ER oxidation is significantly reduced after α-KG treatment, which leads to decreased ER-retained NKA-β and increased NKA cell surface abundance and function. Together with our previously published observation, we propose that α-KG treatment may rescue IDH2 activity and, thus, ATP production. Therefore, this decreases ER oxidation and stabilizes normal NKA trafficking. Of note, recent findings suggest that the mechanism by which α-KG operates is not limited to the TCA cycle but may involve various other metabolic and cellular signaling pathways regulating cellular energy supply donor, epigenetics, and prolyl hydroxylases activity [51–53]. Thus, elucidation of the exact mechanisms of α-KG action in the context of hypercapnia may need further studies.

Our study has some clear limitations. Although we were able to show that elevated CO_2 levels induce ER retention of the NKA-β subunit for up to 24 h that may lead to decreased cell surface abundance and activity of the enzyme, it is also evident that, at later time-points (36–72 h of high CO_2 exposure), elevated levels of NKA-β in the ER are not evident. Our preliminary data (not shown) suggest that this is due to degradation of ER-retained NKA-β. A further study addressing this point is currently a major focus of our laboratory. Additionally, while we demonstrate that, during hypercapnia, an increase in NKA-β is associated with a decrease of the levels of NKA-β in the Golgi apparatus and at the PM, to further strengthen our hypothesis, subsequent studies will be necessary to directly assess trafficking events of both NKA-β and NKA-α from the ER to Golgi and PM. Furthermore, although we demonstrate that ER retention of NKA-β is due to the increased oxidation, we do not know what the primary cause of these reactions is. In addition, despite showing that the formation of carbonyl groups plays a central role in the CO_2-induced protein oxidation reaction, the potential involvement of other oxidation reactions such as thiol oxidation, glutathionylation, or aromatic hydroxylation has not been investigated. Lastly, it will be important that future studies assess the effects of hypercapnia in more complex systems, such as precision-cut lung slices or human alveolar organoids to further enhance the translational relevance of these findings.

Taken together, our study shows for the first time that sustained hypercapnia decreases NKA cell surface abundance and function by inducing ER retention of its β-subunit via oxidative modification, which prevents its assembly with NKA-α. Furthermore, treatment with α-KG that increases ATP production and rescues the high CO_2-induced mitochondrial dysfunction attenuates protein oxidation in the ER and, thus, prevents ER retention of the NKA-β and enhances PM abundance and activity of NKA. Since NKA is both a key driver of alveolar fluid clearance and also a central cell adhesion molecule in the alveolar epithelium that is pivotal for prevention of alveolar edema formation, these novel findings may lead to novel therapeutic options that improve resolution of alveolar edema and restores alveolar epithelial barrier function in patients with ARDS and hypercapnia.

4. Materials and Methods

4.1. Cell Culture

Primary rat alveolar epithelial type II (ATII) cells were isolated as previously described [14]. Isolation of ATII cells from rats was conducted according to the legal regulations of the German Animal Welfare Act and was approved by the regional authority (Regierungspräsidium Gießen, reference number A12/2013 from March 28, 2013 and reference number G41/2018 from July 17, 2018) of the State of Hessen, Germany. ATII, human alveolar epithelial A549 (ATCC, CCL 185), and A549 cells stably expressing Na,K-ATPase α_1-subunit fused to a green fluorescent protein (A549-α_1-GFP) were grown in Dulbecco's modified Eagle's media (DMEM, Thermo Fisher Scientific, Darmstadt, Germany) supplemented with 10% fetal bovine serum (FBS, PAA Laboratories, Egelsbach, Germany), 100 U/mL penicillin, and 100 µg/mL streptomycin, as previously described [14]. For experiments, 600,000 A549 or 2,000,000 ATII cells were grown on 60-mm culture dishes (Sarstedt, Nümbrecht, Germany) in 4 mL of culture media. Alternatively, 200,000 A549 or 1,500,000 ATII cells were seeded on permeable membrane supports (BD Falcon, Heidelberg, Germany) with maintaining a liquid/liquid interface. Subconfluent cell monolayers were used for experiments. Cells were incubated in a humidified atmosphere of 5% CO_2 and 95% air at 37 °C.

4.2. CO_2 Exposure

ATII and A549 cells were exposed to 40 (normocapnia, Ctrl) or 120 mmHg (hypercapnia, CO_2) CO_2 conditions unless otherwise indicated. Normocapnia and hypercapnia media solutions were prepared freshly with DMEM or DMEM/F12, Ham's F12, and MOPS base to obtain a final pH of 7.4 at 40 (5%) or 120 mmHg (15%) of CO_2 while maintaining 21% O_2 balanced with N_2 and were kept overnight in the humidified C-chamber (BioSpherix Ltd., Parish, NY, USA), as described previously [24]. Levels of CO_2 in the chamber were controlled by an RO-CO_2 carbon dioxide controller (BioSpherix Ltd., NY, USA). Before experiments media pH, pCO_2 and pO_2 levels were measured using a Rapid-lab blood gas analyzer (Siemens, Erlangen, Germany).

4.3. Western Blot Analysis

Protein concentrations were determined by using the Bradford assay after lysing the cells. Equal protein concentrations were resolved in 7%–10% polyacrylamide gels and transferred to a nitrocellulose membrane using a semidry apparatus from Bio-Rad (Hercules, Berkeley, CA, USA). Membranes were blocked for one hour in 5% fat-free milk and were subsequently incubated with primary antibodies overnight at 4 °C. For some experiments, loading control was performed by staining of the nitrocellulose membranes with Coomassie brilliant blue 250 (Sigma Aldrich, St. Louis, MO, USA). Densitometric analyses were performed by using the Image J software (NIH, Bethesda, MD, USA).

4.4. Cell Surface Biotinylation

After hypercapnia exposure, PM surface proteins were labeled for 20 min by using 1 mg/mL EZ-Link-NHS-SS-biotin (Pierce Biotechnology, Waltham, MA, USA). Proteins were pulled down with streptavidin-agarose beads (Pierce Biotechnology, Waltham, MA, USA) and analyzed by SDS-PAGE and immunoblotting, as described previously [14].

4.5. Co-Immunoprecipitation

To assess protein-protein interactions, co-immunoprecipitation was used. AEC were exposed to normocapnia or hypercapnia, washed in PBS, and lysed in immunoprecipitation lysis buffer (20 mM

HEPES pH 7.4, 150 mM NaCl, 0.5% NP-40, 2 mM EDTA, 2 mM EGTA, 5% glycerol, protease and phosphatase inhibitors). Afterward, cells were scraped and centrifuged and cell lysates containing 150–300 μg of proteins were incubated with specific antibodies for Na,K-ATPase subunits, GFP, 2,4-DNPH, or IgG negative control and A/G agarose beads (Santa Cruz, Heidelberg, Germany) overnight at 4 °C. Precipitated complexes were eluted from the beads by adding 2X Laemmli buffer, heated at 60 °C for 20 min, and then subjected to SDS-PAGE and Western immunoblotting.

4.6. Antibodies and Chemical Compounds

The following antibodies and reagents were used: mouse anti-Na,K-ATPase β-subunit (clone M17-P5-F11) (Thermo Scientific, Rockford, IL, USA), rabbit anti-GFP (Santa Cruz Biotechnology, Dallas, TX, USA), mouse anti-Na,K-ATPase α-subunit (Merck Millipore, Darmstadt, Germany), rabbit anti-β-actin (Sigma Aldrich, St. Louis, MO, USA), mouse anti-transferrin receptor (Invitrogen, Rockford, IL, USA), rabbit anti-PDI (Cell Signaling, Danvers, MA, USA), rabbit anti-GM130 (Cell Signaling, Danvers, MA, USA), rabbit anti-calnexin (Abcam, Cambridge, UK), rabbit anti-BiP (Cell Signaling, Danvers, MA, USA), HRP-conjugated anti-mouse and anti-rabbit IgG (Cell Signaling, Danvers, MA, USA), and Alexa Fluor 488 and 594 conjugated anti-rabbit, anti-mouse (Thermo Scientific, Eugene, OR, USA). α-ketoglutaric acid was obtained from Sigma Aldrich, St. Louis, MO, USA.

4.7. Immunofluorescent Microscopy

After hypercapnia exposure cells were fixed with 4% paraformaldehyde, permeabilized with 0.1% Triton X-100, blocked by 3% bovine serum albumin (BSA), and incubated overnight with primary antibodies at 4 °C. Immunofluorescent images were captured by using a Carl Zeiss Axio Observer Z1 microscope (Carl Zeiss, Wetzlar, Germany).

4.8. Isolation of Total, Cytosolic Endoplasmic Reticulum and Golgi Cellular Fractions

Isolation of ER and Golgi was performed by adapting a previously described protocol [54]. After normocapnic and hypercapnic exposure cells were collected, homogenized, and centrifuged 10 min at 1400× *g* following supernatant centrifugation for 10 min at 15,000× *g*, 4 °C. Next, a small amount of the supernatant was aspirated and labeled as "total protein" and the rest was loaded on a sucrose gradient (2.0 M, 1.5 M, and 1.3 M) and centrifuged for 70 min at 152,000× *g*. Afterward, the upper 1 mL of the solution was withdrawn and labeled as "Cytosol." The ER fraction was collected from the large band at the interface of the 1.3 M sucrose gradient layer, resuspended in lysis buffer, and centrifuged for 45 min at 126,000× *g*, 4 °C. Afterward, the pellet was collected, resuspended in PBS (pH 7.4), and further analyzed by a Western blot. Since ER and Golgi are morphologically linked and have almost the same density during ultracentrifugation, the obtained ER proteins additionally contained Golgi complexes and, in some experiments, this fraction was named "ER, Golgi".

4.9. Isolation of Soluble Plasma Membrane Proteins

The soluble fractions of PM proteins were obtained by ultracentrifugation, as previously described [55]. After normocapnia or hypercapnia treatment, cells were detached, homogenized in homogenization buffer (10 mM, 1 mM EDTA, 1 mM EGTA, 100 μg/mL N-tosyl-l-phenylalanine chloromethyl ketone, phosphatase, and protease inhibitors), and centrifuged at 500× *g* at 4 °C. Next, supernatants were collected and centrifuged at 100,000× *g* for 1 h at 4 °C. Afterward, the pellet, which contained the crude membrane fraction, was resuspended in homogenization buffer supplemented 1% Triton X-100 and centrifuged at 100,000× *g* for 30 min at 4 °C. After centrifugation, a supernatant containing a soluble membrane fraction was collected and used for the experiments.

4.10. Measurement of Na,K-ATPase Enzymatic Activity

To measure ouabain-sensitive Na,K-ATPase activity, a high-sensitivity ATPase assay kit (Innova Biosciences, Cambridge, United Kingdom) was used, according to the instructions of the manufacturer, and was performed as described previously [55]. After treatment with normocapnia or hypercapnia, cells were detached, homogenized, and the PM fraction was isolated. To measure ouabain-sensitive ATPase activity, ouabain was applied to the soluble PM fractions and absorbance, which was measured at 600 nm by an Infinite M200 Pro reader (TECAN, Männedorf, Switzerland). Na,K-ATPase specific activity was calculated by subtraction of ouabain-sensitive from total ATPase activity.

4.11. Detection of the Protein Oxidation

Total protein oxidation was measured by using the OxyBlot protein oxidation detection kit (Merck Millipore, Darmstadt, Germany), according to instructions of the manufacturer. After normocapnia or hypercapnia treatment, cells were lysed, and an equal amount of proteins were derivatized by adding 1X 2,4-dinitrophenylhydrazine (DNPH) solution for 15 min. Afterward, a neutralization solution was added, samples were subjected to SDS-PAGE and transferred to nitrocellulose membranes. After incubation with antibodies from the kit, protein oxidation was determined by chemiluminescence and the density of detected protein oxidation was calculated by using the Image J software and normalized to the total protein amounts assessed by Coomassie staining.

4.12. Measurement of Intracellular ATP Levels

ATP levels after hypercapnia exposure were measured by an ATP bioluminescence assay kit HSII (Roche Diagnostics, Mannheim, Germany) following the instructions of the manufacturer. Cells were treated with normal or elevated CO_2 levels, detached, and lysed in the lysis buffer provided with the kit. Next, samples were centrifuged at 10,000× g for 60 s and the supernatant was transferred to a fresh tube. Lastly, 50 µL of supernatants were transferred to 96-well plates. Additionally, 50 µL of the luciferase reagent was added to the samples and luminescence was measured immediately by Infinite M200 Pro reader. The obtained values were normalized to the protein amount as assessed by the Bradford assay.

4.13. Measurement of Cellular Viability

Cell viability was assessed by using the CASY cell counter and analyzer model TT (Roche Innovatis AG, Reutlingen, Germany) following the instructions of the manufacturer, as determined by an automatized measurement of plasma membrane integrity via an electric impulse. After exposure to normocapnic or hypercapnic conditions, cells were detached by incubation with 0.25% trypsin-EDTA, resuspended in culture medium, diluted in CASY tone solution, and the membrane integrity measurement was performed.

4.14. Statistics

Data are presented as mean ± SD unless otherwise indicated. Comparison of two groups was performed by paired (dependent) or unpaired (independent) two-tailed Student's t-test. Comparisons between more than two groups were performed by one-way or two-way analysis of variance (ANOVA) with a Dunnet test for multiple comparisons. For statistical analysis and data visualization, GraphPad Prism 6 (GraphPad Software, San Diego, CA, USA) was used. A p-value of <0.05 was considered to be statistically significant.

Author Contributions: Conceptualization, V.K. and I.V. Data curation, V.K., R.E.M., S.H., W.S., O.V., and L.A.D. Formal analysis, V.K., O.V., and L.A.D. Funding acquisition, I.V. Investigation, V.K. and M.W. Methodology, V.K., M.W., O.V., and L.A.D. Project administration, M.W. and I.V. Resources, R.E.M., S.H., W.S., J.I.S., and I.V. Supervision, I.V. Validation, V.K., O.V., L.A.D., and J.I.S. Visualization, V.K. and I.V. Writing—original draft, V.K. and I.V. Writing—review & editing, V.K., R.E.M., S.H., W.S., O.V., L.A.D., J.I.S., and I.V. All authors have read and agreed to the published version of the manuscript.

Abbreviations

α-KG	α-ketoglutaric acid
AEC	alveolar epithelial cell
ALI	acute lung injury
ARDS	acute respiratory distress syndrome
ATII	alveolar epithelial type II
BiP	binding immunoglobulin protein
CO_2	carbon dioxide
ENaC	epithelial sodium channel
ER	endoplasmic reticulum
GFP	green fluorescent protein
IDH2	isocitrate dehydrogenase 2
NKA	Na,K-ATPase
PM	plasma membrane
TCA	tricarboxylic acid
TfR	transferrin receptor

References

1. Clausen, M.V.; Hilbers, F.; Poulsen, H. The Structure and Function of the Na,K-ATPase Isoforms in Health and Disease. *Front. Physiol.* **2017**, *8*, 371. [CrossRef] [PubMed]
2. Kaplan, J.H. Biochemistry of Na,K-ATPase. *Annu. Rev. Biochem.* **2002**, *71*, 511–535. [CrossRef] [PubMed]
3. Tokhtaeva, E.; Sun, H.; Deiss-Yehiely, N.; Wen, Y.; Soni, P.N.; Gabrielli, N.M.; Marcus, E.A.; Ridge, K.M.; Sachs, G.; Vazquez-Levin, M.; et al. The O-glycosylated ectodomain of FXYD5 impairs adhesion by disrupting cell-cell trans-dimerization of Na,K-ATPase beta1 subunits. *J. Cell Sci.* **2016**, *129*, 2394–2406. [CrossRef] [PubMed]
4. Wujak, L.A.; Blume, A.; Baloglu, E.; Wygrecka, M.; Wygowski, J.; Herold, S.; Mayer, K.; Vadasz, I.; Besuch, P.; Mairbaurl, H.; et al. FXYD1 negatively regulates Na(+)/K(+)-ATPase activity in lung alveolar epithelial cells. *Respir. Physiol. Neurobiol.* **2016**, *220*, 54–61. [CrossRef]
5. Flodby, P.; Kim, Y.H.; Beard, L.L.; Gao, D.; Ji, Y.; Kage, H.; Liebler, J.M.; Minoo, P.; Kim, K.J.; Borok, Z.; et al. Knockout Mice Reveal a Major Role for Alveolar Epithelial Type I Cells in Alveolar Fluid Clearance. *Am. J. Respir. Cell Mol. Biol.* **2016**, *55*, 395–406. [CrossRef]
6. Geering, K. Functional roles of Na,K-ATPase subunits. *Curr. Opin. Nephrol. Hypertens.* **2008**, *17*, 526–532. [CrossRef]
7. Tokhtaeva, E.; Sachs, G.; Souda, P.; Bassilian, S.; Whitelegge, J.P.; Shoshani, L.; Vagin, O. Epithelial junctions depend on intercellular trans-interactions between the Na,K-ATPase beta(1) subunits. *J. Biol. Chem.* **2011**, *286*, 25801–25812. [CrossRef]
8. Rajasekaran, S.A.; Palmer, L.G.; Quan, K.; Harper, J.F.; Ball, W.J., Jr.; Bander, N.H.; Peralta Soler, A.; Rajasekaran, A.K. Na,K-ATPase beta-subunit is required for epithelial polarization, suppression of invasion, and cell motility. *Mol. Biol. Cell* **2001**, *12*, 279–295. [CrossRef]
9. Rajasekaran, S.A.; Barwe, S.P.; Rajasekaran, A.K. Multiple functions of Na,K-ATPase in epithelial cells. *Semin. Nephrol.* **2005**, *25*, 328–334. [CrossRef]
10. Vagin, O.; Tokhtaeva, E.; Yakubov, I.; Shevchenko, E.; Sachs, G. Inverse correlation between the extent of N-glycan branching and intercellular adhesion in epithelia. Contribution of the Na,K-ATPase beta1 subunit. *J. Biol. Chem.* **2008**, *283*, 2192–2202. [CrossRef]
11. Cummins, E.P.; Strowitzki, M.J.; Taylor, C.T. Mechanisms and consequences of oxygen- and carbon dioxide-sensing in mammals. *Physiol. Rev.* **2019**. [CrossRef] [PubMed]

12. Vadasz, I.; Hubmayr, R.D.; Nin, N.; Sporn, P.H.; Sznajder, J.I. Hypercapnia: A nonpermissive environment for the lung. *Am. J. Respir Cell Mol. Biol.* **2012**, *46*, 417–421. [CrossRef] [PubMed]
13. Nin, N.; Angulo, M.; Briva, A. Effects of hypercapnia in acute respiratory distress syndrome. *Ann. Transl. Med.* **2018**, *6*, 37. [CrossRef] [PubMed]
14. Vadasz, I.; Dada, L.A.; Briva, A.; Trejo, H.E.; Welch, L.C.; Chen, J.; Toth, P.T.; Lecuona, E.; Witters, L.A.; Schumacker, P.T.; et al. AMP-activated protein kinase regulates CO_2-induced alveolar epithelial dysfunction in rats and human cells by promoting Na,K-ATPase endocytosis. *J. Clin. Investig.* **2008**, *118*, 752–762. [CrossRef]
15. Vadasz, I.; Dada, L.A.; Briva, A.; Helenius, I.T.; Sharabi, K.; Welch, L.C.; Kelly, A.M.; Grzesik, B.A.; Budinger, G.R.; Liu, J.; et al. Evolutionary conserved role of c-Jun-N-terminal kinase in CO_2-induced epithelial dysfunction. *PLoS ONE* **2012**, *7*, e46696. [CrossRef]
16. Dada, L.A.; Trejo Bittar, H.E.; Welch, L.C.; Vagin, O.; Deiss-Yehiely, N.; Kelly, A.M.; Baker, M.R.; Capri, J.; Cohn, W.; Whitelegge, J.P.; et al. High CO_2 Leads to Na,K-ATPase Endocytosis via c-Jun Amino-Terminal Kinase-Induced LMO7b Phosphorylation. *Mol. Cell Biol.* **2015**, *35*, 3962–3973. [CrossRef]
17. Matthay, M.A.; Folkesson, H.G.; Clerici, C. Lung epithelial fluid transport and the resolution of pulmonary edema. *Physiol. Rev.* **2002**, *82*, 569–600. [CrossRef]
18. Brodsky, J.L.; Skach, W.R. Protein folding and quality control in the endoplasmic reticulum: Recent lessons from yeast and mammalian cell systems. *Curr. Opin. Cell Biol.* **2011**, *23*, 464–475. [CrossRef]
19. Tokhtaeva, E.; Sachs, G.; Vagin, O. Assembly with the Na,K-ATPase alpha(1) subunit is required for export of beta(1) and beta(2) subunits from the endoplasmic reticulum. *Biochemistry* **2009**, *48*, 11421–11431. [CrossRef]
20. Tokhtaeva, E.; Sachs, G.; Vagin, O. Diverse pathways for maturation of the Na,K-ATPase beta1 and beta2 subunits in the endoplasmic reticulum of Madin-Darby canine kidney cells. *J. Biol. Chem.* **2010**, *285*, 39289–39302. [CrossRef]
21. Tokhtaeva, E.; Munson, K.; Sachs, G.; Vagin, O. N-glycan-dependent quality control of the Na,K-ATPase beta(2) subunit. *Biochemistry* **2010**, *49*, 3116–3128. [CrossRef] [PubMed]
22. Ellgaard, L.; Helenius, A. Quality control in the endoplasmic reticulum. *Nat. Rev. Mol. Cell Biol.* **2003**, *4*, 181–191. [CrossRef] [PubMed]
23. Araki, K.; Nagata, K. Protein folding and quality control in the ER. *Cold Spring Harb. Perspect. Biol.* **2011**, *3*, a007526. [CrossRef] [PubMed]
24. Vohwinkel, C.U.; Lecuona, E.; Sun, H.; Sommer, N.; Vadasz, I.; Chandel, N.S.; Sznajder, J.I. Elevated CO(2) levels cause mitochondrial dysfunction and impair cell proliferation. *J. Biol. Chem.* **2011**, *286*, 37067–37076. [CrossRef] [PubMed]
25. Fergie, N.; Todd, N.; McClements, L.; McAuley, D.; O'Kane, C.; Krasnodembskaya, A. Hypercapnic acidosis induces mitochondrial dysfunction and impairs the ability of mesenchymal stem cells to promote distal lung epithelial repair. *FASEB J.* **2019**, *33*, 5585–5598. [CrossRef]
26. Schutt, F.; Aretz, S.; Auffarth, G.U.; Kopitz, J. Moderately reduced ATP levels promote oxidative stress and debilitate autophagic and phagocytic capacities in human RPE cells. *Invest. Ophthalmol. Vis. Sci.* **2012**, *53*, 5354–5361. [CrossRef]
27. Esposito, L.A.; Melov, S.; Panov, A.; Cottrell, B.A.; Wallace, D.C. Mitochondrial disease in mouse results in increased oxidative stress. *Proc. Natl. Acad. Sci. USA* **1999**, *96*, 4820–4825. [CrossRef]
28. Huppert, L.A.; Matthay, M.A. Alveolar Fluid Clearance in Pathologically Relevant Conditions: In Vitro and In Vivo Models of Acute Respiratory Distress Syndrome. *Front. Immunol.* **2017**, *8*, 371. [CrossRef]
29. Matalon, S.; Bartoszewski, R.; Collawn, J.F. Role of epithelial sodium channels in the regulation of lung fluid homeostasis. *Am. J. Physiol. Lung Cell Mol. Physiol.* **2015**, *309*, L1229–L1238. [CrossRef]
30. Sznajder, J.I.; Factor, P.; Ingbar, D.H. Invited review: Lung edema clearance: Role of Na(+)-K(+)-ATPase. *J. Appl. Physiol. (1985)* **2002**, *93*, 1860–1866. [CrossRef]
31. Sznajder, J.I. Alveolar edema must be cleared for the acute respiratory distress syndrome patient to survive. *Am. J. Respir Crit. Care Med.* **2001**, *163*, 1293–1294. [CrossRef] [PubMed]
32. Bhattacharya, J.; Matthay, M.A. Regulation and repair of the alveolar-capillary barrier in acute lung injury. *Annu. Rev. Physiol.* **2013**, *75*, 593–615. [CrossRef] [PubMed]
33. Contreras, M.; Masterson, C.; Laffey, J.G. Permissive hypercapnia: What to remember. *Curr. Opin. Anaesthesiol* **2015**, *28*, 26–37. [CrossRef] [PubMed]
34. Nin, N.; Muriel, A.; Penuelas, O.; Brochard, L.; Lorente, J.A.; Ferguson, N.D.; Raymondos, K.; Rios, F.;

Violi, D.A.; Thille, A.W.; et al. Severe hypercapnia and outcome of mechanically ventilated patients with moderate or severe acute respiratory distress syndrome. *Intensive Care Med.* **2017**, *43*, 200–208. [CrossRef] [PubMed]

35. Casalino-Matsuda, S.M.; Nair, A.; Beitel, G.J.; Gates, K.L.; Sporn, P.H. Hypercapnia Inhibits Autophagy and Bacterial Killing in Human Macrophages by Increasing Expression of Bcl-2 and Bcl-xL. *J. Immunol.* **2015**, *194*, 5388–5396. [CrossRef] [PubMed]
36. Gates, K.L.; Howell, H.A.; Nair, A.; Vohwinkel, C.U.; Welch, L.C.; Beitel, G.J.; Hauser, A.R.; Sznajder, J.I.; Sporn, P.H. Hypercapnia impairs lung neutrophil function and increases mortality in murine pseudomonas pneumonia. *Am. J. Respir. Cell Mol. Biol.* **2013**, *49*, 821–828. [CrossRef] [PubMed]
37. Wang, N.; Gates, K.L.; Trejo, H.; Favoreto, S., Jr.; Schleimer, R.P.; Sznajder, J.I.; Beitel, G.J.; Sporn, P.H. Elevated CO_2 selectively inhibits interleukin-6 and tumor necrosis factor expression and decreases phagocytosis in the macrophage. *FASEB J.* **2010**, *24*, 2178–2190. [CrossRef]
38. Gwozdzinska, P.; Buchbinder, B.A.; Mayer, K.; Herold, S.; Morty, R.E.; Seeger, W.; Vadasz, I. Hypercapnia Impairs ENaC Cell Surface Stability by Promoting Phosphorylation, Polyubiquitination and Endocytosis of beta-ENaC in a Human Alveolar Epithelial Cell Line. *Front. Immunol.* **2017**, *8*, 591. [CrossRef]
39. Vagin, O.; Kraut, J.A.; Sachs, G. Role of N-glycosylation in trafficking of apical membrane proteins in epithelia. *Am. J. Physiol. Renal. Physiol.* **2009**, *296*, F459–F469. [CrossRef]
40. Beggah, A.; Mathews, P.; Beguin, P.; Geering, K. Degradation and endoplasmic reticulum retention of unassembled alpha- and beta-subunits of Na,K-ATPase correlate with interaction of BiP. *J. Biol. Chem.* **1996**, *271*, 20895–20902. [CrossRef]
41. Almanza, A.; Carlesso, A.; Chintha, C.; Creedican, S.; Doultsinos, D.; Leuzzi, B.; Luis, A.; McCarthy, N.; Montibeller, L.; More, S.; et al. Endoplasmic reticulum stress signalling - from basic mechanisms to clinical applications. *FEBS J.* **2019**, *286*, 241–278. [CrossRef] [PubMed]
42. Jager, R.; Bertrand, M.J.; Gorman, A.M.; Vandenabeele, P.; Samali, A. The unfolded protein response at the crossroads of cellular life and death during endoplasmic reticulum stress. *Biol. Cell* **2012**, *104*, 259–270. [CrossRef] [PubMed]
43. Braakman, I.; Hebert, D.N. Protein folding in the endoplasmic reticulum. *Cold Spring Harb. Perspect Biol.* **2013**, *5*, a013201. [CrossRef] [PubMed]
44. Marrocco, I.; Altieri, F.; Peluso, I. Measurement and Clinical Significance of Biomarkers of Oxidative Stress in Humans. *Oxid. Med. Cell Longev.* **2017**, *2017*, 6501046. [CrossRef] [PubMed]
45. Wong, C.M.; Marcocci, L.; Liu, L.; Suzuki, Y.J. Cell signaling by protein carbonylation and decarbonylation. *Antioxid Redox Signal.* **2010**, *12*, 393–404. [CrossRef] [PubMed]
46. Dalle-Donne, I.; Aldini, G.; Carini, M.; Colombo, R.; Rossi, R.; Milzani, A. Protein carbonylation, cellular dysfunction, and disease progression. *J. Cell Mol. Med.* **2006**, *10*, 389–406. [CrossRef]
47. Suzuki, Y.J.; Carini, M.; Butterfield, D.A. Protein carbonylation. *Antioxid Redox Signal.* **2010**, *12*, 323–325. [CrossRef]
48. Rasmussen, H.H.; Hamilton, E.J.; Liu, C.C.; Figtree, G.A. Reversible oxidative modification: Implications for cardiovascular physiology and pathophysiology. *Trends Cardiovasc Med.* **2010**, *20*, 85–90. [CrossRef]
49. England, K.; Cotter, T. Identification of carbonylated proteins by MALDI-TOF mass spectroscopy reveals susceptibility of ER. *Biochem Biophys Res. Commun.* **2004**, *320*, 123–130. [CrossRef]
50. Dukan, S.; Farewell, A.; Ballesteros, M.; Taddei, F.; Radman, M.; Nystrom, T. Protein oxidation in response to increased transcriptional or translational errors. *Proc. Natl. Acad. Sci. USA* **2000**, *97*, 5746–5749. [CrossRef]
51. Zdzisinska, B.; Zurek, A.; Kandefer-Szerszen, M. Alpha-Ketoglutarate as a Molecule with Pleiotropic Activity: Well-Known and Novel Possibilities of Therapeutic Use. *Arch. Immunol. Ther. Exp. (Warsz)* **2017**, *65*, 21–36. [CrossRef] [PubMed]
52. Liu, S.; He, L.; Yao, K. The Antioxidative Function of Alpha-Ketoglutarate and Its Applications. *Biomed. Res. Int.* **2018**, *2018*, 3408467. [CrossRef] [PubMed]
53. Chin, R.M.; Fu, X.; Pai, M.Y.; Vergnes, L.; Hwang, H.; Deng, G.; Diep, S.; Lomenick, B.; Meli, V.S.; Monsalve, G.C.; et al. The metabolite alpha-ketoglutarate extends lifespan by inhibiting ATP synthase and TOR. *Nature* **2014**, *510*, 397–401. [CrossRef] [PubMed]
54. Williamson, C.D.; Wong, D.S.; Bozidis, P.; Zhang, A.; Colberg-Poley, A.M. Isolation of Endoplasmic Reticulum, Mitochondria, and Mitochondria-Associated Membrane and Detergent Resistant Membrane Fractions from

Transfected Cells and from Human Cytomegalovirus-Infected Primary Fibroblasts. *Curr. Protoc. Cell Biol.* **2007**, *37*, 3–27. [CrossRef] [PubMed]

55. Magnani, N.D.; Dada, L.A.; Queisser, M.A.; Brazee, P.L.; Welch, L.C.; Anekalla, K.R.; Zhou, G.; Vagin, O.; Misharin, A.V.; Budinger, G.R.S.; et al. HIF and HOIL-1L-mediated PKCzeta degradation stabilizes plasma membrane Na,K-ATPase to protect against hypoxia-induced lung injury. *Proc. Natl. Acad. Sci. USA* **2017**, *114*, E10178–E10186. [CrossRef] [PubMed]

5

Surfactant Protein B Deficiency Induced High Surface Tension: Relationship between Alveolar Micromechanics, Alveolar Fluid Properties and Alveolar Epithelial Cell Injury

Nina Rühl [1], Elena Lopez-Rodriguez [1,2,3,4], Karolin Albert [1], Bradford J Smith [5], Timothy E Weaver [6], Matthias Ochs [1,2,3,4] and Lars Knudsen [1,2,3,*]

1 Institute of Functional and Applied Anatomy, Hannover Medical School, Hannover 30625, Germany
2 Biomedical Research in Endstage and Obstructive Lung Diseases (BREATH), Member of the German Center for Lung Research (DLZ), Hannover 30625, Germany
3 REBIRTH, Cluster of Excellence, Hannover 30625, Germany
4 Institute of Vegetative Anatomy, Charite, Berlin 10117, Germany
5 Department of Bioengineering, University of Colorado Denver, Denver, CO 80045, USA
6 Division of Pulmonary Biology, University of Cincinnati College of Medicine, Cincinnati, OH 45221, USA
* Correspondence: Knudsen.lars@mh-hannover.de

Abstract: High surface tension at the alveolar air-liquid interface is a typical feature of acute and chronic lung injury. However, the manner in which high surface tension contributes to lung injury is not well understood. This study investigated the relationship between abnormal alveolar micromechanics, alveolar epithelial injury, intra-alveolar fluid properties and remodeling in the conditional surfactant protein B (SP-B) knockout mouse model. Measurements of pulmonary mechanics, broncho-alveolar lavage fluid (BAL), and design-based stereology were performed as a function of time of SP-B deficiency. After one day of SP-B deficiency the volume of alveolar fluid V(alvfluid,par) as well as BAL protein and albumin levels were normal while the surface area of injured alveolar epithelium S(AEinjure,sep) was significantly increased. Alveoli and alveolar surface area could be recruited by increasing the air inflation pressure. Quasi-static pressure-volume loops were characterized by an increased hysteresis while the inspiratory capacity was reduced. After 3 days, an increase in V(alvfluid,par) as well as BAL protein and albumin levels were linked with a failure of both alveolar recruitment and airway pressure-dependent redistribution of alveolar fluid. Over time, V(alvfluid,par) increased exponentially with S(AEinjure,sep). In conclusion, high surface tension induces alveolar epithelial injury prior to edema formation. After passing a threshold, epithelial injury results in vascular leakage and exponential accumulation of alveolar fluid critically hampering alveolar recruitability.

Keywords: surfactant protein B; atelectrauma; alveolar fluid; acinar micromechanics; acute lung injury

1. Introduction

The intra-alveolar surfactant is a mixture of 90% lipids (mainly phospholipids) and 10% proteins including surfactant proteins which are produced, stored and secreted by alveolar epithelial type 2 (AE2) cells [1]. Among the protein component the hydrophobic surfactant proteins B (SP-B) and C (SP-C) are both of high relevance for the surface tension lowering properties of alveolar surfactant at the air-liquid interface within the alveolar space. Underneath this interface, a very thin layer of liquid, also referred to as the hypophase, covers the alveolar epithelium [2,3]. This reduction in surface tension is critical to prevent end-expiratory collapse of distal airspaces and to reduce the work of breathing. Comparing quasi-static pressure-volume (PV) loops of air and liquid-filled healthy lungs it becomes obvious that the hysteresis, e.g., the area within the PV-loop, is mainly a feature of the air-liquid interface. The corresponding surface phenomena such as surface tension, moreover, result in larger pressures needed for lung inflation and a loss of energy during the PV-loop as characterized by the hysteresis [4]. The surface active molecules, such as phospholipids, form a dynamic layer at the air-liquid interface. This layer is mechanically challenged by the cyclic intra-tidal changes in the geometry of alveoli and interalveolar septa which expand during inspiration and form pleats at the end of expiration [5]. Accordingly, the surfactant layer at the air-liquid interface is compressed at end-expiration and reduces the surface tension close to 0 mN/m. During inspiration the surface active film of phospholipids is expanded and the surface tension increases at larger lung volumes [6,7]. SP-B, due to its properties to generate phospholipid membrane-membrane contacts, has been suggested to be involved in the formation and stabilization of surface active films so that surface tension lowering properties are critically dependent on the biophysical properties of SP-B [2,8].

The acute respiratory distress syndrome (ARDS) is characterized by a severe failure of the lungs' central function in gas exchange resulting from an injury of the blood-gas barrier. Accordingly, inflammation, alveolar flooding with surfactant inactivation and alveolar collapse are typical features of ARDS [9,10]. The high surface tension itself has effects on the acinar microarchitecture including its dynamic changes during respiration, also known as alveolar micromechanics. Based on the Wilson-Bachofen model, surface tension at the air-liquid interface results in forces which would induce a piling up of interalveolar septal walls and therefore a reduction in surface area [11]. These surface tension-related forces are counter-balanced by the axial system of elastic fibers which usually surround the alveolar entrance. High surface tension induced by lavage of the lung with tween has been shown to result in a diversity of abnormalities in alveolar micromechanics such as intratidal alveolar recruitment/derecruitment [12] but also asynchronous alveolar dynamics such as inverse alveolar ventilation, alveolar stunning or alveolar pendelluft [13].

Clinical studies demonstrated that a reduction in the SP-B level in the alveolar space represents an early event during the time course and can even precede the development of the complete clinical picture of ARDS [14,15]. In established ARDS, moreover, the level of SP-B in broncho-alveolar lavage fluid (BAL) correlated convincingly with the impairment in surfactant function as characterized by the minimum surface tension [16]. However, in the context of clinical ARDS, the relevance of this early SP-B reduction has not been investigated in detail although it has been suggested that surfactant inactivation plays a central role in the development of ARDS [17]. It is well known that high surface tension leads to edema formation [18] and expiratory alveolar derecruitment [19]. In the conditional SP-B knockout mouse model high surface tension results in pulmonary inflammation, respiratory failure and death [20,21]. However, the mechanisms leading to respiratory failure in SP-B deficiency-induced high surface tension are not entirely understood. Several models of pulmonary micromechanics offer realistic scenarios by which SP-B deficiency induced high surface tension can result in progressive lung injury [22–25]. The failure of surfactant to reduce surface tension during expiration results in alveolar instability with derecruitment of alveolar surface area or even complete alveoli which can be recruited if transpulmonary pressure gradients increase again during inspiration [26]. This repetitive intratidal alveolar recruitment/derecruitment has been observed in lavage models of acute lung injury during mechanical ventilation [12]. There is evidence that repetitive recruitment/derecruitment of distal airspaces can be harmful to the alveolar epithelium thereby contributing to ventilation-induced lung injury (VILI) via a mechanism known as atelectrauma [27]. Computational modelling combined with experimental validation in cell culture model systems provided evidence that the opening of a fluid-occluded distal airspace can, in the presence of high surface tension, be associated with potential harmful pressure gradients acting on the epithelial lining [22]. Accordingly, restoring surfactant function and reducing surface tension protected the epithelial lining in models of fluid occluded distal airspace recruitment [22,28]. It has also been shown that the properties of the air-liquid interface are critical for the function of AE2 cells because the surface tension forces exert deforming mechanical stresses (e.g., shear stress and tensile strain) on the AE2 cells [23,24,29]. As a result AE2 cells change gene expression profiles in a way that resembles VILI, cyclic alveolar stretch, and pulmonary fibrosis [23].

Transferring these micromechanical models of atelectrauma [22] and interfacial stresses [23] into the context of SP-B deficiency-induced high surface tension it can be hypothesized that repetitive opening of distal airspaces containing fluid (= hypophase) during breathing might be an initial trigger for injury of the alveolar epithelium. These injuries may represent the initial injurious event that occurs prior to vascular leak and alveolar edema accumulation. On the other hand, high surface tension has also been suggested to result in alveolar edema [18] so that the initial consequence of SP-B deficiency could be alveolar fluid accumulation and heterogeneous alveolar ventilation. Discrete alveolar flooding has been shown to be sufficient to induce epithelial injury characterized by vascular leakage due to overdistension of neighboring alveolar airspaces even during ventilation with quite low tidal volumes [30]. Therefore, injury of the alveolar epithelium and progressive respiratory failure might be the consequence, and not the cause, of edema formation.

Based on these considerations the goal of the present study was to understand the relationship between impaired acinar micromechanics, injury of the alveolar epithelium and the alveolar fluid properties in SP-B deficiency induced high surface tension. For this purpose, the time course of these different pathologies was investigated after depletion of SP-B in a mouse model expressing SP-B under control of a doxycycline dependent promotor [21]. Doxycycline-containing food was withdrawn and animals were investigated 1 (group: Dox off d1) and 3 (group: Dox off d3) days thereafter using lung mechanical and BAL parameters and quantitative morphology based on design-based stereology. The latter included a protocol of vascular perfusion fixation of the lungs at airway opening pressures (Pao) on expiration of 2 and 10 cmH_2O in order to investigate the recruitability of distal airspaces. Alveolar microarchitecture was described by stereological parameters such as the total volume of alveolar airspaces, the number of open alveoli, the total surface area of alveoli and the mean thickness of interalveolar septal walls. For the assessment of lung injury, the surface area of the epithelial basal lamina covered by injured cells (based on ultrastructural criteria) was determined. Finally, the intra-alveolar fluid was characterized by its absolute volume per lung, the mean thickness and the surface area of the alveolar epithelial cells covered by fluid. As additional parameters lung mechanical data and protein levels in BAL were determined. The data of lungs from mice after withdrawal of doxycycline containing food (Dox off) were compared to those of lungs from mice having been fed with the doxycycline containing food (Dox on).

2. Results

2.1. Lung Mechanics

Data describing lung mechanical function are detailed in Figure 1. The quasi-static compliance (Cst) is the slope of the deflation limb of a quasi-static PV-loop at an airway opening pressure of 5 cmH_2O and was significantly reduced in Dox off d3 compared to both the Dox on and the Dox off d1 groups (Figure 1A). However, a difference regarding this parameter was not observed between Dox on and Dox off d1. Quasi-static PV-loops were further investigated and the hysteresis (= area within the PV loop) was determined (Figure 1B). While hysteresis in Dox off d1 was significantly increased compared to Dox on this was not the case considering Dox off d3. Inspiratory capacity (IC) is defined as the volume of displaced air into the lung during a ramp inflation from 3 to 30 cmH_2O over a period of 6 s. Unlike Cst, IC showed a significant decrease in Dox off d1 compared to Dox on (Figure 1C). Dox off d3 was characterized by an even more dramatic reduction in IC compared to Dox on and Dox off d1 (Figure 1C).

As a forth parameter, the tissue elastance H, was determined using the forced oscillation technique (FOT) fit to the constant phase model [31] during ventilation at positive end-expiratory pressures (PEEP) of 2 and 10 cmH_2O. The tissue elastance H reflects the lung mechanics at the different PEEP levels because the onset pressure of the FOT corresponded to the PEEP level and since the FOT volume variations were quite small (3ml/kg bodyweight). As such, tissue elastance H takes the degree of end-expiratory airspace collapse into consideration [19,26,32,33]. At both PEEP levels (2 and 10 cmH_2O) there was no significant difference between Dox on and Dox off d1 Figure 1D). Dox off d3, however, demonstrated a significant increase in H compared to both other groups at both PEEP levels (Figure 1D). The Newtonian resistance (Rn) is also determined from the constant phase model fit to the FOT measurements. This parameter reflects pathologies of the conducting airways and shows a clear dependence on the PEEP at which it was determined (Figure 1E). The decrease of Rn with increasing PEEP can be explained by interdependence of conducting airways and surrounding lung parenchyma [34]. Outward tethering forces of the elastic fiber system which connects the conducting airways and the pleura increase with lung volume (and PEEP) so that the resistance of the conducting airways is reduced. At PEEP = 2 cmH_2O there were no significant differences in Rn between study groups. However, increasing the PEEP from 2 to 10 cmH_2O provided a smaller reduction in Rn for Dox off d3 so that a significant difference became apparent at PEEP 10 cmH_2O compared to Dox on (Figure 1E).

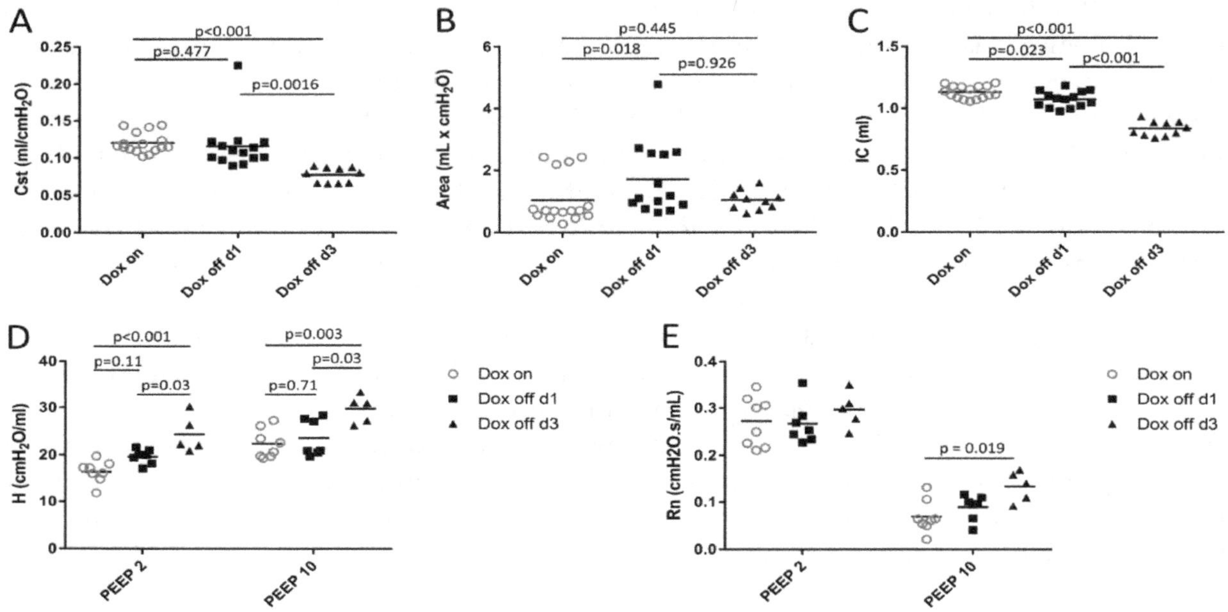

Figure 1. Lung mechanical properties. Quasi-static compliance (**A**), and hysteresis of quasi-static PV loops (**B**), inspiratory capacity (**C**), tissue elastance (**D**), and Newtonian resistance (**E**). PEEP: positive end-expiratory pressure.

2.2. Progressive Disturbances of Acinar Micromechanics in Dox off Groups

Figure 2 illustrates representative light microscopic images of the study groups fixed by vascular perfusion at different end-expiratory airway opening pressures (Pao 2 cmH_2O and 10 cmH_2O). At the time point of fixation the lungs were air-filled so that the air-liquid interface was present and the effects of interfacial surface tension on lung structure could be investigated [26,35]. In general, the blood vessels including the capillary network within the interalveolar septa were free of blood cells and open so that it can be concluded that the perfusion fixation was successful. At lower magnification there were no apparent differences between Dox on (Figure 2) and Dox off d1. At higher magnification both study groups demonstrated signs of collapsed alveoli (microatelectases) and formation of pleats of interalveolar septal walls at Pao = 2 cmH_2O which disappeared at Pao = 10 cmH_2O. On contrary, microatelectases were present at both Pao = 2 cmH_2O and Pao = 10 cmH_2O in Dox off d3. Moreover, the alveolar ducts were widened while the interalveolar septa appeared to be piled up at Pao = 10 cmH_2O (Figure 2).

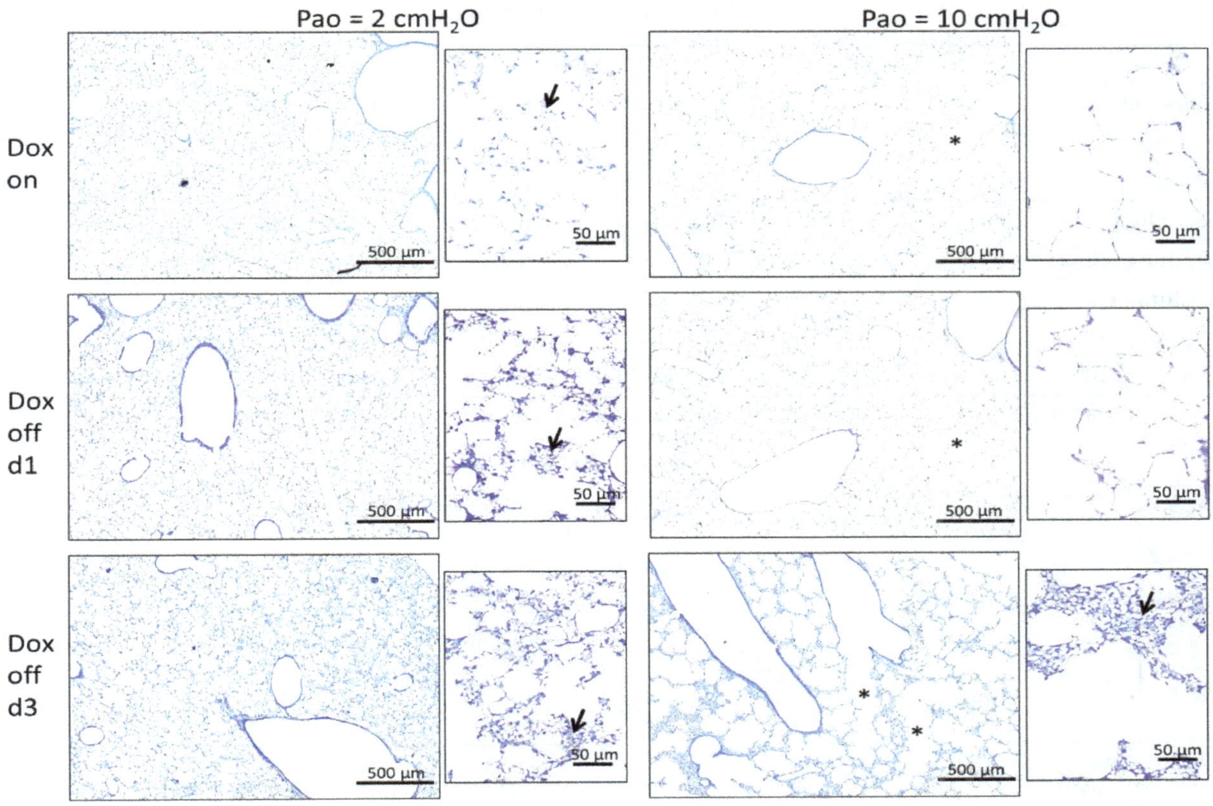

Figure 2. Microatelectases. Representative light microscopic images of Dox on, Dox off d1 and Dox off d3 of lung tissue fixed at end-expiratory airway opening pressure (Pao) of 2 and 10 cmH_2O. The arrows indicate piled septal walls due to microatelectases which can be observed at Pao = 2 cmH_2O in all study groups, while at Pao = 10 cmH_2O microatelectases are present in Dox off d3 but not Dox on or Dox off d1. In addition, the alveolar ducts appear enlarged in some regions (asterisk) in Dox off d3 at Pao = 10 cmH_2O. Arrow: microatelectasis; asterisk: alveolar duct.

The stereological data regarding the acinar microarchitecture are summarized in Table 1. Highly significant effects of the duration of the withdrawal of doxycycline containing food as well as Pao on the total lung volume V(lung) could be identified. Having a closer look at the components of the lung parenchyma elucidated that the total volume of alveolar airspaces V(alvair,lung), (Figure 3A) was affected by the factor Dox off and Pao while the total volume of ductal airspaces V(ductair,lung) (Figure 3B) was effected by Pao only. The total volume of septal wall tissue V(sep,lung) was independent of both Dox off and Pao. At Pao of 2 cmH_2O the differences in V(alvair,lung) between Dox on and the Dox off groups were small and there was only a significance between Dox on and Dox off d3 (Figure 3A). At larger Pao, however, the differences in V(alvair,lung) become more prominent with a highly significant difference between Dox on and Dox off d1 as well as between Dox off d1 and Dox off d3. The total surface area of alveoli S(alv,lung) and the total number of alveoli N(alv,lung) followed similar trends and did not show significant differences between Dox on, Dox off d1 and Dox off d3 at low Pao. At higher Pao, however, the Dox off d3 group was characterized by reduced S(alv,lung) (Figure 3C) and N(alv,lung) (Figure 3D) compared to both Dox on and Dox off d1. Based on the stereological findings illustrated in Figure 3 it can be summarized that one day after induction of SP-B deficiency the lungs have reduced alveolar airspaces at 10 cmH_2O, a finding which is in line with the inspiratory capacity (Figure 1C). This indicates that the alveolar airspaces during inspiration are stiffer in Dox off d1. Three days after induction of SP-B deficiency there is progressive impairment of parenchymal recruitment with increasing Pao as reflected in the reduced alveolar airspace volume, alveolar surface area, and total number of open alveoli. Hence, the Dox off d3 group fails to recruit surface area and collapsed alveoli as Pao is increased.

Table 1. Lung architecture.

Group	Dox on		Dox off d1		Dox off d3		2wayANOVA	
Parameter	Pao 2	Pao 10	Pao 2	Pao 10	Pao 2	Pao 10	group	Pao
V(lung) cm^3	0.52 (0.05)	1.18 (0.10)	0.42 (0.08)	0.95 (0.10)	0.40 (0.05)	0.80 (0.14)	< 0.01	< 0.01
V(alvair,lung) cm^3	0.27 (0.02)	0.72 (0.07)	0.19 (0.05)	0.53 (0.08)	0.16 (0.03)	0.43 (0.08)	< 0.001	< 0.001
V(ductair,lung) cm^3	0.05 (0.02)	0.19 (0.05)	0.04 (0.02)	0.16 (0.03)	0.04 (0.01)	0.14 (0.02)	n.s.	< 0.01
V(sep,lung) cm^3	0.13 (0.02)	0.12 (0.02)	0.12 (0.01)	0.13 (0.03)	0.13 (0.01)	0.12 (0.02)	n.s.	n.s.
S(alv,lung) cm^2	268 (83.0)	374 (110)	272 (55.0)	395 (50.0)	205 (26.7)	254 (72.6)	0.008	0.001
τ (sep) µm	10.3 (2.91)	6.77 (1.04)	9.37 (1.24)	6.53 (1.70)	13.2 (1.19)	10.2 (2.91)	< 0.001	< 0.001
N(alv,lung) 10^6	1.75 (0.81)	2.61 (1.01)	2.31 (0.63)	2.80 (0.39)	1.47 (0.21)	1.47 (0.52)	0.005	n.s.

Data are given as mean (SD). n.s.: not significant. Parameters are detailed in the text and Table 5.

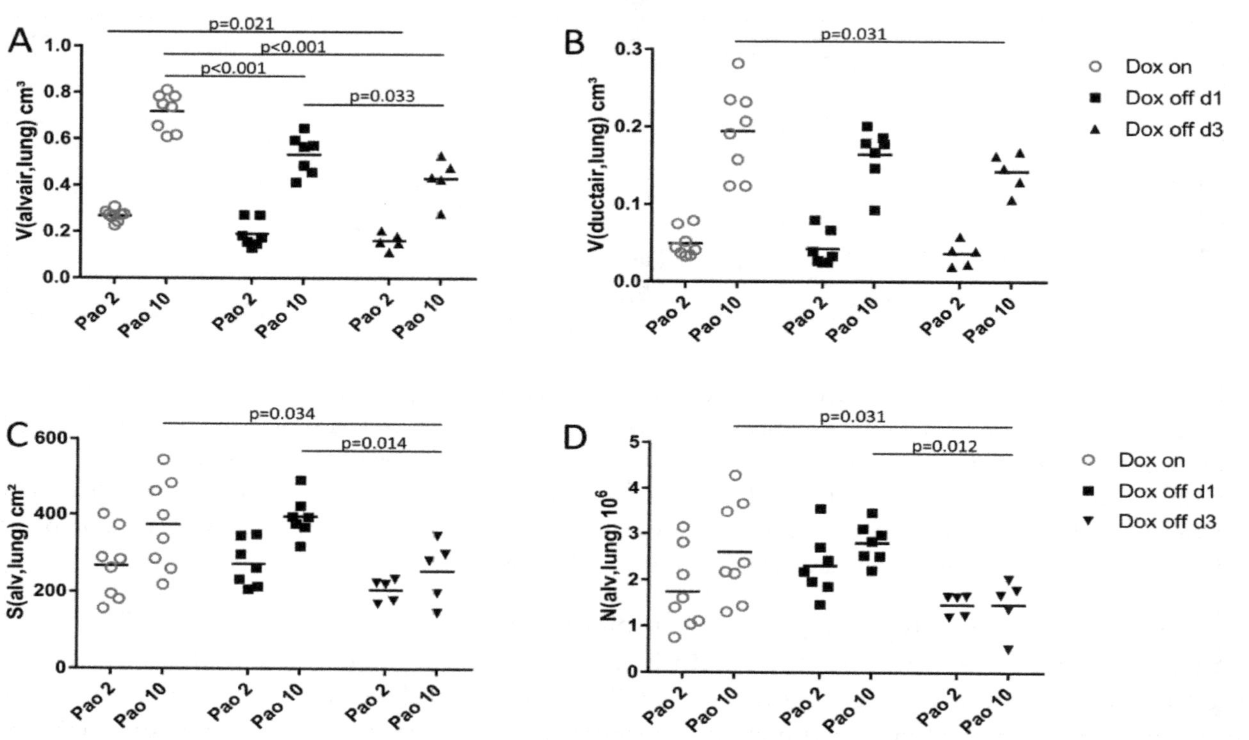

Figure 3. Acinar microarchitecture. The total volumes per lung of alveolar (**A**) V(alvair,lung) and ductal airspaces (**B**) V(ductair,lung) are given. In (**C**) the surface area of alveoli per lung S(alv,lung) and in (**D**) the total number of alveoli per lung N(alv,lung) are illustrated.

2.3. Composition of Inter-alveolar Septa and Intra-alveolar Fluid Properties

The composition of the interalveolar septal walls was analyzed in detail (Table 2) at the electron microscopic level. The factor "group assignment" did not influence total volumes of cellular and extracellular components within the septal walls. This was also the case regarding the total volume of capillary lumen within the interalveolar septa. Effects of Pao were noted in the absolute volumes of extracellular matrix V(ECM,sep) and capillary lumen V(caplumen,sep) as well as the total surface area of the endothelial basal lamina S(endoBL,sep). Higher Pao resulted in a highly significant decrease in V(caplumen,sep) (Table 2) which can be explained by the compression of the septal walls due to higher pressure gradients between the alveolar airspaces and the capillary lumen. The significant increase in S(endoBL,sep) due to higher Pao can be explained by a higher degree of stretch at Pao = 10 cmH_2O compared to Pao = 2 cmH_2O. The behavior of V(ECM,sep), however, which shows larger values at Pao = 10 cmH_2O compared to Pao = 2 cmH_2O, is difficult to understand but might result from alterations in the distribution of water within the interstitial space.

Table 2. Composition of interalveolar septa.

	Dox on		Dox off d1		Dox off d3		2wayANOVA	
Parameter	Pao 2	Pao 10	Pao 2	Pao 10	Pao 2	Pao 10	Group	Pao
V(AE1,sep) mm^3	15.2 (2.01)	15.4 (3.19)	11.6 (2.00)	16.5 (3.14)	14.4 (0.97)	13.0 (1.86)	n.s.	n.s.
V(AE2,sep) mm^3	4.92 (1.36)	7.73 (3.01)	6.24 (1.66)	6.78 (2.20)	5.96 (2.58)	4.67 (2.00)	n.s.	n.s.
V(endo,sep) mm^3	20.8 (1.58)	20.7 (2.94)	18.7 3.42	21.3 (4.97)	20.2 (1.68)	20.1 (2.89)	n.s.	n.s.
V(othercells,sep) mm^3	8.04 (1.95)	9.02 (2.07)	8.01 (1.38)	12.6 (5.49)	9.05 (0.8)	9.12 (1.4)	n.s.	n.s.
V(ECM,sep) mm^3	3.78 (0.95)	4.15 (1.65)	3.60 (0.73)	6.42 (2.99)	3.52 (0.79)	4.69 (2.30)	n.s.	0.024
V(caplumen,sep) mm^3	73.7 (16.3)	63.7 (15.2)	75.3 (8.89)	57.5 (12.5)	73.04 (9.34)	63.05 (10.8)	n.s.	0.009
S(endoBL,sep) cm^2	775 (138)	915 (188)	700 (81.0)	804 (175)	689 (76.3)	739 (83.5)	n.s.	0.049

Data are given as mean (SD). n.s.: not significant. Parameters are defined in the text and in Table 5.

Electron microscopy was further used to study intra-alveolar fluid morphology as a function of the duration of withdrawal of doxycycline containing food and Pao. Figure 4 illustrates representative electron microscopic images of Dox on, Dox off d1 and Dox off d3 from lung tissue fixed at Pao 2 or 10 cmH_2O. At Pao = 2 cmH_20 the formation of pleats of the septal walls was a typical finding in all study groups. A very thin layer of alveolar fluid could be identified between opposing alveolar epithelial cells. In some areas of Dox off d3 these layers of alveolar fluid were much darker and thicker compared to Dox on and Dox off d1. Increasing the Pao to 10 cmH_2O was linked with a dramatic decrease in the frequency of septal wall pleats in Dox on and Dox off d1. The alveolar fluid was concentrated in the corners of alveoli and could be clearly identified at electron microscopic level. In group Dox off d3, however, pleats of septal walls in concert with quite thick layers of dense alveolar fluid interposing the space between the alveolar epithelial cells remained a quite common finding. Protein and albumin concentration in BAL were determined to assess alveolo-capillary barrier disruption [9]. While there were no significant differences in protein content between Dox on and Dox off d1, Dox off d3 demonstrated significantly increased levels compared to the other 2 groups (Figure 5A). These findings were in line with the BAL albumin level which was also significantly higher in Dox off d3 compared to Dox on and Dox off d1 (Figure 5B). Using design-based stereological methods at electron microscopic level, the total volume of alveolar fluid V(alvfluid,par), the arithmetic mean thickness of alveolar fluid τ(alvfluid), and the surface area of alveolar epithelium covered by air S(airAE,par) or by fluid S(fluidAE,par) were quantified. Data regarding the alveolar fluid are provided in Figure 5 and illustrated in Table 3.

Table 3. Alveolar fluid.

	Dox on		Dox off d1		Dox off d3		2wayANOVA	
Parameter	Pao 2	Pao 10	Pao 2	Pao 10	Pao 2	Pao 10	Group	Pao
V(alvfluid,par) mm^3	0.79 (0.32)	1.39 (0.95)	0.92 (0.26)	6.64 (11.4)	8.03 (3.95)	6.63 (3.95)	0.032	n.s.
S(airAE,par) cm^2	401 (103)	717 (112)	320 (76.2)	628 (190)	200 (60.0)	310 (89.2)	< 0.001	< 0.001
S(fluidAE,par) cm^2	353 (58.7)	236 (55.3)	366 (29.4)	280 (113)	483 (39.3)	393 (101)	< 0.001	< 0.001
τ(alvfluid) nm	39.0 (18.6)	89.0 (48.0)	44.2 (16.6)	248 (294)	297 (155)	268 (125)	0.006	n.s.

Data are given as mean (SD). n.s.: not significant. Parameters are defined in Table 5.

The duration of withdrawal of doxycycline containing food but not the Pao demonstrated significant effects on V(alvfluid,par) and therefore Figure 5C illustrates group effects only. Compared to Dox on and Dox off d1 there was a significant increase in V(alvfluid,par) in Dox off d3 (Figure 5C) which was accompanied by a significant increase in the thickness of the fluid layer τ(alvfluid) (Figure 5D). Having a closer look at the Pao effects in the different groups it appeared that there is an increase in τ(alvfluid) with Pao in Dox on and Dox off d1 but not in Dox off d3 (Figure 5D). This observation might be attributed to a redistribution of fluid in Dox on and Dox off d1 during recruitment. Derecruited septal walls or even derecruited alveoli have a thin layer of alveolar fluid between opposing alveolar epithelial cells which, after the recruitment process, is concentrated in the alveolar corners resulting in a thickening of the fluid layer while its total volume remains roughly stable (Figure 4).

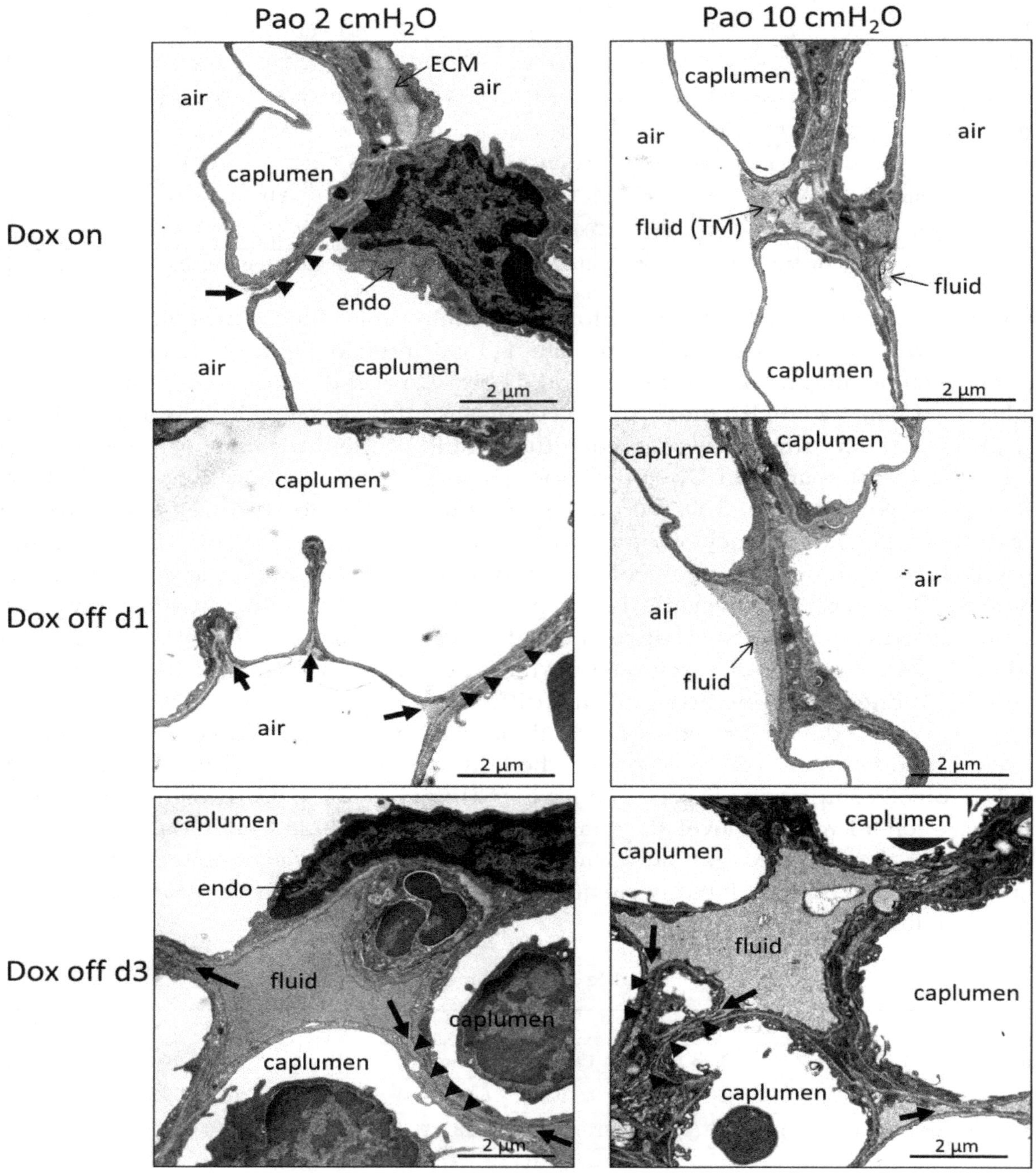

Figure 4. Alveolar fluid and septal wall folding. Electron microscopic images of lungs of Dox on, Dox off d1 and Dox off d3 fixed at positive end-expiratory airway opening pressure (Pao) of 2 and 10 cmH_2O. Septal wall folding can be observed in all study groups at Pao = 2 cmH_2O. The "entrances" to the folds are illustrated by arrows. The opposing septal walls are separated by very thin layers of alveolar fluid (arrowhead). At higher Pao, septal wall folds become less frequent and alveolar fluid can be seen in the corners of the alveoli in Dox on and Dox off d1. In Dox off d3, the amount of alveolar fluid seems to be increased and the occurrence of septal wall folds does not seem to be less frequently at higher Pao. Abbreviations: caplumen: lumen of septal wall capillaries; endo: endothelial cell; ECM: extracellular matrix; TM: tubular myelin, a lattice of membranes corresponding to an active intra-alveolar surfactant component within the hypophase. Black bold arrow: entrance to fold; arrowhead: liquid filled space between opposing epithelial cells.

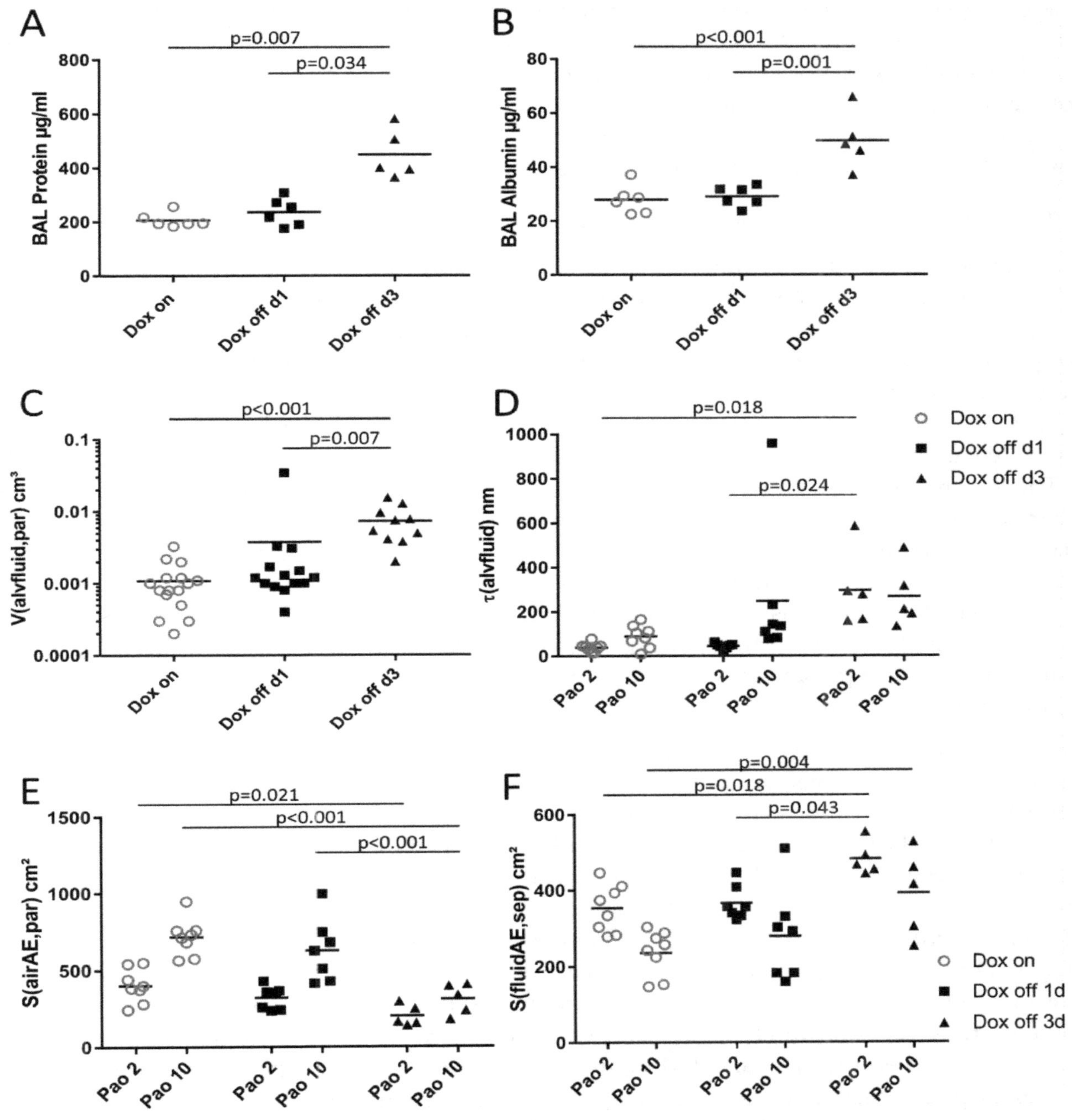

Figure 5. Properties of alveolar fluid. BAL was assessed regarding protein (**A**) and albumin (**B**) concentration. In addition, alveolar fluid was characterized by stereological parameters as follows: Total volume of alveolar fluid per lung (**C**) V(alvfluid,par), arithmetic mean thickness of alveolar fluid (**D**) τ(alvfluid), the surface area of alveolar epithelium covered by air (**E**) S(airAE,par) or covered by alveolar fluid (**F**) S(fluidAE,sep).

In line with these observations were S(airAE,par) and S(fluidAE,par). While S(airAE,par) could be increased by raising Pao from 2 to 10 cmH_2O in Dox on and Dox off d1 this was not the case in Dox off d3 (Figure 5E). The parameter S(fluidAE,par) behaved exactly the other way round (Figure 5F) and decreased with increasing Pao in Dox on and Dox off d1. Accordingly, there were only small differences in S(airAE,par) at Pao 2 cmH_2O between the Dox on and Dox off d3. By contrast, at Pao 10 cmH_2O the surface area of air covered alveolar epithelium was significantly lower in Dox off d3 compared to both Dox on and Dox off d1 (Figure 5E). A similar trend was observed with S(fluidAE,par). By increasing Pao from 2 to 10 cmH_2O, the differences between Dox off d3 and the other groups became larger (Figure 5F). In summary, the data obtained at electron microscopic level show a failure in the

Dox off d3 group to recruit air covered alveolar epithelium with increasing Pao. This finding is in line with the light microscopic data. Moreover, the electron microscopical data demonstrate an increase in the volume and thickness of alveolar fluid in Dox off d3. Since the thickness and the surface area of alveolar epithelium covered by fluid show hardly any Pao effects in Dox off d3 it can be concluded that high surface tension or viscosity is linked with a failure to redistribute with changing Pao. These structural observations correlate with the increased BAL levels of protein and albumin in Dox off d3.

2.4. Ultrastructural Evaluation of Alveolar Epithelial Injury

The increase in BAL albumin in Dox off d3 can be attributed to disruption of the blood-gas barrier consisting of the alveolar epithelial cells, the basal lamina (= interstitium) and the endothelial cells. Previous studies have shown that the surfactant dysfunction in this animal model is present at 1 day after doxycycline withdrawal and remains consistent through day four [21]. High surface tension, moreover, has been shown to result in interfacial stress linked to injury of alveolar epithelial cells [22,36,37]. In order to understand whether Dox off d1 group shows in absence of elevated BAL protein alveolar epithelial injury the further ultrastructural investigation focused on alveolar epithelial cells. There were no obvious alterations in the ultrastructure of AE2 cells including the morphology of lamellar bodies. However, subtle abnormalities were observed regarding the AE1 cells. In Dox off d1 AE1 cells occasionally showed swelling and clearing of the cytoplasmic ground substance (Figure 6C). In healthy controls the AE1 cells were usually not swollen and the cytoplasmic ground substance was characterized by the same density as the endothelial cells or interstitial cells (Figure 6A,B). Furthermore, there were signs of rupture of the apical plasma membrane of AE1 cells in Dox off d1 (Figure 6D). Ruptures of the apical plasma membrane, swelling, and clearing of cytoplasmic ground substance were also observed in Dox off d3 AE1 cells (Figure 6E,F).

Hence, a quantification of alveolar epithelial injury was performed (Table 4 and Figure 7). The total surface area of the alveolar epithelial basal lamina S(alvBL,sep) was found to increase with Pao (Figure 7A). This observation can be explained by Pao-induced stretching of alveolar septal walls. The surface fraction of the basal lamina covered either by injured epithelial cells S_S(AEinjure/alvBL), healthy appearing AE1 cells S_S(AE1/alvBL), or healthy appearing AE2 cells S_S(AE2/alvBL) was determined in order to describe injury severity. Surface fractions were independent of Pao effects and influenced by group assignment. Dox off d1 showed increased S_S(AEinjure/alvBL); the injured fraction increased further in Dox off d3 (Figure 7B). This increase in S_S(AEinjure/alvBL) occurred in concert with decreased S_S(AE1/alvBL) while S_S(AE2/alvBL) remained stable (Table 4). In order to avoid the reference trap, the surface fractions and S(alvBL,sep) were used to calculate absolute values of basal lamina covered by injured epithelial cells [S(AEinjure,sep)], AE1 cells S(AE1,sep) and AE2 cells S(AE2,sep). S(AEinjure,sep) and S(AE1,sep) were greater at higher Pao (Figure 7C,F). Moreover, S(AEinjure,sep) increased progressively from Dox on to Dox off d1 and Dox off d3 (Figure 7C). In order to describe the relationship between V(alvfluid,par) and S(AEinjure,sep) these data were plotted against each other. Since Pao influenced S(AEinjure,sep) this relationship was investigated for Pao = 2 cmH_2O (Figure 7D). The distribution of points argued against a linear relationship. Hence, curve fitting was tested for an exponential or second order quadratic relationship between these two parameters using GraphPad PRISM statistic software (Version 7). The best curve fitting was achieved by an exponential growth equation:

$$Y(x) = Y0 \times e^{kx} \quad (1)$$

where Y(x) is the volume of alveolar fluid as a function of surface area of injured alveolar epithelium (x), Y0 is the volume of alveolar fluid with no injured alveolar surface, and k is the rate constant. In this equation best fit (R^2 = 0.77) was calculated for Y0 = 0.00028 cm^3 and k = 0.044, suggesting an exponential relationship between V(alvfluid,par) and S(AEinjure,sep). Finally, S(AE2,sep) was not effected by Pao (Figure 7E). Although the factor group assignment was significantly influencing S(AE2,sep), the Tukey post-hoc adjustment of the p-level failed to reveal significant differences (Figure 7E).

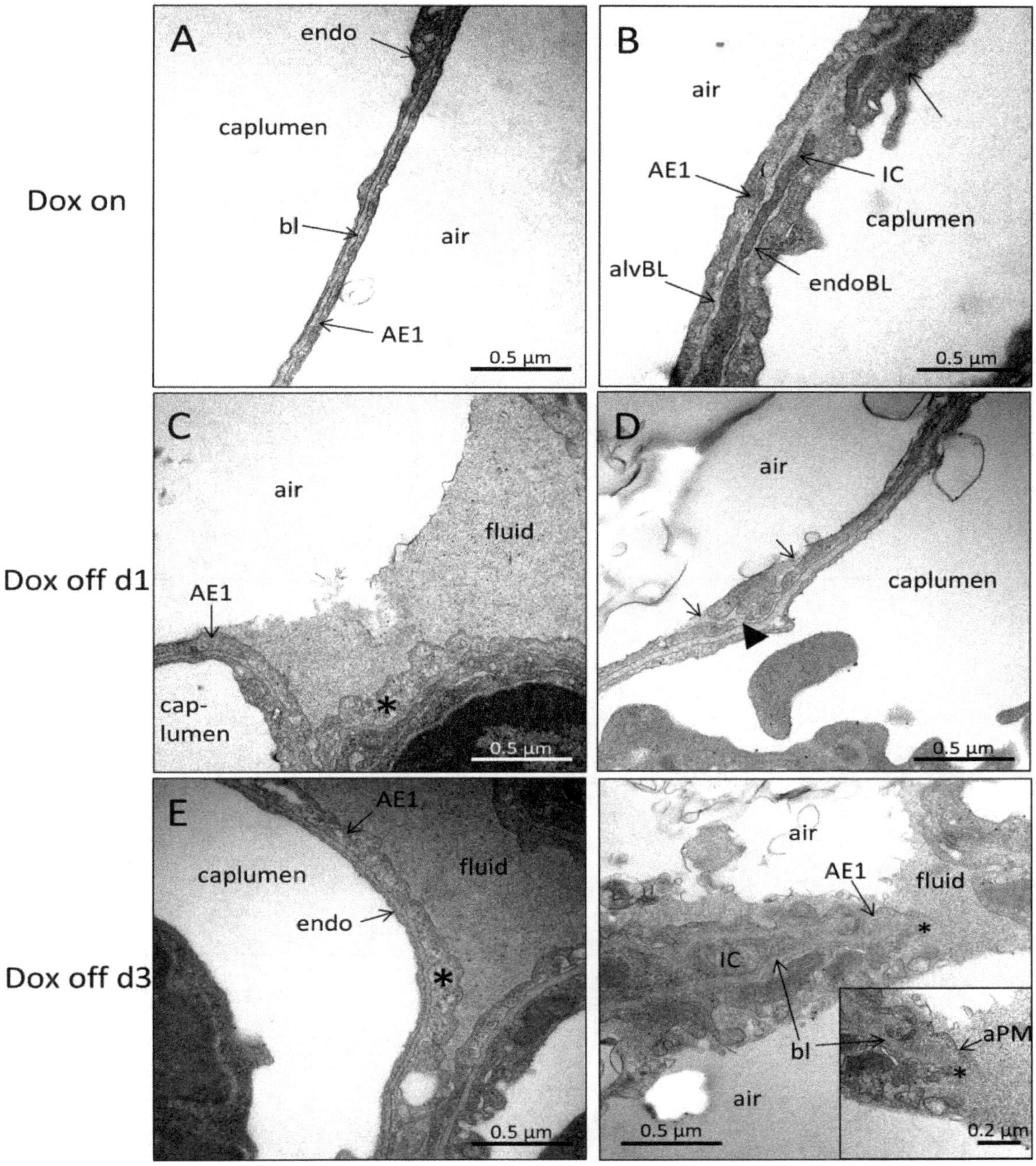

Figure 6. Injury of alveolar epithelial cells. Normal alveolar epithelial cells can be found in Dox on (**A**) and (**B**). In Dox off d1, swelling and clearance of cytoplasmic ground substance (asterisk) and ruptures in alveolar epithelial cell lining (arrowhead) could be found (**C**) and (**D**). In Dox off d3, similar observations as in Dox off d1 were present (**E**) and (**F**). Abbreviations: AE1: alveolar epithelial type 1 cell; endo: endothelial cell; caplumen: lumen of septal wall capillary; bl: basal lamina (junction of alvBL and endoBL); alvBL: alveolar epithelial basal lamina; endoBL: endothelial basal lamina; IC: interstitial cell; aPM: apical plasma membrane; air: alveolar airspace; fluid: alveolar fluid. Arrowhead: rupture of alveolar epithelial cell; asterisk: swollen AE1 cell.

Table 4. Injury of alveolar epithelium.

	Dox on		Dox off d1		Dox off d3		2wayANOVA	
Parameter	Pao 2	Pao 10	Pao 2	Pao 10	Pao 2	Pao 10	Group	Pao
S(alvBL,sep) cm^2	775 (129)	954 (181)	686 (82.4)	879 (206)	660 (76.3)	727 (105)	0.034	0.006
S_S(AEinjure/alvBL)%	0.97 (0.76)	0.86 (0.55)	2.78 (0.99)	4.03 (1.39)	6.83 (2.54)	8.94 (4.12)	< 0.001	n.s.
S_S(AE1/alvBL)%	93.3 (1.27)	94.0 (2.15)	90.1 (2.10)	89.4 (2.30)	88.0 (3.44)	86.4 (3.45)	< 0.001	n.s.

Table 4. *Cont.*

	Dox on		Dox off d1		Dox off d3		2wayANOVA	
Parameter	**Pao 2**	**Pao 10**	**Pao 2**	**Pao 10**	**Pao 2**	**Pao 10**	**Group**	**Pao**
S_S(AE2/alvBL)%	5.16 (1.31)	5.09 (2.37)	7.15 (2.21)	6.59 (1.70)	5.21 (1.18)	4.67 (1.73)	0.033	n.s.
S(AEinjure,sep) cm^2	7.31 (5.48)	7.87 (5.13)	19.0 (4.07)	34.4 (14.1)	44.1 (14.4)	67.7 (37.6)	< 0.001	0.025
S(AE1,sep) cm^2	728 (126)	900 (184)	617 (62.6)	786 (188)	582 (84.9)	626 (78.2)	0.004	0.011
S(AE2,sep) cm^2	39.5 (9.99)	46.4 (22.7)	50.1 (20.1)	58.4 (20.1)	33.7 (4.97)	33.5 (12.0)	0.03	n.s.

Data are given as mean (SD). n.s.: not significant. S_S: surface fraction. Parameters are defined in the text and in Table 5.

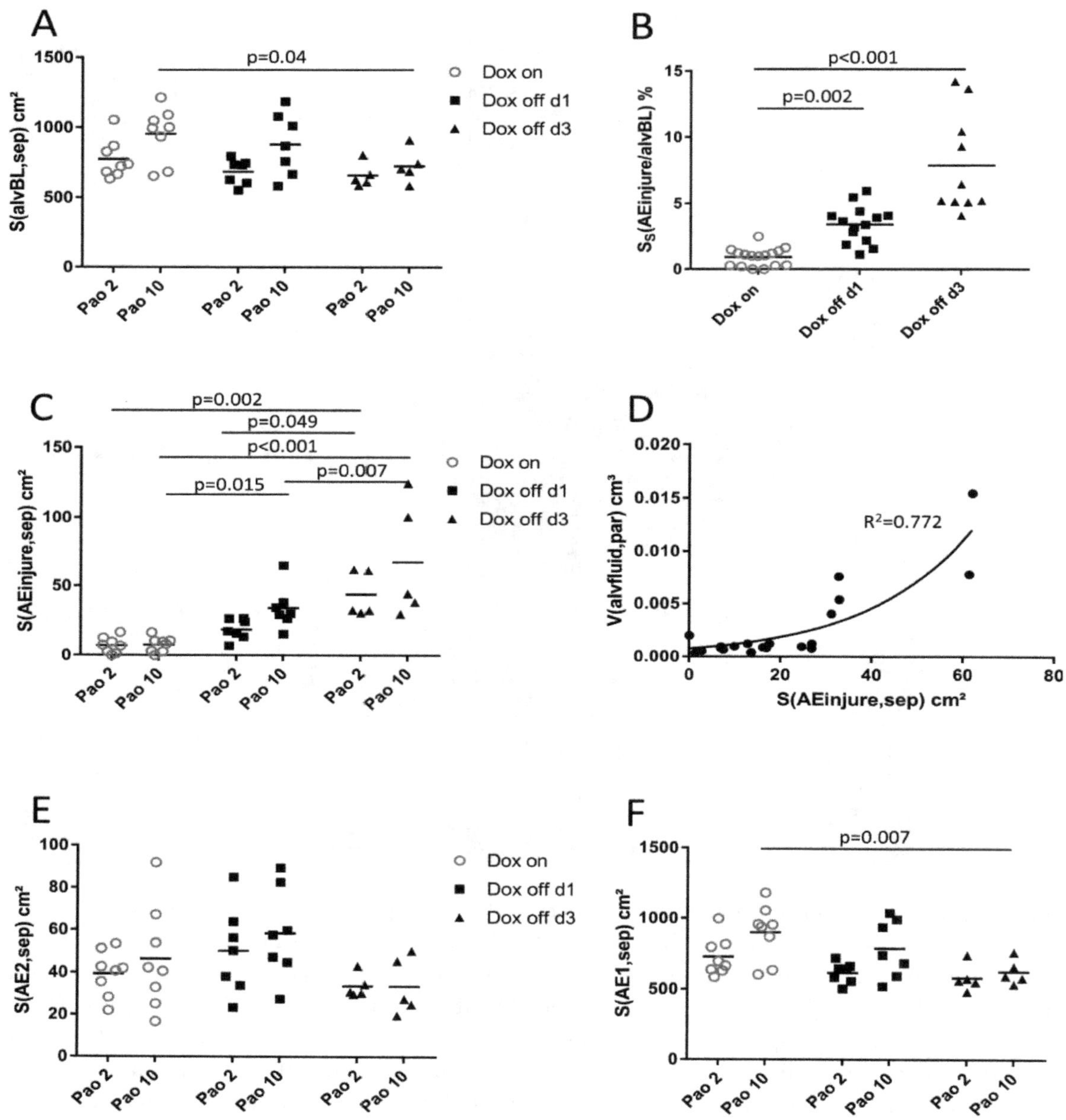

Figure 7. Stereological parameters of alveolar epithelial cell injury. Data were related to the total surface area of the alveolar epithelial basal lamina within septal walls (**A**) S(alvBL,sep). In (**B**), the surface fraction of the basal lamina covered by injured alveolar epithelial cells S_S(AEinjure/alvBL) shows an increase in Dox off d1 and Dox off d3. Multiplication of the surface fraction and S(alvBL,sep) resulted in absolute surface areas within the septal walls of injured alveolar epithelial cells (**C**), normal appearing alveolar epithelial type 2 (**E**) and alveolar epithelial type 1 (**F**) cells. (**D**) demonstrates the relationship between the total surface area of injured alveolar epithelial cells S(AEinjure,sep) and the total volume of alveolar fluid V(alvfluid,par) which can be described by an exponential growth function.

2.5. Structure-function Relationships

In order to establish structure-function relationships, correlation analyses between structural and lung mechanical parameters were performed. The increase in H during PEEP = 2 cmH_2O were correlated with S(AEinjure,sep) ($r = 0.646$, $p = 0.002$) but showed also correlations with parameters related to alveolar fluid such as V(alvfluid,par) ($r = 0.548$, $p = 0.012$), S(fluidAE,par) ($r = 0.559$, $p = 0.01$) and τ(alvfluid) ($r = 0.54$, $p = 0.014$). Cst (quasi-static compliance) and IC (inspiratory capacity) were characterized by an inverse correlation with S(AEinjure,sep) and the alveolar fluid related parameters. Hence, the more injured alveolar epithelial cells and the more alveolar fluid the less were Cst and IC. These relationships indicate mechanical stiffening and volume loss is associated with alveolar injury and fluid accumulation. In addition, V(alvair,par) was inversely correlated with H at PEEP = 2 cmH_2O ventilation ($r = -0.535$, $p = 0.015$). During PEEP = 10 cmH_2O ventilation the association of V(alvair,par) with lung mechanical parameters became stronger compared to PEEP = 2 cmH_2O. For example, IC and V(alvair,par) were highly correlated with each other (r = 0.783, p < 0.001) while H and V(alvair,par) were inversely correlated ($r = -0.516$, $p = 0.02$). The central airway resistance Rn demonstrated a strong inverse correlation with V(alvair,par) ($r = -0.596$, $p = 0.009$) and S(airAE,sep) ($r = -0.539$, $p = 0.014$) and a positive correlation with S(AEinjure,sep) ($r = 0.522$, $p = 0.018$). These relationships indicate that the failure to recruit distal airspaces is linked to the abnormalities observed in the mechanical properties during PEEP = 10 cmH_2O ventilation.

3. Discussion

The decrease in SP-B levels in BAL of patients represents an early event during the development of an ARDS [14] and correlates to the dysfunction of BAL-derived alveolar surfactant [16]. The contribution of this early decrease in BAL SP-B levels to lung injury is not entirely understood but it has been discussed that surfactant dysfunction represents a crucial step in the development of ARDS within a process known as ventilation induced lung injury (VILI) [17,38]. With this regard the repetitive opening of fluid occluded folds of alveolar walls in presence of high surface tension has been suggested to impose harmful forces on epithelial cells [22,39], a mechanism which can be referred to as microatelectrauma.

Mice expressing SP-B under the control of a doxycycline-dependent promotor demonstrated a decline in BAL SP-B levels within 24 h after withdrawal of doxycycline, a finding which correlated with a dramatic increase in minimum surface tension of BAL-derived surfactant [21]. In the present study we did not measure the surface function directly, e.g., by determining the minimum surface tension of BAL derived surfactant. At lung mechanical level, however, we observed an increase in hysteresis of the quasi-static PV-loop (Figure 1B) in Dox off d1 which occurred independently from signs of acute lung injury such as interstitial or alveolar edema formation. This finding can be interpreted as a result of increased surface tension. It has been well known for decades that the properties at the air-liquid interface are the main source of hysteresis related energy-loss during a PV-loop since the pressures to overcome surface tension during inspiration are increased with surface tension related elastic recoil pressure [4,7]. This finding is in line with the decrease in the inspiratory capacity (Figure 1C). Hence, the present study provides indirect evidence of high surface tension under quasi-static conditions during inspiration but we were not able to investigate whether or not high surface tension was present during dynamic breathing.

Further investigations in previous studies taking different time points after the induction of the knockout into account illustrated the occurrence of alveolar inflammation and increased BAL protein levels at day 3 [21] so that important criteria of acute lung injury were fulfilled in this animal model [9]. One goal of the present study was to investigate the time course of high surface tension related pathologies and their relationships, such as the link between alveolar micromechanics, alveolar fluid accumulation, and alveolar epithelial injury. In this context, the conditional SP-B knockout mouse model had a clear advantage compared to other models of direct or indirect lung injury [40]. Isolated high surface tension is the primary event and not a downstream consequence of an injurious trigger so this animal model allows investigation of the pure effect of high surface tension on disease initiation and progression. An important aspect of this study was that the recruitability of distal airspaces was investigated by examining morphometry at different airway pressures (Pao) using vascular perfusion fixation. With this approach, the effects of high surface tension on acinar microarchitecture could be investigated since the lung was air-filled at the time of fixation [35]. Although this is a static evaluation, the comparison of stereological parameters at different Pao provided information on the pressure-dependent dynamic changes in the recruitability of distal airspaces, an aspect of the so-called alveolar micromechanics, and the distribution and thickness of alveolar fluid [26].

3.1. Alveolar Micromechanics

One day after induction of SP-B deficiency discrete abnormalities in alveolar micromechanics were observed independent of an accumulation of alveolar fluid. These abnormalities did not significantly affect the organ-scale lung mechanical properties such as tissue elastance or quasi-static compliance but coincided with a modest decrease in the inspiratory capacity (Figure 1C). Abnormal alveolar micromechanics were characterized at a structural level by a significant reduction of volumes of alveolar airspaces at a Pao of 10 cmH_2O in Dox off d1 compared to Dox on (Figure 3A), although, the number of open alveoli per lung did not differ between these two study groups (Figure 3D). Pressure-dependent alveolar volume changes can be attributed to septal wall stretching, changes in alveolar shape, septal wall folding and alveolar recruitment/derecruitment [5,35,41]. Since the surface area of the alveolar epithelial basal lamina (Table 4, Figure 7A), alveolar number and alveolar surface area (Figure 3) did not differ significantly between Dox on and Dox off d1 at Pao = 10 cmH_2O there was no evidence of changes in alveolar septal wall stretching, folding, or alveolar derecruiment. Hence, it appeared to be likely that differences in alveolar shape were responsible for the high surface tension induced reduction in total volume of alveolar airspaces at Pao = 10 cmH_2O.

Reducing the Pao from 10 to 2 cmH_2O was linked with a substantial loss of alveolar surface area (p = 0.001) and total volume of alveolar airspace (p < 0.001) in all study groups while the number of open alveoli per lung was independent of Pao (Table 1, Figure 3D). In addition, the surface area of the alveolar epithelial basal lamina, a parameter used to quantify stretching of septal walls [6,42], was significantly affected by the factor Pao (Figure 7A, Table 4). Therefore, the alveolar-scale micromechanical mechanisms occurring with a drop in Pao from 10 to 2 cmH_2O include folding of septal walls (Figure 2), alveolar shape changes and de-stretching of septal walls. Alveolar derecruitment seemed to play a minor role in volume changes and this was quite unexpected since the effect of surface tension on lung structure has been suggested to become most evident at low lung volumes, when surfactant function is critical for stabilization of distal airspaces [43]. Although surfactant dysfunction has been demonstrated to be present 24h after withdrawal of Doxycycline in this animal model [21] the loss of alveolar surface area at Pao = 2 cmH_2O did not differ between Dox on and Dox off d1 in the present study. The absence of a relevant increase of alveolar instability in Dox off d1 was confirmed by the measurements of tissue elastance H which did not differ from data measured in Dox on during PEEP = 2 cmH_2O ventilation (Figure 1D). An increase in H during low PEEP ventilation has been linked to alveolar derecruitment in previous studies [26,33,44,45].

Three days after induction of SP-B deficiency more severe abnormalities were observed compared to Dox on. A further reduction of the volume of alveolar airspaces was observed at both Pao = 2 cmH_2O and 10 cmH_2O. But the most striking observation in this group was that both the surface area of alveoli and the number of open alveoli were significantly reduced and this change was most pronounced at Pao = 10 cmH_2O. Comparing Dox off d3 against Dox on and Dox off d1 it is evident that the increase in Pao from 2 to 10 cmH_2O is associated with a failure to increase both the alveolar surface area and the number of open alveoli per lung (Figure 3C,D). This failure to recruit distal airspaces in Dox off d3 (Figure 2) occurs even though the minimum surface tension of BAL-derived, purified surfactant (so-called large aggregates) has been shown to remain constant in this time period [21]. Of note, the hysteresis of the quasi-static PV-loop in Dox off d3 did not differ from Dox on so that it can be speculated that the surface tension related increase in hysteresis in Dox off d1 is linked to recruitment of surface area, a process which is markedly impaired in a progressive state of lung injury at day 3 in this model.

3.2. Alveolar Fluid Properties and the Relationship to Alveolar Micromechanics

At ultrastructural level, the main difference between Dox off d3 and the other two groups was the dramatic increase in the volume of alveolar fluid per lung (Figure 5C). This increase was accompanied by higher BAL concentrations of protein and albumin (Figure 5A,B). The protein level in BAL fluid increased by the factor 2.2 (Figure 5A) while the stereological parameter, the absolute volume of alveolar fluid, increased by the factor 8.1 (Figure 5C). During vascular perfusion fixation of the lung for electron microscopy glutaraldehyde crosslinks the proteins which are located in the alveolar fluid so that the fluid becomes visible. In Dox off d3 the alveolar fluid was much darker in some areas of the lung compared to Dox on so that it can be concluded that the fluid was enriched with proteins. Taking the 8.1-fold increase in the volume of alveolar fluid into account the increase in BAL protein levels appears to be disproportionally low. While the stereological parameter is unbiased taking also the reference space into account, this is not the case regarding the protein level in BAL since the recovery of BAL fluid varied between 2 and 2.5 mL. Moreover, it can be speculated that during broncho-alveolar lavage the derecruited and edema filled distal airspaces could not be opened so that only recruitable parts were reached. This would result in a higher degree of dilution of alveolar proteins in Dox off d3 and therefore an underestimation of the increase in the amount of proteins within the alveolar space since for all lungs the same volume of fluid was instilled into the lungs.

Of note, the accumulation of alveolar fluid volume from 0.0009 cm^3 in Dox on to 0.00734 cm^3 in Dox off d3 was not clearly detectable at light microscopic level so that electron microscopic resolution was necessary for detailed quantitative assessments. In Dox off d3 the failure of recruitment of lung parenchyma could be observed at ultrastructural level in the surface area of alveolar epithelium covered by air (Figure 5E) or alveolar fluid (Figure 5F). In both Dox on and Dox off d1 a shift of surface areas from fluid covered to air covered alveolar epithelium was observed as Pao increased from 2 to 10 cmH_2O. These pressure-dependent differences in alveolar airspace fluid distribution was coupled with an increase in the mean thickness of alveolar fluid (Figure 5D). At ultrastructural level, septal wall folds filled with a very thin leaflet of alveolar fluid were typical findings at low Pao while at higher Pao the fluid was concentrated in the corners of the alveoli. These observations suggest a pressure-dependent redistribution of fluid within the alveolar space, a mechanism which was linked with an unfolding of septal walls and therefore a recruitment of air-covered surface area. In Dox off d3, however, this pressure-dependent re-distribution of alveolar fluid was severely impaired as shown by the failure to shift the surface area of fluid-covered to air-covered alveolar epithelium with increase in Pao. In line with this observation was the fact that Pao had virtually no effect on the mean thickness of the alveolar fluid located on top of the alveolar epithelium in that group. Based on these observations it can be inferred that the surface tension and viscoelastic properties of the alveolar fluid differs substantially at day 3 of conditional SP-B knockout, leading to severe effects on alveolar micromechanics such as impaired alveolar recruitment. These alterations coincided with the increase in protein and albumin levels in BAL. It has been shown that distal airspace recruitability is impaired by increased alveolar protein [46] and fibrin levels [47], a finding which is in line with the structural data illustrated in the present study. In addition, the degradation of lung mechanical properties correlated with stereological data describing alveolar fluid and derecruitment of distal airspaces. This was also the case regarding the airway resistance (Rn) which usually decreases with PEEP due to outward tethering forces of elastic fibers that connect the conducting airways and the pleura [34,48]. In Dox off d3 the effect of increasing PEEP on airway resistance was less pronounced compared to the other groups (Figure 1E), an observation which can be explained by impaired recruitability of alveolar airspaces and therefore a reduction in the tethering forces on the conducting airways.

3.3. Injury of Alveolar Epithelium in the Context of impaired Alveolar Micromechanics and Fluid Accumulation

In both the Dox on and Dox off d1 groups the formation of septal wall pleats filled with a thin layer of fluid were observed with decreasing incidence with increasing Pao (Figure 4) so that it is possible that folding and unfolding of septal walls occurs during ventilation within the physiological range [5,41].

Computational simulations and in vitro experiments provided evidence that a finger-shaped bubble of air penetrating a fluid occluded airway is associated with harmful shear stresses resulting in necrosis of lining epithelial cells, an injurious event which can be prevented by addition of surfactant [22,49]. In the current study, an increase in the surface area of the basal lamina covered by injured epithelial cells was observed in Dox off d1 compared to Dox on (Figure 7C) and this was present even though the volume of alveolar fluid had not increased significantly (Figure 5C). Based on these observations we infer that the recruitment of airspaces by septal wall unfolding is an injurious event in Dox off d1 but not in Dox on, where the epithelium is protected from injury by functional surfactant. The injury of epithelial cells progresses in Dox off d3 to affecting approximately 6 to 8% of the surface area. A previous study using the LPS model of acute lung injury and light microscopic staining for AE1 cell markers found a loss of AE1 cells in 3% of the surface area [50]. In the present study, a complete denudation of the alveolar epithelial basal lamina was rarely observed and the main features related to injury were swelling and clearing of cytoplasmic ground substance, blebbing, and rupture of apical membranes (Figure 6). Among the structural parameters, the surface area of epithelial basal lamina covered by injured cells demonstrated a strong correlation with lung mechanical impairment, a finding which confirms observation in models of VILI where epithelial injury observed with scanning electron microscopy was strongly correlated with elastance [51]. Based on the presented data, the primary effects of induced SP-B deficiency are subtle alterations in alveolar micromechanics and alveolar epithelial injury that initially occur without abnormalities in the ultrastructural features of the alveolar fluid. The relationship between injury of the alveolar epithelial lining and the volume of alveolar fluid could best be described by an exponential growth function. The volume of alveolar fluid increased exponentially with the surface area of injured alveolar epithelium (Figure 7D). Similar relationships have been observed in a model of VILI between histologic injury scores and BAL protein levels [46] or after LPS injury during alveolar epithelial regeneration, plotting the percentage of regenerated alveolar epithelium against the BAL albumin level [50].

3.4. Limitations

In the present study assessment of lung structure was performed under "quasi-static" conditions at different airway pressures with the goal to characterize micromechanical aspects [26]. Also, fixed lung tissue was used for this purpose. While the microarchitecture was investigated by a robust methodology, the design-based stereology, up to the ultrastructural level, we did not study micromechanics directly. Instead, conclusions on the micromechanical behavior were made based on the comparison between parameters of microarchitecture at different airway pressures. Since the lung has viscoelastic properties the micromechanical behavior under dynamic breathing conditions is likely to differ from "quasi-static" conditions. For example nothing is known regarding the time scales at which folding and unfolding or fluid redistribution occurs. In vivo microscopy offers a powerful tool to study alveolar micromechanics under dynamic conditions [12,13]. However, it has to be pointed out that currently available imaging methods of in vivo microscopy are only able to study subpleural alveoli which might be not representative and do not have the appropriate resolution to investigate dynamics in fluid shift and unfolding of interalveolar septa since these aspects would require electron microscopic resolution [5]. In addition, female mice were used in the present study so that it cannot be excluded that a study using male mice would end up with different results and conclusion.

3.5. Summary

The presented data suggest that a kind of microatelectrauma might be the initial injurious event during spontaneous breathing in this animal model (Figure 8). We investigated the lung structure at low airway opening pressures and within a range of transpulmonary pressure gradients which is known to occur physiologically during quite breathing [52]. Hence, we consider the recruitment of pleats as a possible mechanism during spontaneous breathing. The unfolding of septal walls in the absence of SP-B might be responsible for alveolar epithelial cell injury in a manner similar to the reopening of fluid-occluded compliant airway models [22,36,49]. In the current study, the tissue strains resulting from peeling apart of septal pleats may be elevated by the same fluid-mechanical mechanisms that increase tissue strains during compliant airway reopening with high surface tension [39]. This injury of alveolar epithelium may occur prior to fluid accumulation and, in turn, increase alveolo-capillary permeability and lead to the observed exponential increase in alveolar fluid with increased alveolar protein and albumin levels. The combination of high surface tension and fluid accumulation results in a progressive alveolar derecruitment linked with a severely reduced recruitability of alveoli and increased ventilation heterogeneity. Alveolar interdependence with derecruited or edema filled alveoli next to ventilated alveoli has been shown to be a mechanism responsible for injurious overdistension of neighboring alveoli even at ventilation with low tidal volumes and pressures [30,53,54]. With this regard the forces acting on lung parenchyma are a consequence of the pressure gradient between the acinar airspaces and the pleural space, also known as elastic recoil pressure [25,55]. The elastic recoil pressure can be elevated during mechanical ventilation (high airway opening pressure), during spontaneous breathing (high negative pressure in pleural space) but also locally within a network of airspaces in the presence of stress concentrators. In principle, the latter can occur within a range of physiological pressure gradients at the organ scale and under spontaneous breathing. Hence, we consider non-recruitable distal airspaces as stress concentrators [25,56] which could end-up in a fatal vicious cycle following induction of SP-B deficiency. A similar scenario as we suggest for these spontaneously breathing SP-B deficient mice has been postulated as a rich-get-richer process in a model of alveolar leak during VILI. Accordingly, microatelectrauma represents the initial injurious trigger followed by a positive feedback mechanism of vascular leakage, edema formation, tethering-induced volutrauma, and further vascular leakage [46,57].

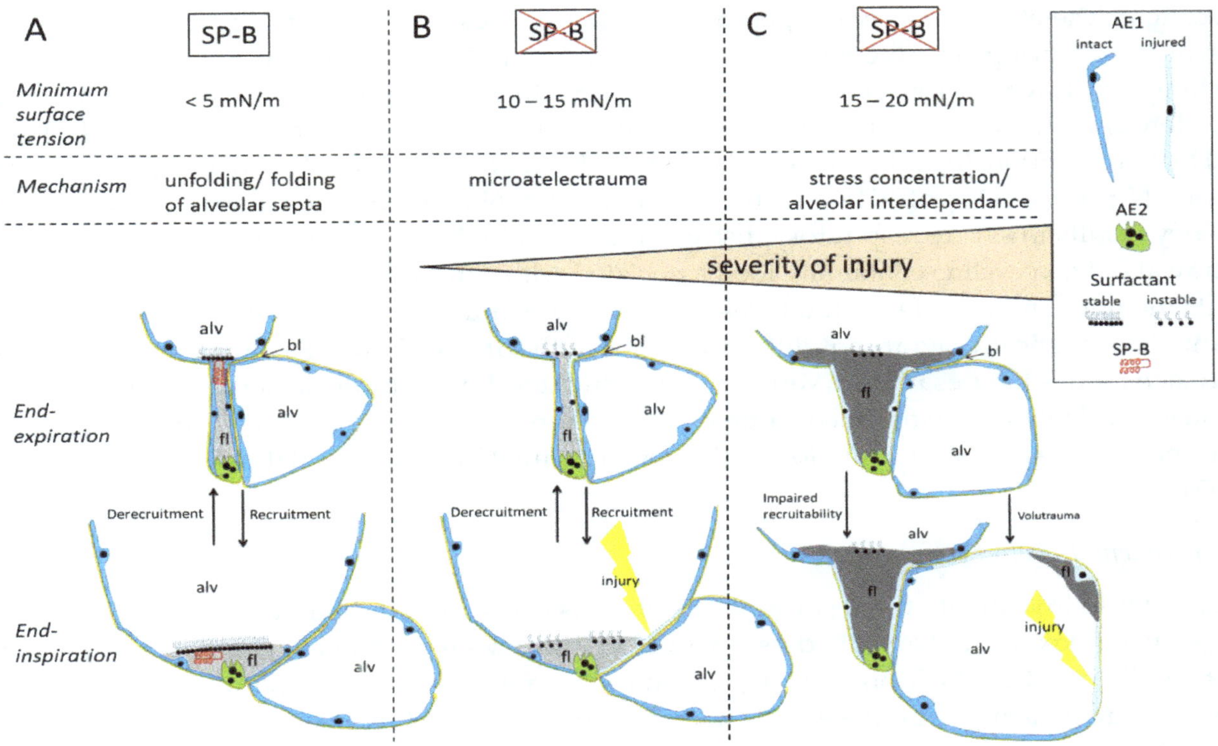

Figure 8. Proposed mechanism of lung injury in SP-B deficiency: Under physiological conditions (**A**) volume changes during ventilation include recruitment and derecruitment of folds. At low lung volumes folds are filled with a very thin leaflet of alveolar fluid (fl), the surfactant monolayer is compressed at the air-liquid interface and stabilized by SP-B. With increasing lung volume the folds are recruited and the fluid is pressed into the corners of the alveoli. The fluid-mechanical stress during this opening process acting on the alveolar epithelium is reduced by surface lowering properties of surfactant [22,39]. In absence of SP-B (indicated in B and C by the red cross) the monolayer is unstable,

the minimum surface tension increases within 24 h [21]. The opening process of folds (**B**) is linked with harmful stresses acting on the alveolar epithelial cells (microatelectrauma) [22,39]. The blood-gas barrier is compromised by the progressing injury and the volume of alveolar fluid and plasma protein levels increase. High surface tension combined with increased viscosity of alveolar fluid reduces the recruitability of folds (**C**). Heterogeneous ventilation with overdistension of neighboring alveoli (alveolar interdependence) occurs with leakage of the blood-gas barrier in adjacent alveoli. Abbreviations: AE1: alveolar epithelial type 1 cell, AE2: alveolar epithelial type II cell, fl: alveolar fluid, bl: basal lamina, alv: alveolar airspace.

4. Materials and Methods

4.1. Animal Model and Study Groups

For pulmonary structural and mechanical investigations 40 female conditional Surfactant Protein B (SP-B) knock out mice [CCSP-rtTA, $(tetO)_7$ *SFTPB/Sftpb*$^{-/-}$] aged between 10 and 13 weeks were included. SP-B expression was under control of a doxycycline dependent promotor as has been described before [20,21]. The mice were randomly assigned to 3 groups. The control group (Dox on) was continuously fed with doxycycline containing food (625mg per kg standard diet, Altromin 1324, Lage, Germany). The experimental groups were deprived of doxycycline containing food for 1 and 3 days, respectively (Dox off d1 or Dox off d3) in order to investigate time effects of SP-B deficiency on lung structure and function. Animals assigned to Dox off d1 were transferred to cages with standard food on Mondays at 8:00 am. Lung mechanical properties were measured on Tuesdays between 8 and 10 am. The interval for Dox off d3 groups was from Monday 8:00 am to Thursday 8:00 am. In order to investigate the effects of airway opening pressures in these study groups, respiratory mechanics was evaluated during positive end-expiratory pressure (PEEP) ventilation with 2 and 10 cmH_2O while lung structure was assessed at corresponding positive end-expiratory airway opening pressures (Pao). Hence, within each group animals were randomized to PEEP 2/Pao 2 cmH_2O or PEEP 10/Pao 10 cmH_2O. In addition, broncho-alveolar lavage (BAL) fluid was obtained from additional 17 animals (Dox on: $N = 6$ vs. Dox off d1: $N = 6$ vs. Dox off d3: $N = 5$). Since it is well-known that SP-B deficiency results in severe respiratory distress and death in this animal model starting at day 4 after withdrawal of Doxycycline containing food associated with a mortality rate of 40% [21], the number of subjects included in group Dox off d3 was reduced to the minimum, necessary to detect biologically relevant and statistically significant differences. The authorities of Lower Saxony, Germany (= LAVES: Niedersächsisches Landesamt für Verbraucherschutz und Lebensmittelsicherheit), which house the German equivalent of an institutional animal care and use committee, approved all animal experiments performed in this study according to the European Animal Welfare Regulations (Approval number: 16/2245).

4.2. Experimental Protocol

In order to investigate the respiratory mechanics during controlled ventilation in the different study groups (Dox on vs. Dox off 1d vs. Dox off 3d), mice were invasively ventilated by a FlexiVent rodent ventilator (SCIREQ, Montreal, PQ, Canada). The animals were anesthetized by intraperitoneal administration of 80 mg/kg bodyweight ketamine (Anesketin, Dechra Veterinary Products, Aulendorf, Germany), 5 mg/kg bodyweight xylazine (Rompun, Leverkusen, Germany) and 2mg/kg bodyweight midazolam. After disappearance of pain reflexes a tracheotomy was performed and the airways were connected to the FlexiVent rodent ventilator via a cannula (Braun cannula, 21 G, Diameter 0.8mm, Melsungen, Germany). Baseline ventilation parameters were as follows: tidal volume 10 mg/kg bodyweight, respiratory rate 150/min, inspiratory-to-expiratory time ratio 1:2 and PEEP 3 cmH_2O. After a run-in phase of 5 min two deep inflations followed by three pressure-controlled pressure-volume (PV) loops were recorded to determine the inspiratory capacity, the quasi-static compliance of the respiratory system and the area within the PV-loop as a parameter of hysteresis [26]. Afterwards, PEEP was either adjusted to 2 cmH_2O or 10 cmH_2O followed by derecruitability tests as described elsewhere [19,26]. In brief, the derecruitability tests consisted of 2 recruitment manoeuvres (deep inflation with a pressure plateau at 30 cmH_2O) and subsequent repetitive measurements of respiratory mechanics every 30 s using the forced oscillation technique. By fitting the constant phase model to impedance spectra obtained during forced oscillation technique, tissue elastance (H) and Newtonian resistance (Rn) were calculated. Tissue elastance is a parameter reflecting the mechanical properties of the fine lung parenchyma while Newtonian resistance is affected by alterations of the conducting airways and therefore the more central parts of the respiratory system. After recording tissue elastance for 5 min, the abdomen and chest wall was opened by a median laparo-thoracotomy. The lung was inflated to a plateau pressure of 30 cmH_2O for 3 s two times (deep inflation) and airway opening pressure (Pao) was adjusted at either Pao of 2 or 10cmH_2O on expiration, corresponding to the PEEP at which lung mechanics were assessed in each case [26].

4.3. Perfusion Fixation, Preparation and Sampling

The lungs were fixed by vascular perfusion at either Pao 2 or 10 cmH_2O. The trachea was ligated at the corresponding Pao and flow of zero. The abdominal aorta was immediately incised and the right ventricle was punctured. The lungs were first flushed with a hydrostatic pressure of 40 cmH_2O with Heparin (12,500 IU/l) in 0.9% sodium chloride solution to prevent coagulation in the pulmonary vasculature. Then, the fixative, consisting of 1.5% paraformaldehyde (PFA), 1.5% glutaraldehyde (GA) and 0.15 mM HEPES buffer, was perfused [45]. Finally, the organ package consisting of heart, lung, thymus and esophagus were carefully removed from the thoracic cavity and stored in the above mentioned fixation solution at 4 °C for at least 24 h.

For preparation and sampling, the lungs had to be carefully removed from the organ block using surgical scissors and tweezers. During the preparation, it was crucial to avoid compression of the lung to prevent contusing artifacts and artificial manipulation of the sensitive lung parenchyma. The heart, thymus, esophagus and fatty tissue were removed and the lungs were re-inserted in the fixation solution for at least 3 h.

The total lung volume [V(lung)] was determined based on the principle of Archimedes by the fluid displacement method as described by Scherle [58]. After measuring the lung volume, the whole lung was embedded in 4% agar and cut with a tissue slicer into slices of equal thickness from the apex to the base, enabling a “systematic uniform random sampling” [59]. The aim of “systematic uniform random sampling” was to give every part of the lung tissue the same chance of being selected for stereological investigation [60]. The tissue slicer generated 7 lung slices of an approximate thickness of 2 mm. Slices were randomly allocated to light (LM) or electron microscopy (EM).

Since the EM samples were limited in size, a subsampling of the slices assigned to EM was used to obtain 6-8 small cubes eligible to be further processed [59]. A point grid was thrown onto the lung slices. The lung tissue hit by the test points was selected and cut into cubes of 1 mm edge length with a scalpel knife and used for further EM embedding.

4.4. Embedding for Light Microscopy

The LM samples were embedded in hydroxyethylmethacrylate (Technovit 8100, Heraeus Kulzer, Wehrheim, Germany) in accordance to the user’s instructions. After washing in 0.2 mol Na-cacodylate buffer and osmification of the samples, the lungs were vented in a vacuum desiccator. After incubation in uranyl acetate overnight, dehydration was followed by an ascending acetone dilution series (70%, 90%, 100%). Then, the polymerization by the Technovit 8100 resulted in the curing of the samples. The rotation microtome (Leica, RM2265, Nussloch, Germany) was used for the slicing of the 1.5 µm thin sections. The first and the forth of a consecutive series of slices were placed on a glass slide, with Toluidine blue and capped with a cover glass [61].

4.5. Embedding for Electron Microscopy

The samples were washed in 0.15 HEPES buffer, post-fixed in osmium and contrasted *en-bloc* with uranyl acetate. Afterwards, dehydration was performed with an ascending acetone dilution series (70%, 90%, 100%). The probes were embedded in epoxy resin (Epon, Serva, Germany) in order to cut the samples into 60 nm thin slices employing the ultramicrotome (Leica, Nussloch, Germany),. Both the light microscopic and the electron microscopic embedding are based on the common procedures use in design-based stereological analyses [61].

4.6. Design-based Stereology

The methodology of stereology was applied to determine structural changes in the lungs as a function of the duration of SP-B deficiency (Dox on vs. Dox off d1 vs. Dox off d3) as well as the end-expiratory airway opening pressure (Pao = 2 cmH_2O vs. Pao = 10 cmH_2O). All methods for quantitative morphology used in the present study were based on the American Thoracic Society (ATS)/European Respiratory Society (ERS) joint statement for quantitative assessment of lung structures [62]. Design-based stereology provides information on 3-dimensional structures based on 2-dimensional sections which are combined with tests systems such as test points, test lines or counting frames interacting with the structures of interest in a stochastic manner [63]. The parameters determined at light and electron microscopic level are defined in Table 5.

Table 5. Definition of stereological parameters.

Definition	Abbreviation	Test System	Magnification
Volume of parenchyma	V(par,lung)	Point counting (P)	5 ×
Volume of non-parenchyma (conducting airways, larger vessels, connective tissue)	V(nonpar,lung)	Point counting (P)	5 ×
Volume of alveolar airspaces within lung parenchyma	V(alvair,lung)	Point counting(P)	20 ×
Volume of ductal airspaces within lung parenchyma	V(ductair,lung)	Point counting (P)	20 ×
Volume of interalveolar septa within lung parenchyma	V (sep,lung)	Point counting (P)	20 ×
Surface area of alveoli within lung parenchyma	S (alv,lung)	Intersection counting (I)	20 ×
Arithmetic mean septal wall thickness	τ(sep)	Volume-to-surface ratio	20 ×
Number alveoli within lung parenchyma	N(alv,lung)	Physical disector	10 ×
Volume of alveolar epithelial type 1 cells within septal walls	V(AE1,sep)	Point counting (P)	11.000 ×
Volume of alveolar epithelial type 2 cells within septal walls	V(AE2,sep)	Point counting (P)	11.000 ×
Volume of endothelial cell within septal walls	V(endo,sep)	Point counting (P)	11.000 ×
Volume of other cells (e.g., macrophages, fibroblasts)	V(othercells,sep)	Point counting (P)	11.000 ×
Volume of extracellular matrix within septal walls	V(ECM,sep)	Point counting (P)	11.000 ×
Volume of capillary lumen within septal walls	V(cap,sep)	Point counting (P)	11.000 ×
Volume of alveolar fluid within parenchyma	V(alvfluid,par)	Point counting (P)	11.000 ×

Table 5. *Cont.*

Definition	Abbreviation	Test System	Magnification
Surface area of the alveolar epithelial basal lamina within septal walls	S(alvBL,sep)	Intersection counting (I)	11.000 ×
Surface area of the basal lamina covered by AE1 cells	S(AE1,sep)	Intersection counting (I)	11.000 ×
Surface area of the basal lamina covered by AE2 cells	S(AE2,sep)	Intersection counting (I)	11.000 ×
Surface area of the basal lamina covered by injured alveolar epithelial cells	S(AEinjure,sep)	Intersection counting (I)	11.000 ×
Surface area of the endothelial basal lamina within septal walls	S(endoBL,sep)	Intersection (I) counting	11.000 ×
Surface area of the alveolar epithelium covered by air within parenchyma	S(airAE,par)	Intersection (I) counting	11.000 ×
Surface area of alveolar epithelium covered by alveolar fluid within parenchyma	S(fluidAE,par)	Intersection (I) counting	11.000 ×
Arithmetic mean thickness of alveolar fluid	τ(alvfluid)	Volume-to-surface ratio	11.000 ×

The light microscopic assessments were carried out using a light microscope (Leica 6000, Wetzlar, Germany) equipped the computer-controlled stage and the NewCAST stereology software (Visiopharm A/S, Horshorm, Denmark) for systematic uniform area sampling and generation of an appropriate unbiased test-system for counting. The test system specified by the examiner was projected onto the sampled fields of view. The counting of events, defined as a stochastic interaction of the structures of interest with the test system was carried out by the blinded investigator. In order to ensure sufficient precision the unbiased test system was adjusted in a way that at least 100-200 counting events per parameter and organ were generated on 100 to 200 fields of view [64].

During the whole procedure, a cascade sampling design was applied [65]. In a first step, the lung was examined with a primary magnification of 5 × with the goal to distinguish between parenchymal and non-parenchymal components. Parenchyma was defined as fine lung structures which are directly involved in gas exchange while non-parenchyma was represented by conducting airways, larger vessels (excluding septal wall capillaries) and perivascular connective tissue. Test points were projected on fields of view. If a point hit structures involved in gas exchange (alveolar and ductal airspaces, interalveolar septa) it was counted as parenchyma [P(par)]. Points hitting bronchi, bronchiole, vessels or connective tissue were counted as non-parenchyma [P(nonpar)]. The following formula describes the volume density of parenchyma within the lung as a function of the total of all points hitting the lung (= reference space):

$$Vv\left(\frac{par}{lung}\right) = \frac{\Sigma}{\Sigma P(par) + \Sigma P\ (nonpar)} \tag{2}$$

A final statement about the volume V of parenchymal and non-parenchymal components can only be taken if the result is related to the total lung volume. Otherwise there is a risk of falling into the "reference trap", defined by Braendgaard and Gundersen [66]. Generally speaking, all generated densities must always be related to their reference volume in order to obtain absolute data, e.g., the total volume of lung parenchyma per lung. This avoids misinterpretations of densities or volume fractions due to differences in the reference space (= reference trap) [59].

$$V(par,\ lung)\left(cm^3\right) = Vv\left(\frac{par}{lung}\right) \times V(lung)\left(cm^3\right) \tag{3}$$

In a second step of the cascade sampling design, the reference space was the lung parenchyma which was now assessed at higher magnification (primary magnification: 20 ×). The lung parenchyma was further differentiated into volumes of alveolar airspace V(alvair,lung), ductal airspaces V(ductair,lung) and interalveolar septa V(sep,lung) via point counting. The alveolar surface area S(alv,lung) was determined by counting the intersection points between a defined test line $\left(\frac{l}{p}\right)$ and the septa.

For example, the volume density of alveolar airspace within lung parenchyma was calculated using the following formula:

$$Vv\left(\frac{alvair}{par}\right) = \frac{\sum P(alvair)}{\sum P(alvair) + \sum P(ductair) + \sum P(sep)} \tag{4}$$

The total volume of alveolar airspace was accordingly calculated by multiplication of the volume density with the reference space:

$$V(alvair, lung)\left(cm^3\right) = Vv\left(\frac{alvair}{par}\right) \times V(par,\ lung)\left(cm^3\right) \tag{5}$$

The surface density of the alveoli within reference space (= lung parenchyma) was calculated as follows:

$$Sv\left(\frac{alv}{par}\right)\left(cm^{-1}\right) = \frac{2 \times \sum I}{\left(\frac{l}{p}\right)(\mu m) \times P(line)} \times 10.000 \tag{6}$$

$$\frac{l}{p}(\mu m) = 30.84 \tag{7}$$

$$P(line) = Points\ of\ the\ testline = reference\ points \tag{8}$$

The total surface area of alveoli at light microscopic level was accordingly determined by multiplication with the reference space:

$$S(alv,\ lung)\left(cm^2\right) = Sv\left(\frac{alv}{Par}\right)\left(cm^{-1}\right) \times V(par, lung)\left(cm^3\right) \tag{9}$$

In addition, the mean thickness of the septa was calculated from the ratio of the volume of the septa to the surface area.

$$\tau(sep)(\mu m) = \frac{2 \times V(sep, lung)\left(cm^3\right) \times 10.000}{S(alv, lung)(cm^2)} \tag{10}$$

Furthermore, the number of open alveoli per lung N(alv,lung) [67,68] was calculated by employing the physical disector which consisted of a pair of section, corresponding to the first and the forth section of a consecutive series with a sections thickness of 1.5 μm. Hence, the distance from the top of the first to the top of the forth section was 4.5 μm representing the disector height. Using a counting frame with a defined area A(frame) a test volume for counting was generated. Whenever an alveolar mouth was present in one section and absent in the other, a counting event was recorded [67,69]. The estimate of the number of alveoli is based on the Euler number; a mathematical parameter (named after the swiss mathematician Leonard Euler), that quantifies the connectivity of an object. The Euler number [x_3] represents the number of alveolar openings (B).

$$x_3 = \sum B \tag{11}$$

$$N(alv, lung) = \frac{\sum B}{disector\ height\ x\ A(frame)x \sum P(reference\ counting\ frame)} \times V(par, lung) \tag{12}$$

In the third step of the cascade sampling design, the volume of the interalveolar septa V(sep,lung) represented the reference space for further analyses at electron microscopic resolution. A transmission electron microscope (Morgani, FEI, Eindhoven, The Netherlands) equipped with an integrated camera (Olympus Soft Imaging Solution, Münster, Germany) was used to perform a systematic uniform area sampling at electron microscopic level. The section was traced meander-shaped via a coordinate system in x and y direction at a distance of 50 × 50 μm [59]. The septal wall was imaged every 50 μm using a primary magnification of 11,000x. Afterwards the sampled images were examined with the STEPanizer stereology tool [70]. The volume and surface densities were measured using unbiased test systems consisting of tests points for volume fractions of different structures and test lines for surface densities within the septal walls. The total volume of alveolar epithelial type I cells V(AE1,sep) and the total surface area of the alveolar epithelial basal lamina S(alvBL,sep) within the septal wall volume were for example calculated with the following equations:

$$V(AE1, sep)\left(cm^3\right) = \frac{\sum P(AE1)}{\sum P(all\ counts)} \times V(sep, lung)\left(cm^3\right) \tag{13}$$

$$S(alvBL, sep)\left(cm^2\right) = \frac{2\ x\ I\ x\ 10.000}{l(t)x\ \sum P(all\ counts)}\left(cm^{-1}\right) \times V(sep, lung)\left(cm^3\right) \tag{14}$$

$$test\ line = l(t)(\mu m) = 1.066\ \mu m \tag{15}$$

$$Intersection\ point\ between\ test\ line\ and\ interface\ of\ BL\ and\ AE = I \tag{16}$$

In addition, test lines were used to determine the surface area of the alveolar epithelial basal lamina (alvBL) covered by healthy AE1 or alveolar epithelial type 2 (AE2) cells or injured alveolar epithelial cells [19,71]. At the intersection of the test line with the alveolar epithelial basal lamina the topping epithelial cell was categorized as healthy appearing AE1 or AE2 cell or injured cell. The later was identified according the following criteria: swelling with formation of small vacuoles and clearing of the cytoplasmic ground substance, or fragmentation such as disruption of the apical plasma membrane, formation of vesicles up to denudation of the basal lamina. Data were calculated as surface fractions (in %) and absolute surface areas (in cm^2).

4.7. Analyses of Broncho-alveolar Lavage Fluid

Animals were anaesthetized by intraperitoneal administration of 80 mg/kg bodyweight ketamine (Anesketin, Dechra Veterinary Products, Aulendorf, Germany), 5 mg/kg bodyweight xylazine (Rompun, Leverkusen, Germany) and 2 mg/kg bodyweight midazolam. After cessation of pain reflexes, the abdomen was opened and the abdominal aorta incised. Afterwards, a tracheotomy was carried out and the chest opened. For harvest of broncho-alveolar lavage (BAL) fluid three aliquots of 1 mL 0.9% sodium chloride solution were successively instilled and suctioned out of the lung. The range of recovery per lung was 2–2.5 mL. In order to separate cellular components and debris from fluid, a centrifugation with 1000g was carried out for 10 min. The supernatant was removed and snap frozen in liquid nitrogen and stored at –80 °C till further assessments of protein and albumin concentration as described previously [72]. In brief, albumin concentrations in BAL fluid were assessed with the albumin ELISA kit (Bethyl Laboratories, Montgomery, AL) according to the manufacturer's instructions. Protein and albumin concentrations in BAL fluid served as indicators of vascular leak.

4.8. Statistical Analyses

A descriptive statistics was performed to calculate the mean and standard deviation of each parameter. A two-way ANOVA on ranks was carried out taking the factors "group" and the end-expiratory airway opening pressure (PEEP for lung mechanics and Pao for structural assessments) into account. In case of statistically significant differences, a Tukey´s post-hoc adjustment of the p-level for multiple testing was added. Regarding quasi-static compliance (Cst), hysteresis (area), inspiratory capacity (IC) and BAL data (protein and albumin) a one-way ANOVA was used followed by Tukey´s post-hoc test in case data were normally distributed according to Shapiro-Wilk normality test. Otherwise, a Kruskal-Wallis test followed by Dunn´s test for multiple comparisons was used. Pearson´s correlation analyses were performed between structural and lung mechanical parameters. V(alvfluid,par) and S(AEinjure,sep) were plotted against each other and the best fit curve was interpolated to describe the relationship between these parameters. Data are provided in the Tables as means and standard deviations while the graphs in the figures show dot blots of individual data for each group. Statistical assessments were performed using GraphPad Prism (Version 7.0, GraphPad Software, La Jolla, CA, USA) or in case of correlation analyses SPSS (Version 25, IBM, Armonk, NY, USA).

Author Contributions: Conceptualization: N.R., E.L.-R., and L.K.; methodology: N.R., E.L.-R., K.A., T.E.W., B.J.S., M.O. and L.K.; formal analysis: N.R., K.A., and L.K.; investigation, N.R., E.L.-R., K.A., T.E.W., B.J.S., M.O. and L.K.; resources, N.R., E.L.-R., K.A., T.E.W., B.J.S., M.O. and L.K.; data curation, N.R., E.L.-R., K.A., T.E.W., B.J.S., M.O. and L.K.; writing—original draft preparation, N.R., and L.K.; writing—review and editing, N.R., E.L.-R., K.A., T.E.W., B.J.S., M.O. and L.K.; visualization, N.R., K.A., and L.K.; supervision, E.L.-R., M.O. and L.K.; project administration, L.K.; funding acquisition, M.O. and L.K.

Acknowledgments: The authors thank Karin Westermann and Susanne Fassbender for their excellent technical assistance.

References

1. Lopez-Rodriguez, E.; Gay-Jordi, G.; Mucci, A.; Lachmann, N.; Serrano-Mollar, A. Lung surfactant metabolism: Early in life, early in disease and target in cell therapy. *Cell Tissue Res.* **2017**, *367*, 721–735. [CrossRef] [PubMed]
2. Schürch, D.; Ospina, O.L.; Cruz, A.; Pérez-Gil, J. Combined and independent action of proteins SP-B and SP-C in the surface behavior and mechanical stability of pulmonary surfactant films. *Biophys. J.* **2010**, *99*, 3290–3299. [CrossRef] [PubMed]
3. Ochs, M. The closer we look the more we see? Quantitative microscopic analysis of the pulmonary surfactant system. *Cell Physiol. Biochem.* **2010**, *25*, 27–40. [CrossRef] [PubMed]
4. Mead, J. Mechanical properties of lungs. *Physiol. Rev.* **1961**, *41*, 281–330. [CrossRef] [PubMed]
5. Knudsen, L.; Ochs, M. The micromechanics of lung alveoli: Structure and function of surfactant and tissue components. *Histochem. Cell Biol.* **2018**, *150*, 661–676. [CrossRef] [PubMed]
6. Bachofen, H.; Schürch, S.; Urbinelli, M.; Weibel, E. Relations among alveolar surface tension, surface area, volume, and recoil pressure. *J. Appl. Physiol. (1985)* **1987**, *62*, 1878–1887. [CrossRef] [PubMed]
7. Schürch, S.; Bachofen, H.; Possmayer, F. Surface activity in situ, in vivo, and in the captive bubble surfactometer. *Comp. Biochem. Physiol. A Mol. Integr. Physiol.* **2001**, *129*, 195–207. [CrossRef]
8. Almlén, A.; Stichtenoth, G.; Linderholm, B.; Haegerstrand-Björkman, M.; Robertson, B.; Johansson, J.; Curstedt, T. Surfactant proteins B and C are both necessary for alveolar stability at end expiration in premature rabbits with respiratory distress syndrome. *J. Appl. Physiol. (1985)* **2008**, *104*, 1101–1108. [CrossRef]
9. Matute-Bello, G.; Downey, G.; Moore, B.B.; Groshong, S.D.; Matthay, M.A.; Slutsky, A.S.; Kuebler, W.M.; Group, A.L.I.i.A.S. An official American Thoracic Society workshop report: Features and measurements of experimental acute lung injury in animals. *Am. J. Respir. Cell Mol. Biol.* **2011**, *44*, 725–738. [CrossRef]
10. Cabrera-Benítez, N.E.; Parotto, M.; Post, M.; Han, B.; Spieth, P.M.; Cheng, W.E.; Valladares, F.; Villar, J.; Liu, M.; Sato, M.; et al. Mechanical stress induces lung fibrosis by epithelial-mesenchymal transition. *Crit. Care Med.* **2012**, *40*, 510–517. [CrossRef]
11. Wilson, T.A.; Bachofen, H. A model for mechanical structure of the alveolar duct. *J. Appl. Physiol. (1985)* **1982**, *52*, 1064–1070. [CrossRef] [PubMed]
12. Schiller, H.J.; McCann, U.G.; Carney, D.E.; Gatto, L.A.; Steinberg, J.M.; Nieman, G.F. Altered alveolar mechanics in the acutely injured lung. *Crit. Care Med.* **2001**, *29*, 1049–1055. [CrossRef] [PubMed]
13. Tabuchi, A.; Nickles, H.T.; Kim, M.; Semple, J.W.; Koch, E.; Brochard, L.; Slutsky, A.S.; Pries, A.R.; Kuebler, W.M.

Acute Lung Injury Causes Asynchronous Alveolar Ventilation That Can Be Corrected by Individual Sighs. *Am J. Respir. Crit. Care Med.* **2016**, *193*, 396–406. [CrossRef] [PubMed]
14. Greene, K.; Wright, J.; Steinberg, K.; Ruzinski, J.; Caldwell, E.; Wong, W.; Hull, W.; Whitsett, J.; Akino, T.; Kuroki, Y.; et al. Serial changes in surfactant-associated proteins in lung and serum before and after onset of ARDS. *Am. J. Respir Crit. Care Med.* **1999**, *160*, 1843–1850. [CrossRef] [PubMed]
15. Gregory, T.J.; Longmore, W.J.; Moxley, M.A.; Whitsett, J.A.; Reed, C.R.; Fowler, A.A.; Hudson, L.D.; Maunder, R.J.; Crim, C.; Hyers, T.M. Surfactant chemical composition and biophysical activity in acute respiratory distress syndrome. *J. Clin. Investig.* **1991**, *88*, 1976–1981. [CrossRef]
16. Schmidt, R.; Markart, P.; Ruppert, C.; Wygrecka, M.; Kuchenbuch, T.; Walmrath, D.; Seeger, W.; Guenther, A. Time-dependent changes in pulmonary surfactant function and composition in acute respiratory distress syndrome due to pneumonia or aspiration. *Respir. Res.* **2007**, *8*, 55. [CrossRef] [PubMed]
17. Albert, R.K. The role of ventilation-induced surfactant dysfunction and atelectasis in causing acute respiratory distress syndrome. *Am. J. Respir. Crit. Care Med.* **2012**, *185*, 702–708. [CrossRef]
18. Nieman, G.F.; Bredenberg, C.E. High surface tension pulmonary edema induced by detergent aerosol. *J. Appl. Physiol.* **1985**, *58*, 129–136. [CrossRef]
19. Lutz, D.; Gazdhar, A.; Lopez-Rodriguez, E.; Ruppert, C.; Mahavadi, P.; Gunther, A.; Klepetko, W.; Bates, J.H.; Smith, B.; Geiser, T.; et al. Alveolar Derecruitment and Collapse Induration as Crucial Mechanisms in Lung Injury and Fibrosis. *Am. J. Respir. Cell Mol. Biol.* **2015**, *52*, 232–243. [CrossRef]
20. Nesslein, L.L.; Melton, K.R.; Ikegami, M.; Na, C.L.; Wert, S.E.; Rice, W.R.; Whitsett, J.A.; Weaver, T.E. Partial SP-B deficiency perturbs lung function and causes air space abnormalities. *Am. J. Physiol. Lung Cell Mol. Physiol.* **2005**, *288*, L1154–L1161. [CrossRef]
21. Ikegami, M.; Whitsett, J.A.; Martis, P.C.; Weaver, T.E. Reversibility of lung inflammation caused by SP-B deficiency. *Am. J. Physiol. Lung Cell Mol. Physiol.* **2005**, *289*, L962–L970. [CrossRef] [PubMed]
22. Bilek, A.M.; Dee, K.C.; Gaver, D.P. Mechanisms of surface-tension-induced epithelial cell damage in a model of pulmonary airway reopening. *J. Appl. Physiol. (1985)* **2003**, *94*, 770–783. [CrossRef] [PubMed]
23. Hobi, N.; Ravasio, A.; Haller, T. Interfacial stress affects rat alveolar type II cell signaling and gene expression. *Am J. Physiol. Lung Cell Mol. Physiol.* **2012**, *303*, L117–L129. [CrossRef] [PubMed]
24. Ravasio, A.; Hobi, N.; Bertocchi, C.; Jesacher, A.; Dietl, P.; Haller, T. Interfacial sensing by alveolar type II cells: A new concept in lung physiology? *Am. J. Physiol. Cell Physiol.* **2011**, *300*, C1456–C1465. [CrossRef] [PubMed]
25. Mead, J.; Takishima, T.; Leith, D. Stress distribution in lungs: A model of pulmonary elasticity. *J. Appl. Physiol.* **1970**, *28*, 596–608. [CrossRef]
26. Knudsen, L.; Lopez-Rodriguez, E.; Berndt, L.; Steffen, L.; Ruppert, C.; Bates, J.H.T.; Ochs, M.; Smith, B.J. Alveolar Micromechanics in Bleomycin-induced Lung Injury. *Am. J. Respir. Cell Mol. Biol.* **2018**, *59*, 757–769. [CrossRef]
27. Slutsky, A.S.; Ranieri, V.M. Ventilator-induced lung injury. *N. Engl. J. Med.* **2013**, *369*, 2126–2136. [CrossRef]
28. Glindmeyer, H.W.; Smith, B.J.; Gaver, D.P. In situ enhancement of pulmonary surfactant function using temporary flow reversal. *J. Appl. Physiol.* **2012**, *112*, 149–158. [CrossRef]
29. Ramsingh, R.; Grygorczyk, A.; Solecki, A.; Cherkaoui, L.S.; Berthiaume, Y.; Grygorczyk, R. Cell deformation at the air-liquid interface induces Ca^{2+}-dependent ATP release from lung epithelial cells. *Am. J. Physiol. Lung Cell Mol. Physiol.* **2011**, *300*, L587–L595. [CrossRef]
30. Wu, Y.; Kharge, A.B.; Perlman, C.E. Lung ventilation injures areas with discrete alveolar flooding, in a surface tension-dependent fashion. *J. Appl. Physiol. (1985)* **2014**, *117*, 788–796. [CrossRef]
31. Hantos, Z.; Daroczy, B.; Suki, B.; Nagy, S.; Fredberg, J.J. Input impedance and peripheral inhomogeneity of dog lungs. *J. Appl. Physiol.* **1992**, *72*, 168–178. [CrossRef] [PubMed]
32. Allen, G.B.; Pavone, L.A.; DiRocco, J.D.; Bates, J.H.; Nieman, G.F. Pulmonary impedance and alveolar instability during injurious ventilation in rats. *J. Appl. Physiol. (1985)* **2005**, *99*, 723–730. [CrossRef] [PubMed]
33. Massa, C.B.; Allen, G.B.; Bates, J.H. Modeling the dynamics of recruitment and derecruitment in mice with acute lung injury. *J. Appl. Physiol.* **2008**, *105*, 1813–1821. [CrossRef] [PubMed]
34. Paré, P.D.; Mitzner, W. Airway-parenchymal interdependence. *Compr. Physiol.* **2012**, *2*, 1921–1935. [CrossRef] [PubMed]
35. Gil, J.; Bachofen, H.; Gehr, P.; Weibel, E. Alveolar volume-surface area relation in air- and saline-filled lungs fixed by vascular perfusion. *J. Appl. Physiol. (1985)* **1979**, *47*, 990–1001. [CrossRef] [PubMed]

36. Gaver, D.P.; Halpern, D.; Jensen, O.E.; Grotberg, J.B. The steady motion of a semi-infinite bubble through a flexible-walled channel. *J. Fluid Mech.* **1996**, *319*, 25–65. [CrossRef]
37. Kay, S.S.; Bilek, A.M.; Dee, K.C.; Gaver, D.P. Pressure gradient, not exposure duration, determines the extent of epithelial cell damage in a model of pulmonary airway reopening. *J. Appl. Physiol.* **2004**, *97*, 269–276. [CrossRef]
38. Nieman, G.F.; Gatto, L.A.; Habashi, N.M. Impact of mechanical ventilation on the pathophysiology of progressive acute lung injury. *J. Appl. Physiol. (1985)* **2015**, *119*, 1245–1261. [CrossRef]
39. Naire, S.; Jensen, O.E. Epithelial cell deformation during surfactant-mediated airway reopening: A theoretical model. *J. Appl. Physiol. (1985)* **2005**, *99*, 458–471. [CrossRef]
40. Matute-Bello, G.; Frevert, C.W.; Martin, T.R. Animal models of acute lung injury. *Am. J. Physiol. Lung Cell Mol. Physiol.* **2008**, *295*, L379–L399. [CrossRef]
41. Roan, E.; Waters, C.M. What do we know about mechanical strain in lung alveoli? *Am. J. Physiol. Lung Cell Mol. Physiol.* **2011**, *301*, L625–L635. [CrossRef] [PubMed]
42. Tschumperlin, D.J.; Margulies, S.S. Alveolar epithelial surface area-volume relationship in isolated rat lungs. *J. Appl. Physiol. (1985)* **1999**, *86*, 2026–2033. [CrossRef] [PubMed]
43. Bachofen, H.; Schürch, S. Alveolar surface forces and lung architecture. *Comp. Biochem. Physiol. A Mol. Integr. Physiol.* **2001**, *129*, 183–193. [CrossRef]
44. Smith, B.J.; Grant, K.A.; Bates, J.H. Linking the development of ventilator-induced injury to mechanical function in the lung. *Ann. Biomed. Eng.* **2013**, *41*, 527–536. [CrossRef] [PubMed]
45. Beike, L.; Wrede, C.; Hegermann, J.; Lopez-Rodriguez, E.; Kloth, C.; Gauldie, J.; Kolb, M.; Maus, U.A.; Ochs, M.; Knudsen, L. Surfactant dysfunction and alveolar collapse are linked with fibrotic septal wall remodeling in the TGF-β1-induced mouse model of pulmonary fibrosis. *Lab. Investig.* **2019**, *99*, 830–852. [CrossRef]
46. Smith, B.J.; Bartolak-Suki, E.; Suki, B.; Roy, G.S.; Hamlington, K.L.; Charlebois, C.M.; Bates, J.H.T. Linking Ventilator Injury-Induced Leak across the Blood-Gas Barrier to Derangements in Murine Lung Function. *Front. Physiol.* **2017**, *8*, 466. [CrossRef] [PubMed]
47. Allen, G.B.; Leclair, T.; Cloutier, M.; Thompson-Figueroa, J.; Bates, J.H. The response to recruitment worsens with progression of lung injury and fibrin accumulation in a mouse model of acid aspiration. *Am. J. Physiol. Lung Cell Mol. Physiol.* **2007**, *292*, L1580–L1589. [CrossRef]
48. Weibel, E. What makes a good lung? *Swiss Med. Wkly.* **2009**, *139*, 375–386.
49. Ghadiali, S.; Huang, Y. Role of airway recruitment and derecruitment in lung injury. *Crit. Rev. Biomed. Eng.* **2011**, *39*, 297–317. [CrossRef]
50. Jansing, N.L.; McClendon, J.; Henson, P.M.; Tuder, R.M.; Hyde, D.M.; Zemans, R.L. Unbiased Quantitation of Alveolar Type II to Alveolar Type I Cell Transdifferentiation during Repair after Lung Injury in Mice. *Am. J. Respir. Cell Mol. Biol.* **2017**, *57*, 519–526. [CrossRef]
51. Hamlington, K.L.; Smith, B.J.; Dunn, C.M.; Charlebois, C.M.; Roy, G.S.; Bates, J.H.T. Linking lung function to structural damage of alveolar epithelium in ventilator-induced lung injury. *Respir. Physiol. Neurobiol.* **2018**, *255*, 22–29. [CrossRef] [PubMed]
52. Fredberg, J.J.; Kamm, R.D. Stress transmission in the lung: Pathways from organ to molecule. *Annu. Rev. Physiol.* **2006**, *68*, 507–541. [CrossRef] [PubMed]
53. Perlman, C.E.; Lederer, D.J.; Bhattacharya, J. Micromechanics of alveolar edema. *Am. J. Respir. Cell Mol. Biol.* **2011**, *44*, 34–39. [CrossRef] [PubMed]
54. Schirrmann, K.; Mertens, M.; Kertzscher, U.; Kuebler, W.M.; Affeld, K. Theoretical modeling of the interaction between alveoli during inflation and deflation in normal and diseased lungs. *J. Biomech.* **2010**, *43*, 1202–1207. [CrossRef] [PubMed]
55. Loring, S.H.; Topulos, G.P.; Hubmayr, R.D. Transpulmonary Pressure: The Importance of Precise Definitions and Limiting Assumptions. *Am. J. Respir. Crit. Care Med.* **2016**, *194*, 1452–1457. [CrossRef]
56. Albert, R.K.; Smith, B.; Perlman, C.E.; Schwartz, D.A. Is Progression of Pulmonary Fibrosis due to Ventilation-induced Lung Injury? *Am. J. Respir. Crit. Care Med.* **2019**, *200*, 140–151. [CrossRef]
57. Hamlington, K.L.; Bates, J.H.T.; Roy, G.S.; Julianelle, A.J.; Charlebois, C.; Suki, B.; Smith, B.J. Alveolar leak develops by a rich-get-richer process in ventilator-induced lung injury. *PLoS ONE* **2018**, *13*, e0193934. [CrossRef]
58. Scherle, W. A simple method for volumetry of organs in quantitative stereology. *Mikroskopie* **1970**, *26*, 57–60.

59. Tschanz, S.; Schneider, J.P.; Knudsen, L. Design-based stereology: Planning, volumetry and sampling are crucial steps for a successful study. *Ann. Anat.* **2014**, *196*, 3–11. [CrossRef]
60. Ochs, M.; Mühlfeld, C. Quantitative microscopy of the lung: A problem-based approach. Part 1: Basic principles of lung stereology. *Am. J. Physiol. Lung Cell Mol. Physiol.* **2013**, *305*, L15–L22. [CrossRef]
61. Muhlfeld, C.; Knudsen, L.; Ochs, M. Stereology and morphometry of lung tissue. *Methods in Mol. Biol. (Clifton, N.J.)* **2013**, *931*, 367–390. [CrossRef]
62. Hsia, C.; Hyde, D.; Ochs, M.; Weibel, E. An official research policy statement of the American Thoracic Society/European Respiratory Society: Standards for quantitative assessment of lung structure. *Am. J. Respir. Crit. Care Med.* **2010**, *181*, 394–418. [CrossRef] [PubMed]
63. Weibel, E.; Hsia, C.; Ochs, M. How much is there really? Why stereology is essential in lung morphometry. *J. Appl. Physiol.* **2007**, *102*, 459–467. [CrossRef]
64. Gundersen, H.; Jensen, E. The efficiency of systematic sampling in stereology and its prediction. *J. Microsc.* **1987**, *147*, 229–263. [CrossRef] [PubMed]
65. Ochs, M. A brief update on lung stereology. *J. Microsc.* **2006**, *222*, 188–200. [CrossRef] [PubMed]
66. Braendgaard, H.; Gundersen, H.J. The impact of recent stereological advances on quantitative studies of the nervous system. *J. Neurosci. Methods* **1986**, *18*, 39–78. [CrossRef]
67. Ochs, M.; Nyengaard, L.R.; Lung, A.; Knudsen, L.; Voigt, M.; Wahlers, T.; Richter, J.; Gundersen, H.J.G. The number of alveoli in the human lung. *Am. J. Respir. Crit. Care Med.* **2004**, *169*, 120–124. [CrossRef]
68. Gundersen, H.; Bagger, P.; Bendtsen, T.; Evans, S.; Korbo, L.; Marcussen, N.; Møller, A.; Nielsen, K.; Nyengaard, J.; Pakkenberg, B. The new stereological tools: Disector, fractionator, nucleator and point sampled intercepts and their use in pathological research and diagnosis. *APMIS* **1988**, *96*, 857–881. [CrossRef]
69. Hyde, D.; Tyler, N.; Putney, L.; Singh, P.; Gundersen, H. Total number and mean size of alveoli in mammalian lung estimated using fractionator sampling and unbiased estimates of the Euler characteristic of alveolar openings. *Anat. Rec. A Discov. Mol. Cell Evol. Biol.* **2004**, *277*, 216–226. [CrossRef]
70. Tschanz, S.A.; Burri, P.H.; Weibel, E.R. A simple tool for stereological assessment of digital images: The STEPanizer. *J. Microsc.* **2011**, *243*, 47–59. [CrossRef]
71. Fehrenbach, H.; Schepelmann, D.; Albes, J.; Bando, T.; Fischer, F.; Fehrenbach, A.; Stolte, N.; Wahlers, T.; Richter, J. Pulmonary ischemia/reperfusion injury: A quantitative study of structure and function in isolated heart-lungs of the rat. *Anat. Rec.* **1999**, *255*, 84–89. [CrossRef]
72. Steffen, L.; Ruppert, C.; Hoymann, H.G.; Funke, M.; Ebener, S.; Kloth, C.; Mühlfeld, C.; Ochs, M.; Knudsen, L.; Lopez-Rodriguez, E. Surfactant replacement therapy reduces acute lung injury and collapse induration-related lung remodeling in the bleomycin model. *Am. J. Physiol. Lung Cell Mol. Physiol.* **2017**, *313*, L313–L327. [CrossRef] [PubMed]

6

The Three-Dimensional Ultrastructure of the Human Alveolar Epithelium Revealed by Focused Ion Beam Electron Microscopy

Jan Philipp Schneider [1,2,*], Christoph Wrede [1,2,3] and Christian Mühlfeld [1,2,3]

1 Institute of Functional and Applied Anatomy, Hannover Medical School, Carl-Neuberg-Straße 1, 30625 Hannover, Germany; wrede.christoph@mh-hannover.de (C.W.); muehlfeld.christian@mh-hannover.de (C.M.)

2 Biomedical Research in Endstage and Obstructive Lung Disease Hannover (BREATH), Member of the German Center for Lung Research (DZL), Hannover Medical School, Carl-Neuberg-Straße 1, 30625 Hannover, Germany

3 Research Core Unit Electron Microscopy, Hannover Medical School, Carl-Neuberg-Straße 1, 30625 Hannover, Germany

* Correspondence: schneider.jan@mh-hannover.de

Abstract: Thin type 1 alveolar epithelial (AE1) and surfactant producing type 2 alveolar epithelial (AE2) cells line the alveoli in the lung and are essential for normal lung function. Function is intimately interrelated to structure, so that detailed knowledge of the epithelial ultrastructure can significantly enhance our understanding of its function. The basolateral surface of the cells or the epithelial contact sites are of special interest, because they play an important role in intercellular communication or stabilizing the epithelium. The latter is in particular important for the lung with its variable volume. The aim of the present study was to investigate the three-dimensional (3D) ultrastructure of the *human* alveolar epithelium focusing on contact sites and the basolateral cell membrane of AE2 cells using focused ion beam electron microscopy and subsequent 3D reconstructions. The study provides detailed surface reconstructions of two AE1 cell domains and two AE2 cells, showing AE1/AE1, AE1/AE2 and AE2/AE2 contact sites, basolateral microvilli pits at AE2 cells and small AE1 processes beneath AE2 cells. Furthermore, we show reconstructions of a surfactant secretion pore, enlargements of the apical AE1 cell surface and long folds bordering grooves on the basal AE1 cell surface. The functional implications of our findings are discussed. These findings may lay the structural basis for further molecular investigations.

Keywords: lung; alveolus; type 1 alveolar epithelial cell; type 2 alveolar epithelial cell; focused ion beam scanning electron microscopy; 3D reconstruction

1. Introduction

Type 1 alveolar epithelial (AE1) and type 2 alveolar epithelial (AE2) cells form the epithelial lining of alveoli in the *human* lung. Both are essential for normal lung function: AE1 cells cover the majority of the alveolar surface with thin cytoplasmic extensions that participate in a very thin blood gas barrier and AE2 cells serve as the regeneration source for the alveolar epithelium and secrete the pulmonary surfactant, which lowers the surface tension at the air liquid interface and, thus, prevents alveolar collapse [1], see also [2]. In the past, it was suggested that these cells may show complex morphological properties, such as having more than one apical surface for serving different alveoli or branching of AE1 cells [3,4]. Sirianni et al. [5] described basolateral microvilli on AE2 cells for contacting interstitial fibroblasts and AE1 cells that extend both above and underneath AE2 cells. In a recent study, three entire AE1 cells were modeled in three dimensions (3D) by manual segmentation of a serial block-face

(SBF) scanning electron microscopic data set of a *human* lung sample. Both the branching capability and the chance of having more than one apical surface could be confirmed for AE1 cells by this method. Additionally, the 3D data set revealed that different branches of the same cell can form cellular junctions between each other [6]. During this study the questions arose how the sites of contacts both between AE1 and AE1 and between AE1 and AE2 cells as well as the lateral borders of AE2 cells are configured in 3D. The SBF data suggested a complex morphology of AE1/AE2 cell contacts, variable overlap of adjacent AE1 cells and the existence of numerous microvilli that may appear clustered in small niches of the basolateral AE2 cell surface, findings in line with those of Sirianni et al. [5] and Mercurio and Rhodin [7,8]. A special 3D organization of the contact sites may be of relevance for the mechanical stability (or behavior) and integrity of the alveolar epithelium during breathing or the migration of cells from the interstitial space into the alveolus. Knowledge about the detailed 3D organization of the basolateral cell membrane of AE2 cells may help to understand the crosstalk between AE2 and other cells of the septal wall.

While the SBF scanning electron microscope (SEM) used by Schneider et al. [6] has the advantage that it can image rather large fields of view (FOV) and, thus, volumes with entire AE1 cells, it has to live with a compromise in lateral and axial resolution. A high resolution combined with a large FOV tremendously increases the scanning duration (see [9]) and/or may lead to beam damage at the specimen because of exposure to the electron beam. The latter is in particular significant for lung samples because of the small amount of conducting tissue in the epoxy resin block since the lung primarily "consists of air". Using lower section thicknesses fortifies this problem, cf. [10], so the minimal section thickness as the major determinant of the z-resolution is also a limiting factor of SBF SEM. Thus, for 3D evaluation of structural details, such as cellular junctions or microvilli, focused ion beam (FIB) SEM with both a higher x-/y- and in particular higher z-resolution, appeared to be more appropriate (consider the dimensions of microvilli and the section thicknesses in the aforementioned studies: 80 nm in Schneider et al. [6], 100 nm in Sirianni et al. [5] and unknown in Mercurio and Rhodin [7,8], for review of SBF SEM and FIB SEM, see [10–12]). As a consequence, after having reconstructed entire AE1 cells by SBF SEM, we conducted the current study to explore the complexity of the AE1 cell contact sites and the structure of the basolateral AE2 cell membrane using FIB SEM. It was expected that the new insights into AE1 and AE2 cell ultrastructure would enhance our functional understanding of the alveolar epithelium.

2. Results

2.1. Generation of the Data Set for 3D Reconstructions

After export, the data set comprised 2297 images with a size of $6663 \times 4635\,px^2$ and a pixel size of 5 nm. Based on the number of images and the penetration depth into the z-direction, an average section thickness of 9.94 nm could be calculated, which is less than 1 % deviation from the desired thickness of 10 nm. Since the milling process and, thus, the section thickness, is an undulation around an average and because the system needs a stabilization period after initiation of the image acquisition, the first 139 images were not accounted for in the calculation. This cut off was determined by qualitative inspection of the z-advance at the beginning of the data set.

2.2. Segmentation and 3D Reconstructions

Two AE1 cell domains and parts of two AE2 cells in immediate topographic relationship were segmented and reconstructed in 3D for the current work. The part of the dataset underlying the segmentations comprises the images 378 to 1624 of the dataset. A global overview of the models is given in Figure 1 and Table 1 indicates how many outlines per AE1 cell domain and AE2 cell were manually segmented (12,623 in total). It should be noted at this point, that AE1 cells are obviously capable of making cellular junctions with themselves [6], so it cannot be excluded that the two "AE1 models" are parts of one and the same cell. To account for this, we stick to the term AE1 cell domain(s) instead of AE1 cell(s), when we refer to the particular models. Apart from a few, very small portions, the pink AE2 cell is completely included in the dataset and, thus, the model also comprises almost the entire AE2 cell. The small "defects" because of missing portions can be seen in Figure 3.

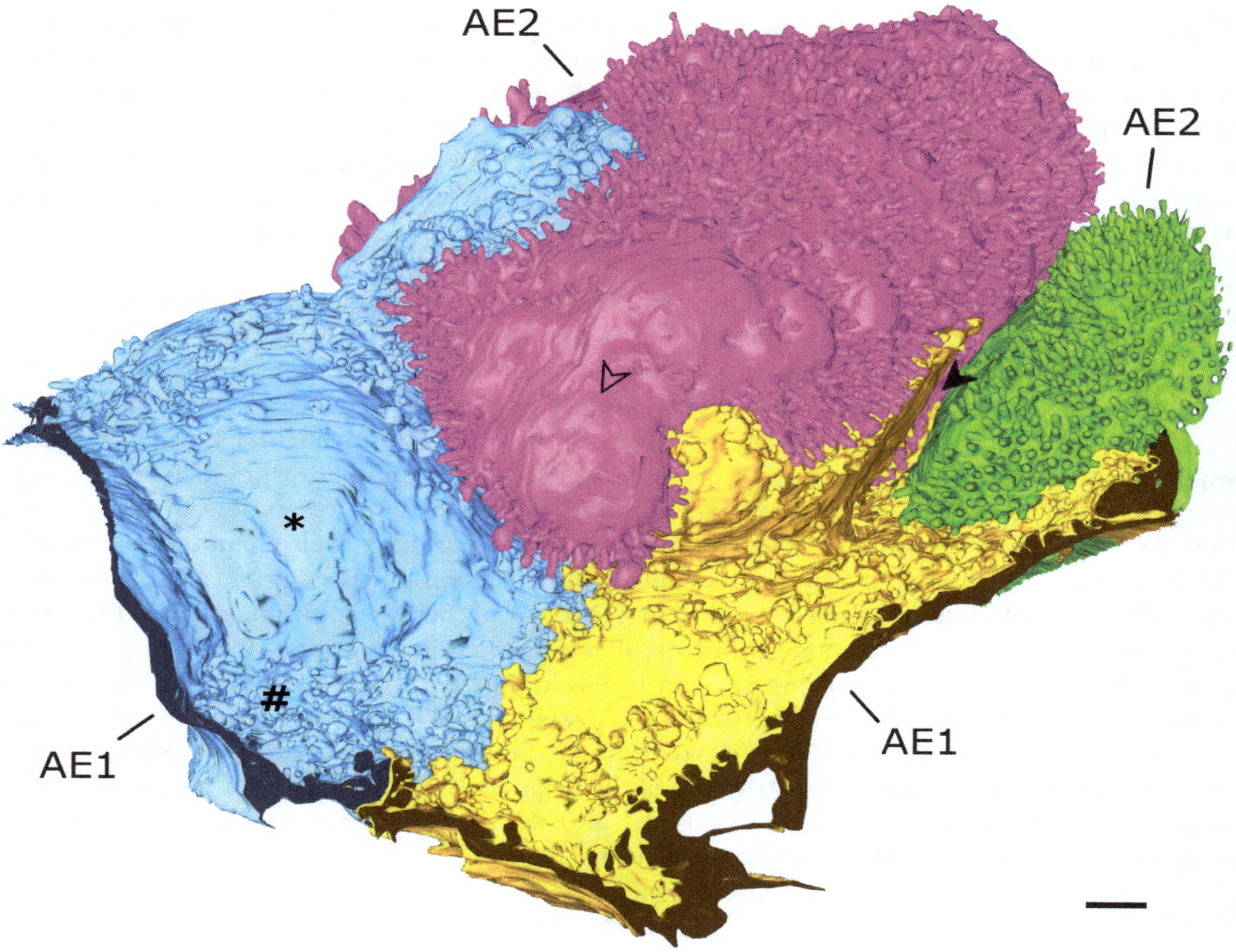

Figure 1. Overview of the 3D model. The figure shows an overview of the 3D model from an alveolar viewing direction. The model includes an almost complete type 2 alveolar epithelial (AE2) cell (pink) and parts of another AE2 cell (green) as well as two type 1 alveolar epithelial (AE1) cell domains (blue and yellow), which are labeled as AE2 and AE1, respectively. The filled arrowhead indicates a deep recess between the pink and green AE2 cells as well as the yellow AE1 cell. The AE2 cells show abundant microvilli on their surfaces but also plain parts (empty arrowhead on the pink AE2 cell, for example). The luminal AE1 cell surface may also be plain at a certain spot (asterisk) or enlarged somewhere else (hash key). Scale bar: 1 μm.

Table 1. Number of outlines manually segmented for modeling.

Structure	Number of Outlines
AE1 cell domain 1 (yellow)	2439
AE1 cell domain 2 (blue)	2683
AE2 cell 1 (pink)	5772
AE2 cell 2 (green)	1729
Total amount of outlines	12,623

2.3. Epithelial Surface

The apical AE2 cell surface exhibits smooth areas surrounded by microvilli as described previously [1]. The pink cell has two larger plain areas and one of them shows an open surfactant secretion pore (Figure 2). (At this stage of exocytosis) the pore has a smaller diameter than the vesicle under secretion, cf. [1]. The green AE2 cell shows a larger plain surface area in the recess between the adjacent AE2 cells (Figure 1). Also the basolateral AE2 cell surface shows abundant microvilli. In contrast to the luminal microvilli, they may appear clustered in small groups, located in small niches of the cell surface. These microvilli are found both between adjacent epithelial cells (AE2 and AE2 or AE2 and AE1), but also at gaps in the basal lamina, where they may reach interstitial cells (Figure 3). They are even found above a continuous basal lamina (not shown).

The AE1 cell domains also exhibit a combination of smooth surface areas with surface enlargements (Figures 1 and 4). In contrast to the AE2 cells, this enlargement is realized primarily by protrusions of the plasma membrane filled with cytoplasm. However, some microvilli are found here as well, which can be identified by their regular structure and inner architecture of the cytoskeleton. Some microvilli may share a common basis and some seem to rest on surface protrusions. Both AE1 cell domains show grooves bordered by cellular folds on their basal surface. These grooves stretch across the cells in a relatively orientated fashion along space. Beneath the groove of the yellow AE1 cell domain primarily extracellular matrix is found while it is primarily capillary endothelium beneath the blue cell domain (Figure 5). Additionally, the AE1 cells show abundant caveolae and it is the basal compartment that seems to house most of them (Figure 5B).

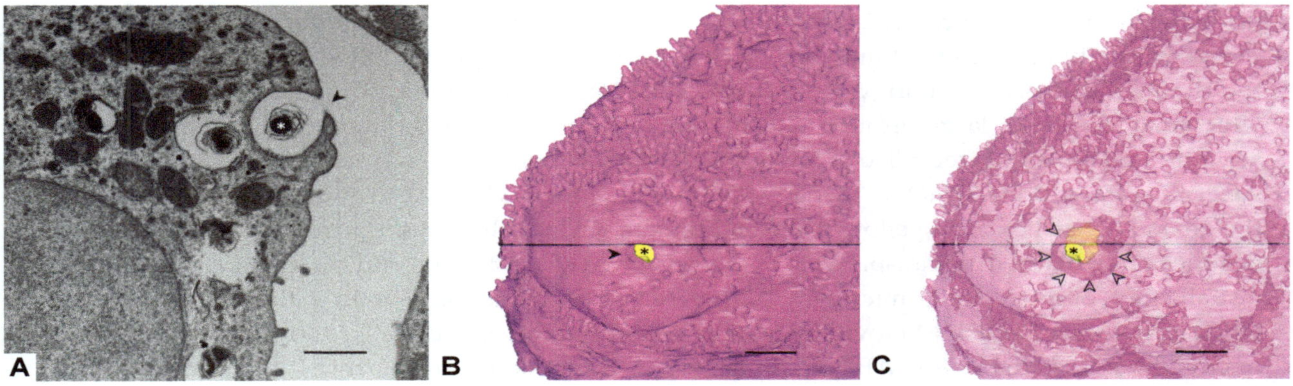

Figure 2. Luminal AE2 cell surface and surfactant secretion pore. (**A**) Detail from image 884 which shows an open surfactant secretion pore (arrowhead) and remnants of a lamellar body inside (asterisk). In this image the opening is much smaller than the profile diameter of the vesicle under secretion. (**B**) 3D model of the AE2 cell with the secretion pore (arrowhead) and the remnants of the lamellar body inside (yellow, asterisk). Note the plain cell surface in this area. (**C**) Same image content as in B but with a transparent cell body, which reveals the entire remnant of the lamellar body and indicates the size of the secretory vesicle (circumference marked by arrowheads), the projection of which is much larger than the secretion pore. Scale bars: 1 μm. The black lines in B and C indicate the position of the section plane of A.

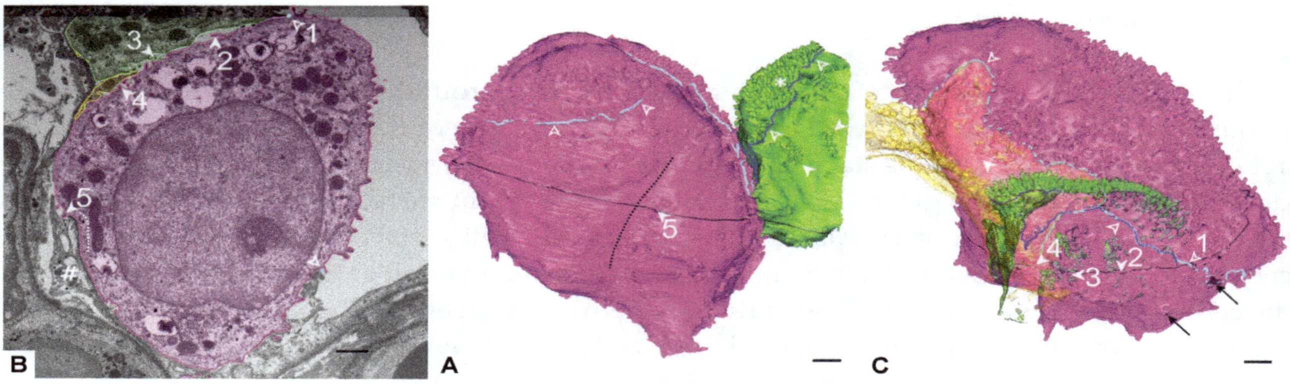

Figure 3. Basolateral surface of AE2 cells. (**A**) Segmented electron micrograph (image 988 of the data set). The micrograph shows the segmentations of the pink and green AE2 cell as well as of the yellow AE1 cell domain with opaque outlines and transparent filling. Microvilli can be found at different sites of the AE2 cell, three of them are indicated on the micrograph: towards the adjacent green AE2 cell, which also shows microvilli at this site (filled arrowheads 2 and 3), towards the yellow AE1 cell domain (filled arrowhead 4), towards an interstitial cell (hash key) through a hole in the basal lamina (filled arrowhead 5). Turquoise circles indicate the lateral luminal cell border of the pink AE2 cell (empty arrowheads). The position at empty arrowhead 1 is found in the 3D model in C. The dotted line indicates the profile of the groove depicted in B. (**B**) 3D Model of the pink and green AE2 cells. The position of the segmented electron microscopic (EM) plane in A is indicated in black and the lateral luminal cell borders of the pink and green AE2 cells are indicated by turquoise and blue delineations, respectively (empty arrowheads; note that the positions do not correspond to the empty arrowheads in A). The pink AE2 cell has only one luminal surface. Note the abrupt appearance of a dense microvilli lawn on the luminal surface in some areas (asterisk). Filled arrowhead 5 indicates the region of the corresponding arrowhead 5 in A. Note also the surrounding basolateral microvilli, which may appear in larger groups. Two sites of basolateral groups of microvilli on the green cell are indicated (unnumbered filled arrowheads). Note the long and mostly smooth groove of the pink AE2 cell surface (dotted line). (**C**) Opaque 3D model of the pink AE2 cell and transparent models of the green AE2 cell and the yellow AE1 cell domain. The position of the segmented EM plane in A is indicated in black. The transparency of the yellow AE1 cell domain and the green AE2 cell enable visualization of intercellular microvilli. Numbered arrowheads correspond to the arrowheads in A: Filled arrowhead 2 and 3: Microvilli between the pink and green AE2 cells. Filled arrowhead 4: AE2 microvilli towards the yellow AE1 cell domain. The unnumbered filled arrowhead indicates another region with AE2 microvilli under the yellow AE1 cell domain. The lateral luminal AE2 cell borders are indicated by turquoise and blue delineations (cf. B). Empty arrowhead 1 refers to the corresponding empty arrowhead in A. Black arrows indicate the small parts of the cell where the cell extends beyond the available dataset. Scale bars: 1 μm.

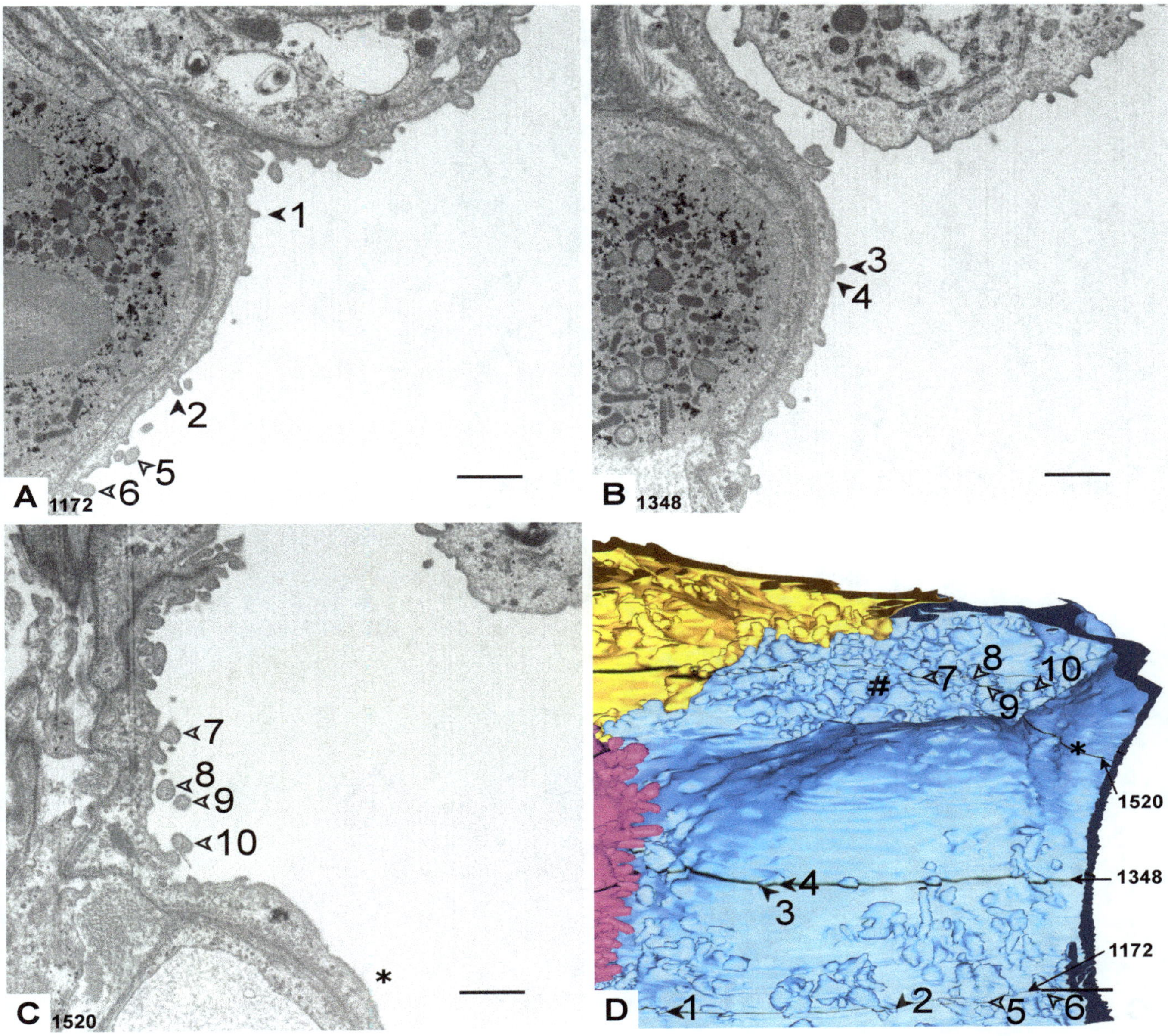

Figure 4. Luminal surface of AE1 cells. (**A–C**) Images 1172, 1348 and 1520 of the dataset. Filled arrowheads 1 and 2 (**A**) indicate profiles of microvilli. Filled arrowheads 3 and 4 (**B**) indicate microvilli with a shared basis. Empty arrowheads 5 and 6 (**A**) and 7–10 (**C**) indicate profiles of plasma membrane protrusions filled with cytoplasm. The hash key indicates a region with smooth AE1 luminal surface. (**D**) Detail of the 3D model. Arrowheads and hash key refer to the particular profiles in A–C. The particular section planes 1172, 1348 and 1520 are labeled and emphasized by black color in the model. The different thickness of these black markings is caused by different segmentation intervals in these regions. Note the smooth surface of the cell in the center of the image and the surface enlargements around. Some of them seem to be concentrated in a surface cavity (asterisk). Scale bars: 1 μm.

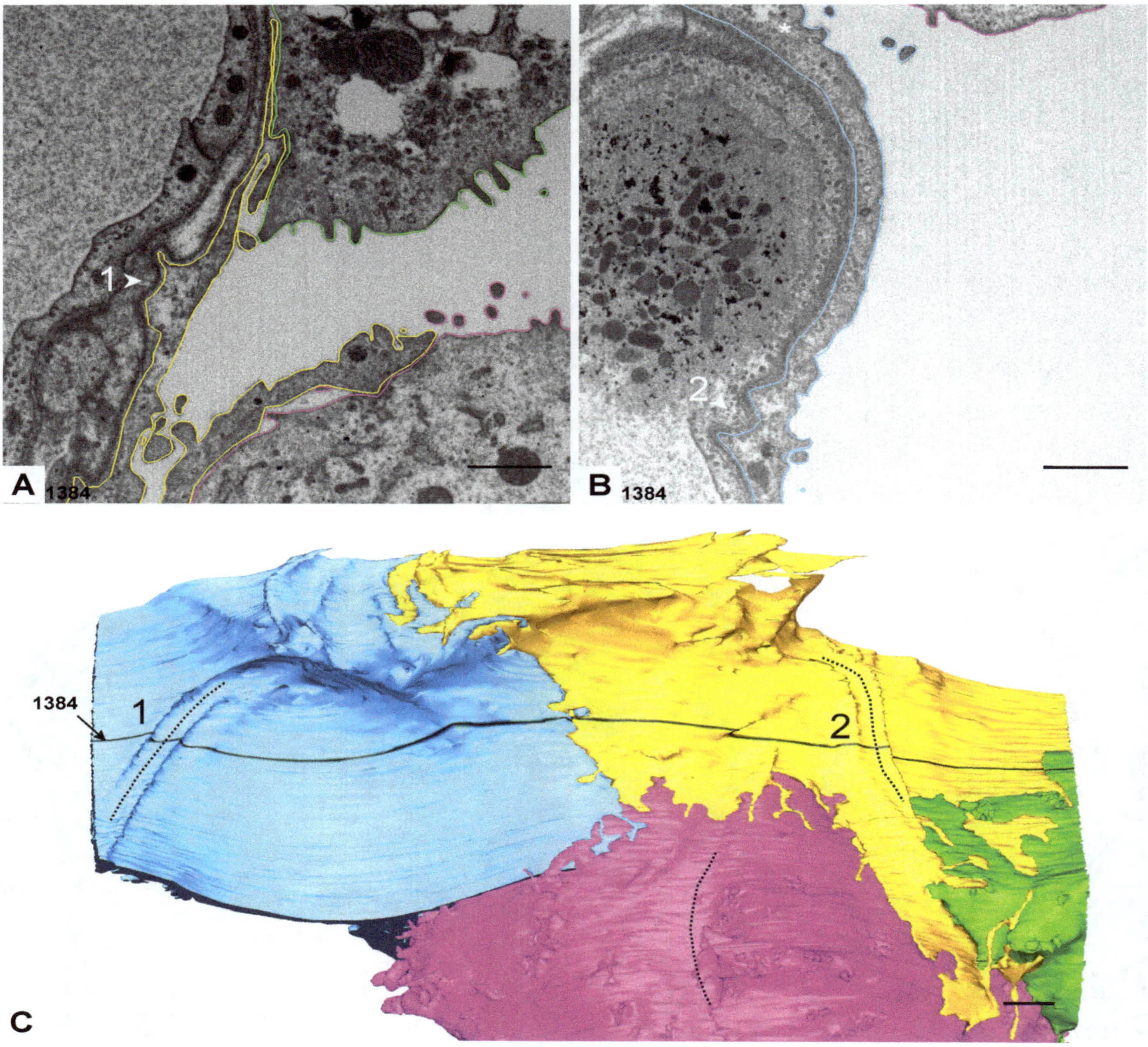

Figure 5. Basolateral surface of AE1 cells. (**A**) Detail of the segmented EM plane 1384 including parts of the yellow AE1 cell domain. At the basal side, small folds may appear which create a groove-like profile with the concavity pointing towards the interstitial space. The groove beyond the epithelium is filled with extracellular matrix (arrowhead 1). (**B**) A similar situation is found at the basal side of the blue AE1 cell domain, but here the groove is filled with capillary endothelium (arrowhead 2). Note the densely packed caveolae, which appear to be predominantly located in the basal compartment of the cell (asterisk). (**C**) View on the basal side of the 3D model. The model reveals that indeed the AE1 cell domains form grooves on their basal side, which are bordered by cellular folds. The groove in the AE2 cell surface, which has been already described in Figure 3, is also indicated by a dotted line. The EM plane 1384 is indicated by black color. Scale bars: 1 µm.

2.4. *Sites of Cell Contacts*

The AE1 cell domains contact each other with or without overlap. At a certain point, they may simply prod against each other (edge to edge), while a few micrometers further one cell domain slips under the other. Directly at the site of contact they may bulge out into the alveolus (Figures 6–8). On the basolateral side, cellular processes may interdigitate with the neighbor cell domain, while the luminal edges appear more regular (Figure 9).

At the contact site to AE2 cells, AE1 cells may simultaneously both crawl up and beneath AE2 cells. This is achieved by a y-shaped branching pattern with one branch crawling up and the other branch crawling beneath the AE2 cell. In 3D, this behavior reminds of a bowl partially enwrapping the AE2 cell (Figure 10). Additionally, the AE1 cells may send out thin, finger-like processes into the space between the AE2 cells and the underlying basal lamina. Such processes can be found in close proximity to AE2 microvilli (Figure 11).

The two AE2 cells contact each other edge to edge, with niches of microvilli facing each other (Figure 12).

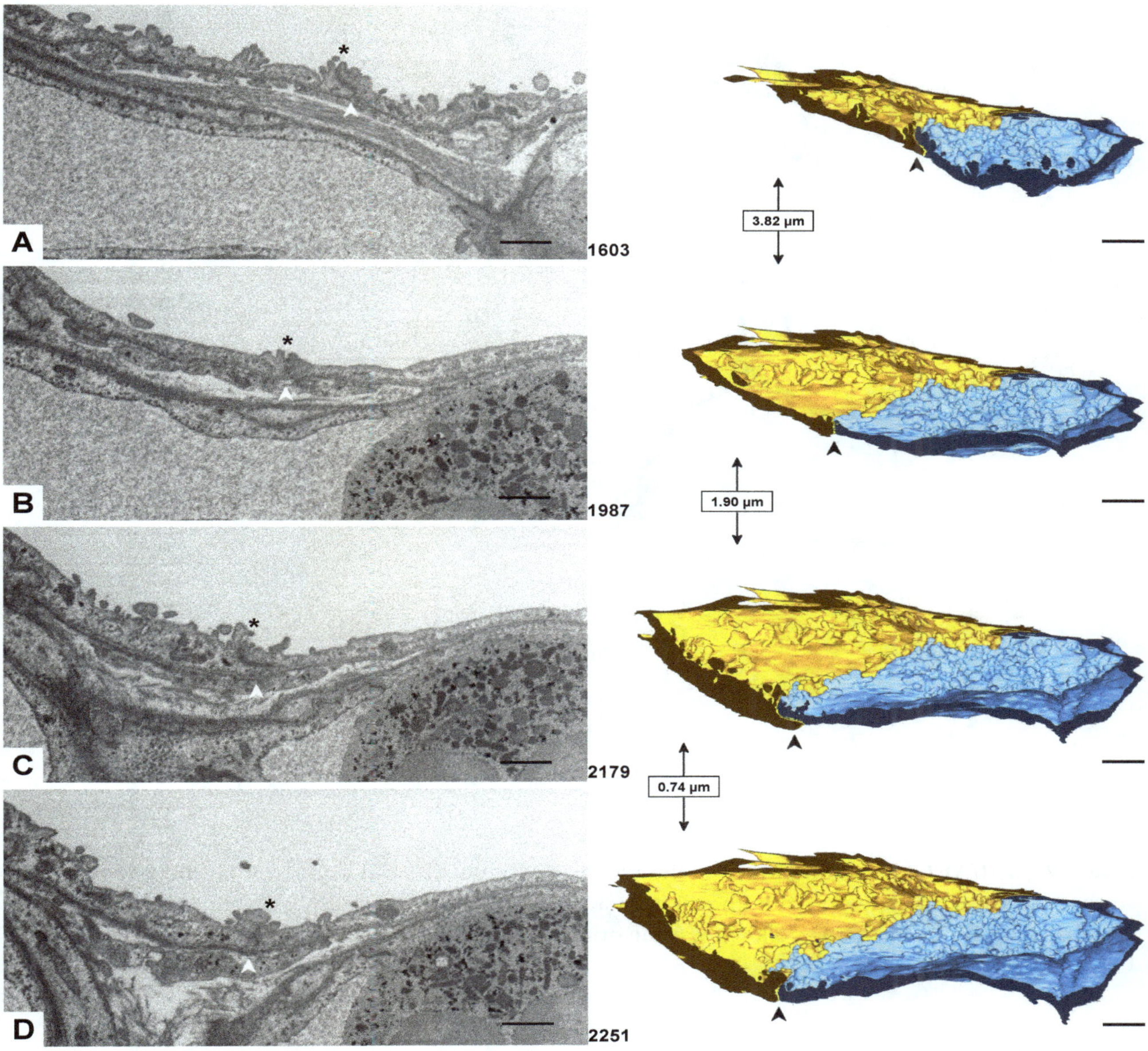

Figure 6. AE1/AE1 contact. (**A–D**) show the x-plane reconstructions 1603, 1987, 2179 and 2251 of the data set (lateral view on the dataset) on the left side of the panel and a clipped model of the yellow and blue AE1 cell domains on the right side of the panel. The transect plane in the foreground corresponds to the EM plane on the left side. The site of cell contact is indicated by arrowheads. The distance between the different transect planes is indicated in micrometers between the models. Note how the yellow AE1 cell domain slips under the blue cell domain in A and C while the cell domains in B and D meet each other just edge to edge. Note also the bulging of the cell domains into the alveolar lumen at the contact site (asterisks on the EM images). Scale bars: 1 µm.

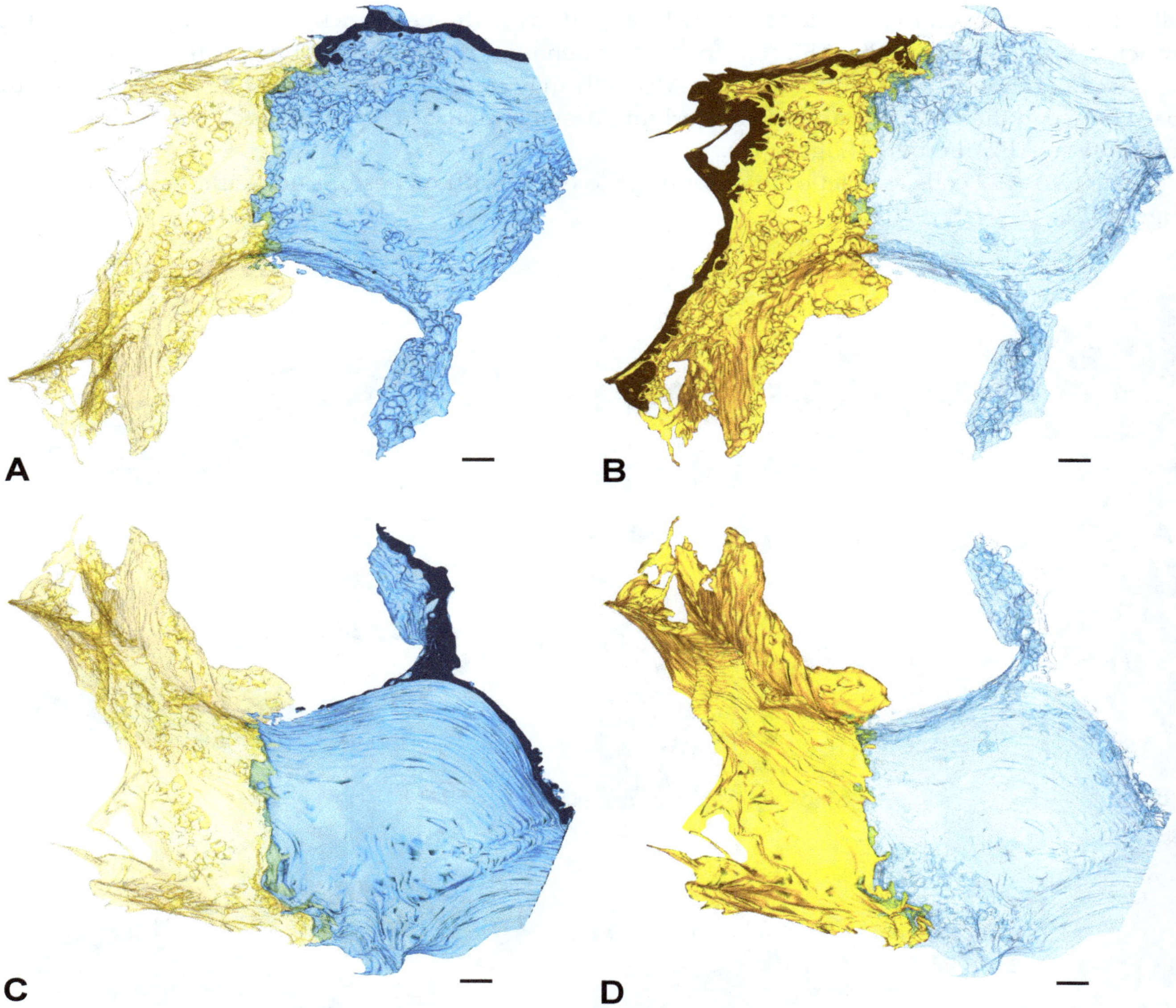

Figure 7. AE1/AE1 contact. (**A**,**B**) show the yellow and blue AE1 cell domain with their alveolar surfaces. On each image one of both cell domains is shown transparently (A: yellow, B: blue) to visualize overlap. Images (**C**,**D**) follow the same principle but show the basolateral surfaces. Scale bars: 1 μm.

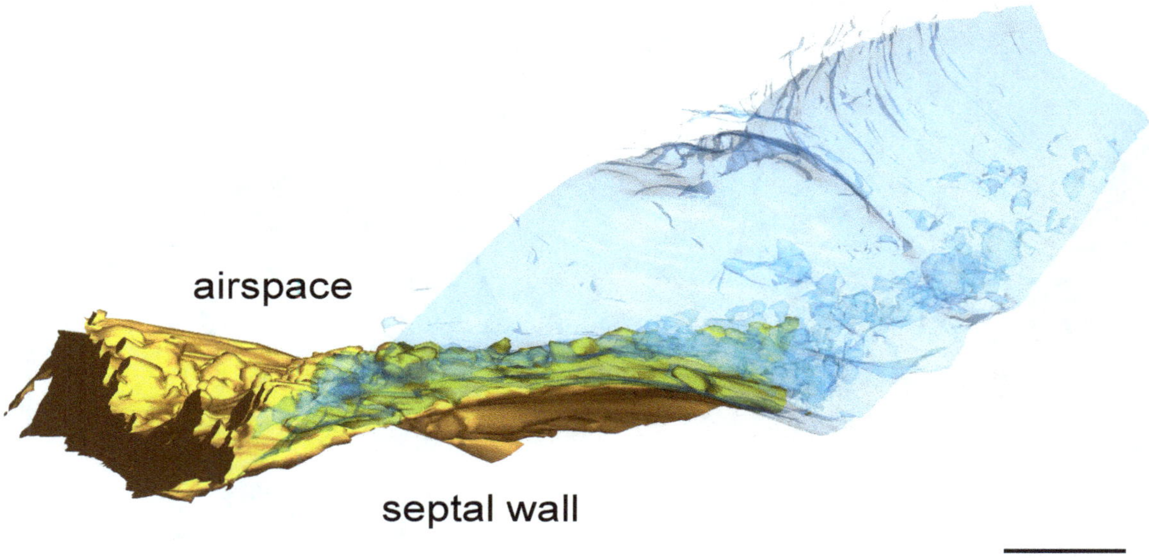

Figure 8. AE1/AE1 contact. The image shows the contact of parts of the yellow and blue AE1 cell domains. The blue cell domain in the foreground is displayed transparently to enable visualization of the yellow AE1 cell domain. Note how the yellow AE1 cell domain slips beneath the blue cell domain. Scale bar: 1 μm.

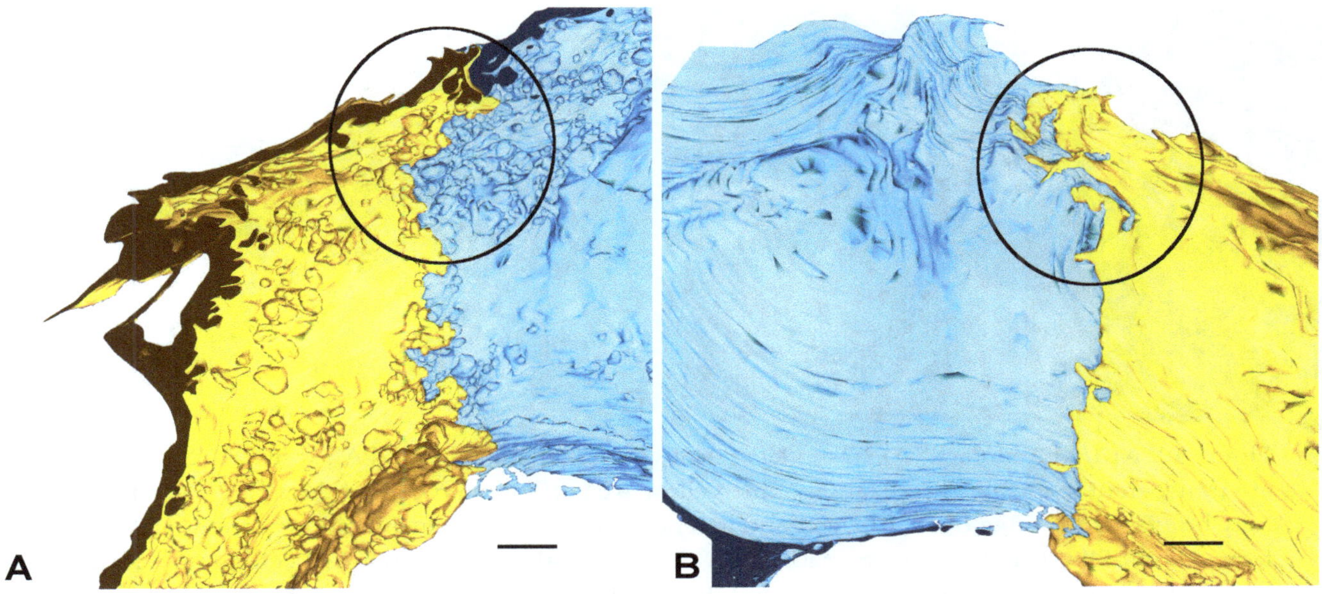

Figure 9. AE1/AE1 contact. (**A**,**B**) again show the yellow and blue AE1 cell domain from a luminal (**A**) and a basolateral (**B**) perspective but without transparency. Note the irregular contact site on the abluminal side compared to the luminal side caused by interdigitating cell processes. Compare in particular the region emphasized by the ellipse. Scale bars: 1 μm.

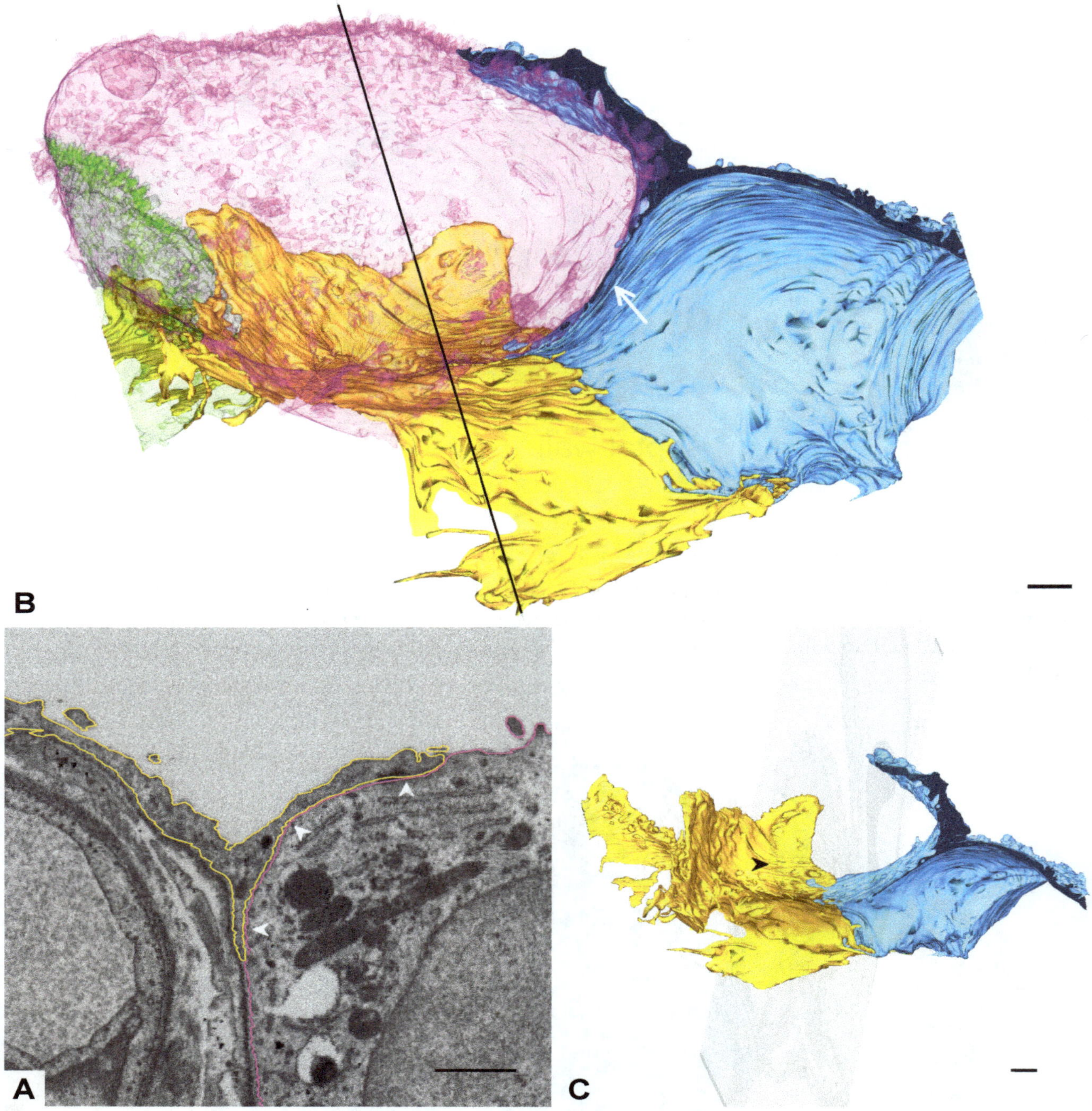

Figure 10. AE1/AE2 contact. (**A**) 3D model of the two AE1 cell domains and AE2 cells. AE2 cell models are transparent to enable visualization of the yellow AE1 cell domain behind the AE2 cells. AE1 cells may branch at the edge of an AE2 cell and extend their branches beneath and over the AE2 cell to form a bowl-like structure that enwraps the AE2 cell partially. The yellow AE1 cell domain forms a bowl at the edge of the pink AE2 cell (behind the transparent AE2 cell model). Note also the y-shaped branching of the blue AE1 cell domain and its extension beneath the pink AE2 cell (arrow). The black line indicates the position of the transect image in B. (**B**) Reconstruction of the y-plane (lateral view on the dataset) at the position indicated by the black line in A. The profiles of the yellow AE1 cell domain and the pink AE2 cell are indicated by yellow and pink outlines. Note the y-shaped profile of the yellow AE1 cell domain. The surface of the yellow AE1 cell domain ("inner surface" of the bowl) looked at in A and C is indicated by arrowheads. (**C**) 3D model of the yellow and blue AE1 cell domain transected by the y-plane shown in B. The different angle of view compared to A facilitates the imagination of a bowl formed by the yellow AE1 cell domain. The arrowhead indicates where the image plane transects the bowl of the yellow AE1 cell domain. Scale bars: 1 μm.

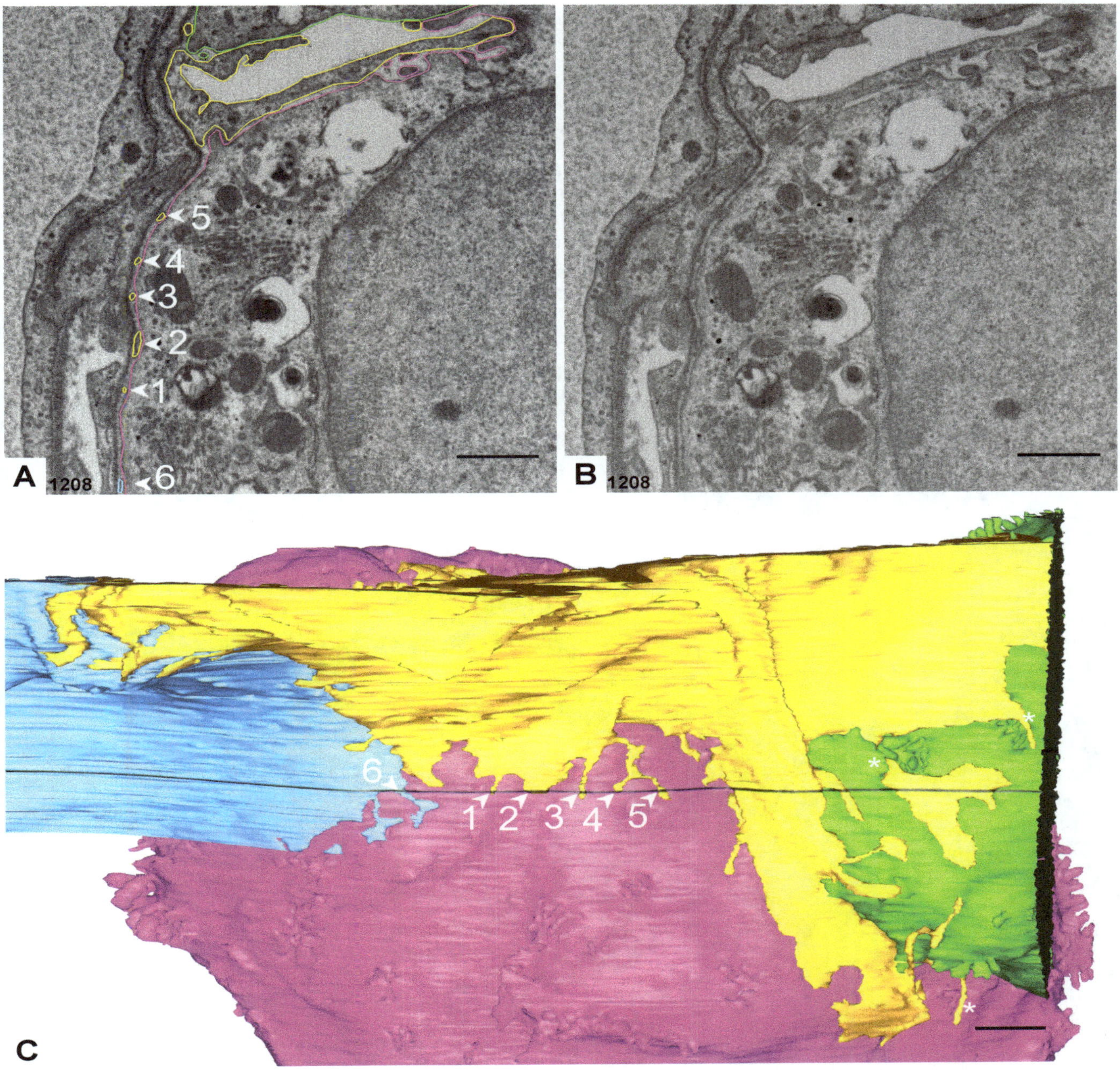

Figure 11. AE1/AE2 contact. (**A**) Detail of segmented image 1208. The image shows the segmentation of the pink and green AE2 cells as well as of the yellow and blue AE1 cell domain. Note the very small profiles of the yellow AE1 cell domain (arrowheads 1–5) and the small profile of the blue AE1 cell domain (arrowhead 6). These will probably be overseen if only single images are investigated. If they are recognized, it will almost be impossible to assign them to different cells (compare B). Only the sequence of images reveals their belonging. (**B**) The same EM image as in A but without segmentations. (**C**) 3D Modell of the yellow and blue AE1 cell domain as well as the pink and green AE2 cell with a view on the basolateral cell surfaces. The 3D model reveals that the labeled profiles in A belong to small and thin AE1 processes that crawl along the surface of the pink AE2 cell. The numbered arrowheads correspond to the arrowheads in A. Note also the processes of the yellow cell domain along the green AE2 cell. Some of the processes are found in close proximity to AE2 cell microvilli (asterisks). Scale bars: 1 μm.

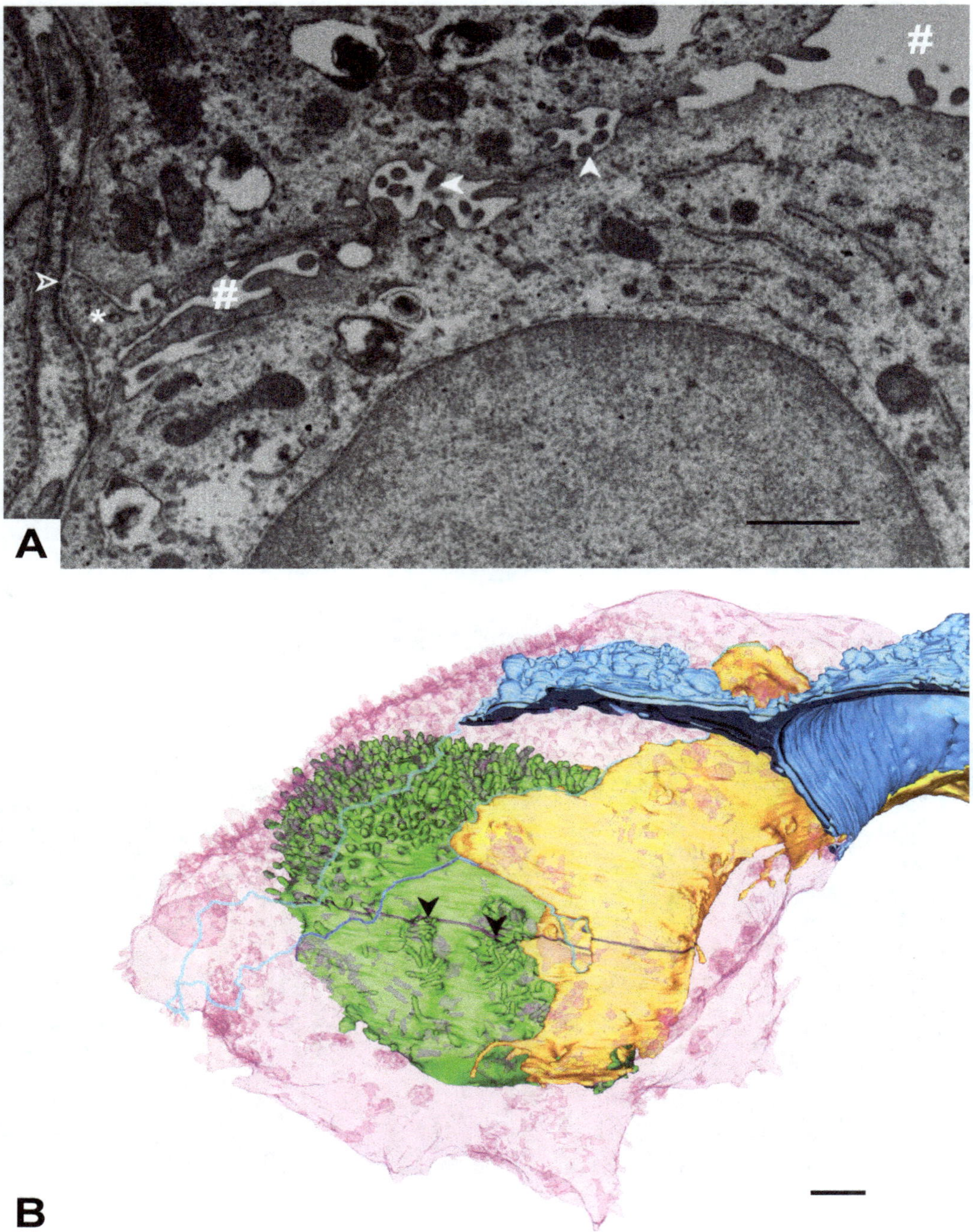

Figure 12. AE2/AE2 contact. (**A**) EM image 1112. The image shows the green (top) and pink (bottom) AE2 cell contacting each other. Both cells show niches with microvilli on their basolateral surface facing each other (filled arrowheads). Between both cells also parts of the yellow AE1 cell domain are found (asterisk). The alveolar lumen is indicated by the hash key and the basal lamina by an empty arrowhead. (**B**) 3D model of the pink and green AE2 cell as well as the yellow and blue AE1 cell domains. The image plane of A is indicated in black. Arrowheads correspond to the arrowheads in A. The borders of the luminal/abluminal surface of the AE2 cells are indicated by turquoise (pink cell) and blue lines (green cell) (cf. Figure 3). The pink AE2 cell and its luminal/abluminal border are displayed transparently to visualize the green AE2 cell and yellow AE1 cell domain behind as well as the luminal/abluminal border of the green AE2 cell. Note the well defined niches with microvilli on the basolateral surface of the green AE2 cell (black arrowheads). Scale bars: 1 μm.

3. Discussion

Volume electron microscopic (EM) techniques for 3D modeling of biological structures, including "conventional" techniques like single sectioning transmission electron microscopy (ssTEM) and "new" techniques like SBF SEM and FIB SEM, have been reviewed extensively recently, e.g., [9–13] and some of them have already been used for 3D reconstructions of lung structure: ssTEM [5,7,8,14]; electron tomography [15]; array tomography [16] and SBF SEM [6,11]. Even FIB SEM has been applied [17–19], but the study of Købler et al. was rather focused on testing an alternative method to diamond knife ultramicrotomy and transmission electron microscopic imaging of nanotubes; the review of Ochs et al. gave an outlook on the potential of this technique in lung research; and Hegermann et al. demonstrated a method for correlative light and electron microscopy. Kremer et al. [11] showed a FIB SEM-based reconstruction of a small part of a *human* A549 cell. Here, to our knowledge, we provide the first extensive study of the alveolar epithelial 3D ultrastructure based on FIB SEM in a *human* lung sample. We were able to reconstruct an almost complete AE2 cell with two adjacent AE1 cell domains as well as a part of a neighboring AE2 cell. The model shows detailed reconstructions of the epithelial surface, including a surfactant secretion pore on an AE2 cell, enlargements of the apical AE1 cell surface, long folds bordering grooves on the basal AE1 cell surface, AE1/AE1, AE1/AE2 and AE2/AE2 contact sites, basolateral microvilli pits at AE2 cells and small AE1 processes beneath AE2 cells. The functional relevance of these findings will be discussed below.

AE1 cells seem to be responsible for the majority of fluid transport across the alveolar epithelium [20–22]. According to Dobbs et al. [20] different sodium channels (highly selective Na^+ channel (HSC), non-selective Na^+ channel (NSC) and cyclic nucleotide-gated channel (CNG)), the cystic fibrosis transmembrane regulator (chloride channel), potassium and water (Aquaporin 5) channels and Na^+/K^+ATPases are involved in that. The surface enlargements of the AE1 cell domains shown here may serve as a membrane compartment housing the particular transport proteins and, thus, be the ultrastructural correlate of liquid absorbtion.

Interestingly, when looking at Figure 4, one gets the idea, that the surface in a septal concavity is rich in these surface enlargements, while they seem to be reduced or even absent on convexities. Concave niches are filled with the (liquid) hypophase of surfactant [1,7] and these "puddles" may be the sites where most of the fluid absorption takes place. Microvilli on AE1 cells have been described previously [20] and were also found during *cat* lung development [8,14].

Fixation (cf. the studies of Gil et al. [23], Oldmixon et al. [24] and Oldmixon and Hoppin Jr. [25] or long-term storage can lead to microscopic artefacts. The following arguments, however, indicate that the non-microvillus surface enlargements are a real biological phenomenon: (1) The cytoplasm within these excrescences is quite electron dense, while lytic cell parts regularly appear electron light. (2) The surface enlargements seem to be concentrated at certain spots, while other areas remain smooth. (3) Microvillus-like surface irregularities without obvious microfilaments have also been described by Mercurio and Rhodin [7] in the *cat*. (4) Surface irregularities on AE1 cells can also be seen on some scanning electron micrographs in textbooks or other articles [1,3,5,26,27].

Another explanation for the surface irregularities was given by Mercurio and Rhodin [7], who suggested that they are incorporated into the cell membrane during inflation. This was concluded, because they also found a cell with a rather smooth surface, where they thought that the flatness was caused by trapped air in the airspaces. If this interpretation is true, however, then also the basolateral cell membrane needs membrane reserves, since the apical and basolateral membranes are separated by tight junctions [28]; Sirianni et al. [5] also mentioned the existence of discontinuous tight junctions. Such reserves could be provided by the cytoplasmic folds of the basolateral cell membrane or by the AE1 cell branches beneath the AE2 cells shown by our models.

The basal AE1 cell membrane folds, however, could also serve as mechanical stabilization, i. e., anchoring the epithelium in the septal wall by interdigitation with the interstitium to resist shearing forces. This principle is well established for the skin, where connective tissue papillae or ridges of the dermal papillary layer interdigitate with the epidermis at the dermal-epidermal junction [29] (p. 147).

With respect to AE1/AE1 cell contacts in the *cat* lung, Mercurio and Rhodin [7,8] described the possibility that adjacent cells may show alternating overlap or meet edge to edge. Our data suggest that this is also true for the *human* lung, even if the images and models shown here only demonstrate a clear overlap with the blue cell domain on top of the yellow cell or edge to edge contacts (Figures 6 and 7). What is the functional relevance of this overlap? Overlap per se enhances mechanical stability but additionally enlarges the contact area; in particular it may enlarge the available "contact area" for important cell junctions like the relatively wide (see [1,30]) tight junctions and/or gap junctions, for review, see [31]. The latter have been described to be in close topographic relation to the occluding junctions [30]. Mercurio and Rhodin [7] suggested that the overlap may change during breathing.

With respect to the AE1/AE2 contacts, we could confirm and extend our SBF-based presumption and Sirianni et al's [5] data that AE1 cells may extend both under and on the AE2 cells. Our data set and model revealed a y-shaped branching pattern in 3D (cf. Figure 2 of [5]) and additionally added that AE1 cells may extend various thin foot processes under AE2 cells.

Branches beneath AE2 cells may serve as membrane reserve during inspiration (see above). This may also be an explanation for the foot processes, but these may also be structural correlate of cellular interaction: Sirianni et al. [5] demonstrated linkage of AE1 and AE2 cells with interstitial fibroblasts via holes in the basal lamina, which seem to be primarily located beneath AE2 cells and Nabhan et al. [32] demonstrated that Wnt signaling between fibroblasts and alveolar epithelial stem cells (a small fraction of distinct AE2 cells) is necessary to maintain their stem cell status. Eventually, the small AE1 processes "look for" those holes for linkage to interstitial fibroblasts. Alternatively, the close proximity of these processes to AE2 microvilli pits in some cases (see Figure 11) could indicate exchange of material (too large for gap junctional transport) from AE1 to AE2 cells or vice versa (or fibroblasts).

These microvilli pits of AE2 cells, however, were also found towards other cell types (i.e. the other AE2 cell or interstitial cells (see Figure 3). Interestingly, they were also found above an intact basal lamina (not shown). Proximity to cells and holes in the basal lamina suggests a role in intercellular communication, material exchange or sensory functions. Localization above a closed basal lamina may be the structural correlate of basal lamina turnover or the initiation of creating a hole for consecutive subepithelial communication.

Summing up, the current FIB SEM study of a *human* lung sample provided new insights into the *human* alveolar epithelial cell morphology and topography. Our model reveals detailed reconstructions of the alveolar epithelial surface, including a surfactant secretion pore on an AE2 cell, enlargements of the apical AE1 cell surface, long folds bordering grooves on the basal AE1 cell surface, AE1/AE1, AE1/AE2 and AE2/AE2 contact sites, basolateral microvilli pits at AE2 cells and small AE1 processes beneath AE2 cells. These data may serve as morphological blueprint for molecular investigations of alveolar epithelial biology.

4. Materials and Methods

4.1. Sample Preparation

An archival sample of a *human* lung [33], kindly provided by Professor Ewald R. Weibel (Institute of Anatomy, University of Berne, Berne, Switzerland), was used for the current study. The sample was prepared as described previously [6] following a modified protocol from Deerinck et al. [34] to enhance membrane contrast, cf. also [16]:

In brief, the fixed sample was rinsed in 0.15 M HEPES buffer followed by 0.1 M cacodylate buffer and subsequently postfixed by reduced osmium tetroxide (OsO_4) (1.5 % hexacyanoferrate II, 1 % OsO_4 in 0.1 M cacodylate buffer) in the dark for half an hour. The sample was then washed in double distilled water (ddH_2O), infiltrated with 1 % thiocarbohydrazide in ddH_2O for 20 min and washed again in ddH_2O before it was once more postfixed by 1 % OsO_4 in ddH_2O in the dark for half an hour. After washing in ddH_2O the sample was block stained overnight in the dark at 4 °C in an aqueous half saturated uranyl acetate solution, followed by a washing step in ddH_2O and block staining by Walton's lead aspartate at 60 °C for half an hour. After washing in ddH_2O, the sample was dehydrated in an ascending series of acetone (70 %, 90 % and 100 %) and finally embedded in Durcupan (Sigma-Aldrich Chemie GmbH, Munich, Germany).

The sample was trimmed and an ultrathin section (60 nm) was generated to look for appropriate regions of interest in a conventional transmission electron microscope (Morgagni 268, FEI, Eindhoven, Netherlands) for imaging with the FIB SEM.

The Durcupan block was mounted in a slotted SEM specimen holder and the sides were covered with conductive silver (Plano, Wetzlar, Germany) before the sample was sputtered with a 20 nm gold layer (Quorum Q150R ES sputter coater; Quorum Technologies Ltd, Laughton, East Sussex, United Kingdom), cf. [17].

4.2. FIB SEM Data Set Acquisition

The prepared specimen with the region of interest (ROI) was approached with a Zeiss Crossbeam 540 (Carl Zeiss Microscopy GmbH, Jena, Germany) at 20 kV acceleration voltage. A deposition of platinum and the generation of carbon-highlighted marks on the area of interest enabled adequate handling, tracking, autofocus and autostigmation during the acquisition process. Finally, using the Inlens Secondary Electron (SE) and the Energy selective Backscattered (EsB) detector (grid voltage 800 V), a z-stack of 2297 images, each showing a ROI of 33 µm × 20 µm was generated (pixel size 2 nm, section thickness 10 nm). Image acquisition was performed at 1.5 kV with 1.0 nA using the ATLAS software package (Carl Zeiss Microscopy GmbH, Jena, Germany) accompanying the microscope, cf. [17]. For later segmentations and 3D reconstructions a cropped data set was exported from the ATLAS software package with a pixel size of 5 nm and an Inlens SE to EsB detector ratio of 80 % to 20 %.

4.3. Segmentations and 3D Reconstructions

For segmentations and 3D reconstructions 3dmod (part of the iMOD package [35]) was used: After import of the data set, the cells or cell parts of interest were segmented by manually tracing their outlines on the FIB SEM images. As a basic algorithm the structures were segmented on every fourth image. If the complexity of structure and/or the modeling, however, required a narrower segmentation interval, also sections in between the first and fourth image (up to every image) were segmented. The stack of contours was then used by 3dmod to generate 3D models of the segmented structures. For the AE2 cells also the luminal-abluminal border as an approximation of the apical/basolateral surface border was segmented by tracing the luminal edges of the alveolar cell surface through the z-Stack, cf. [6].

4.4. Figure Preparation

Figures were prepared in the GNU Image Manipulation Program (gimp 2.10.12; www.gimp.org [accessed on 23 September 2019]) after having created snapshots with 3dmod.

For a general overview of sample preparation techniques and the volume EM workflow, see [10].

Author Contributions: (In alphabetical order) Conceptualization, C.M., C.W. and J.P.S.; Methodology, C.W. and J.P.S.; Investigation, C.W. and J.P.S.; Resources, C.M., C.W. and J.P.S.; data curation, C.W. and J.P.S.; writing—original draft, J.P.S.; writing—review and editing, C.M., C.W. and J.P.S.; Visualization, C.W. and J.P.S.; supervision, C.M.; funding acquisition, C.M. and J.P.S. All authors have read and agreed to the published version of the manuscript.

Acknowledgments: The authors wish to thank Susanne Faßbender for excellent technical assistance, David Mastronarde for outstanding support in using IMOD and his efforts to improve the software continuously and Jan Hegermann, Matthias Ochs, Lars Knudsen, Stephanie Groos and Andreas Schmiedl for valuable discussions with impact on the current work. We acknowledge support by the German Research Foundation (DFG) and the Open Access Publication Fund of Hannover Medical School (MHH).

Abbreviations

The following abbreviations are used in this manuscript:

AE1	Type 1 alveolar epithelial
AE2	Type 2 alveolar epithelial
3D	Three dimensions/-dimensional
SBF	Serial block-face
SEM	Scanning electron microscope/microscopy
FOV	Field of view
FIB	Focused ion beam
EM	Electron microscopic
HSC	Highly selective Na^+ channel
NSC	Non-selective Na^+ channel
CNG	Cyclic nucletide-gated channel
ssTEM	Single sectioning transmission electron microscopy
OsO_4	Osmium tetroxide
ddH_2	Double distilled water
ROI	Region of interest
SE	Secondary electron
EsB	Energy selective Backscattered

References

1. Ochs, M.; Weibel, E.R. Functional design of the human lung for gas exchange. In *Fishman's Pulmonary Diseases and Disorders*, 4th ed.; Fishman, A.P., Elias, J.A., Fishman, J.A., Grippi, M.A., Senior, R.M., Pack, A.I., Eds.; McGraw-Hill Medical: New York, NY, USA, 2008; chapter 2, Volume 1, pp. 23–69.
2. Guillot, L.; Nathan, N.; Tabary, O.; Thouvenin, G.; Le Rouzic, P.; Corvol, H.; Amselem, S.; Clemen, A. Alveolar epithelial cells: Master regulators of lung homeostasis. *Int. J. Biochem. Cell Biol.* **2013**, *45*, 2568–2573. [CrossRef] [PubMed]
3. Weibel, E.R. On the tricks alveolar epithelial cells play to make a good lung. *Am. J. Respir. Crit. Care Med.* **2015**, *191*, 504–513. doi:10.1164/rccm.201409-1663OE. [CrossRef] [PubMed]
4. Weibel, E.R. The mystery of "non-nucleated plates" in the alveolar epithelium of the lung explained. *Acta Anat. (Basel)* **1971**, *78*, 425–443. doi:10.1159/000143605. [CrossRef] [PubMed]
5. Sirianni, F.E.; Chu, F.S.F.; Walker, D.C. Human alveolar wall fibroblasts directly link epithelial type 2 cells to capillary endothelium. *Am. J. Respir. Crit. Care Med.* **2003**, *168*, 1532–1537. doi:10.1164/rccm.200303-371OC. [CrossRef]
6. Schneider, J.P.; Wrede, C.; Hegermann, J.; Weibel, E.R.; Mühlfeld, C.; Ochs, M. On the topological complexity of human alveolar epithelial type 1 cells. *Am. J. Respir. Crit. Care Med.* **2019**, *199*, 1053–1056. doi:10.1164/rccm.201810-1866LE. [CrossRef]
7. Mercurio, A.R.; Rhodin, J.A.G. An electron microscopic study on the type I pneumocyte in the cat: Postnatal morphogenesis. *J. Morphol.* **1984**, *182*, 169–178. doi:10.1002/jmor.1051820205. [CrossRef]
8. Mercurio, A.R.; Rhodin, J.A.G. An electron microscopic study on the type I pneumocyte in the cat: Pre-natal morphogenesis. *J. Morphol.* **1978**, *156*, 141–156. doi:10.1002/jmor.1051560203. [CrossRef]
9. Knott, G.; Genoud, C. Is EM dead? *J. Cell Sci.* **2013**, *126*, 4545–4552. doi:10.1242/jcs.124123. [CrossRef]
10. Titze, B.; Genoud, C. Volume scanning electron microscopy for imaging biological ultrastructure. *Biol. Cell* **2016**, *108*, 307–323. doi:10.1111/boc.201600024. [CrossRef]
11. Kremer, A.; Lippens, S.; Bartunkova, S.; Asselbergh, B.; Blanpain, C.; Fendrych, M.; Goossens, A.; Holt, M.; Janssens, S.; Krols, M.; et al. Developing 3D SEM in a broad biological context. *J. Microsc.* **2015**, *259*, 80–96. doi:10.1111/jmi.12211. [CrossRef]

12. Peddie, C.J.; Collinson, L.M. Exploring the third dimension: Volume electron microscopy comes of age. *Micron* **2014**, *61*, 9–19. doi:10.1016/j.micron.2014.01.009. [CrossRef] [PubMed]
13. Miranda, K.; Girard-Dias, W.; Attias, M.; De Souza, W.; Ramos, I. Three dimensional reconstruction by electron microscopy in the life sciences: An introduction for cell and tissue biologists. *Mol. Reprod. Dev.* **2015**, *82*, 530–547. doi:10.1002/mrd.22455. [CrossRef] [PubMed]
14. Mercurio, A.R.; Rhodin, J.A.G. An electron microscopic study on the type I pneumocyte of the cat: Differentiation. *Am. J. Anat.* **1976**, *146*, 255–271. doi:10.1002/aja.1001460304. [CrossRef] [PubMed]
15. Burgoyne, T.; Lewis, A.; Dewar, A.; Luther, P.; Hogg, C.; Shoemark, A.; Dixon, M. Characterizing the ultrastructure of primary ciliary dyskinesia transposition defect using electron tomography. *Cytoskeleton (Hoboken)* **2014**, *71*, 294–301. doi:10.1002/cm..21171. [CrossRef]
16. Beike, L.; Wrede, C.; Hegermann, J.; Lopez-Rodriguez, E.; Kloth, C.; Gauldie, J.; Kolb, M.; Maus, U.A.; Ochs, M.; Knudsen, L. Surfactant dysfunction and alveolar collapse are linked with fibrotic septal wall remodeling in th TGF-ß1-induced mouse model of pulmonary fibrosis. *Lab. Invest.* **2019**, *99*, 830–852. doi:10.1038/s41374-019-0189-x. [CrossRef]
17. Hegermann, J.; Wrede, C.; Fassbender, S.; Schliep, R.; Ochs, M.; Knudsen, L.; Mühlfeld, C. Volume-CLEM: A method for correlative light and electron microscopy in three dimensions. *Am. J. Physiol. Lung Cell Mol. Physiol.* **2019**, *317*, L778–L784. doi:10.1152/ajplung.00333.2019. [CrossRef]
18. Købler, C.; Thoustrup Saber, A.; Raun Jacobsen, N.; Wallin, H.; Vogel, U.; Ovortrup, K. Mølhave, K. FIB-SEM imaging of carbon nanotubes in mouse lung tissue. *Anal. Bioanal. Chem.* **2014**, *406*, 3863. doi:10.1007/s00216-013-7566-x. [CrossRef]
19. Ochs, M.; Knudsen, L.; Hegermann, J.; Wrede, C.; Grothausmann, R.; Mühlfeld, C. Using electron microscopes to look into the lung. *Histochem. Cell Biol.* **2016**, *146*, 695–707. doi:10.1007/s00418-016-1502-z. [CrossRef]
20. Dobbs, L.G.; Johnson, M.D.; Vanderbilt, J.; Allen, L.; Gonzalez, R. The great big alveolar TI cell: Evolving concepts and paradigms. *Cell Physiol. Biochem.* **2010**, *25*, 55–62. doi:10.1159/000272063. [CrossRef]
21. Flodby, P.; Kim, Y.H.; Beard, L.L.; Gao, D.; Ji, Y.; Kage, H.; Liebler, J.M.; Minoo, P.; Kim, K.J.; Borok, Z.; et al. Knockout mice reveal a major role for alveolar epithelial type I cells in alveolar fluid clearance. *Am. J. Respir. Cell Mol. Biol.* **2016**, *55*, 395–406. doi:10.1165/rcmb.2016-0005OC. [CrossRef]
22. Ridge, K.M.; Olivera, W.G.; Saldias, F.; Azzam, Z.; Horowitz, S.; Rutschman, D.H.; Dumasius, V.; Factor, P.; Sznajder, J.I. Alveolar type 1 cells express the $\alpha 2$ Na,K-ATPase, which contributes to lung liquid clearance. *Circ. Res.* **2003**, *92*, 453–460. doi:10.1161/01.RES.0000059414.10360.F2. [CrossRef]
23. Gil, J.; Bachofen, H.; Gehr, P.; Weibel, E.R. Alveolar volume-surface area relation in air- and saline-filled lungs by vascular perfusion. *J. Appl. Physiol. Respir. Environ. Exerc. Physiol.* **1979**, *47*, 990–1001. doi:10.1152/jappl.1979.47.5.990. [CrossRef] [PubMed]
24. Oldmixon, E.H.; Suzuki, S.; Butler, J.P.; Hoppin, F.G., Jr. Perfusion dehydration fixes elastin and preserves lung air-space dimensions. *J. Appl. Physiol.* **1985**, *58*, 105–113. doi:10.1152/jappl.1985.58.1.105. [CrossRef] [PubMed]
25. Oldmixon, E.H.; Hoppin, F.G., Jr. Alveolar septal folding and lung inflation history. *J. Appl. Physiol.* **1991**, *71*, 2369–2379. doi:10.1152/jappl.1991.71.6.2369. [CrossRef] [PubMed]
26. Fawcett, D.W.; Raviola, E. *Bloom and Fawcett. A Textbook of Histology*, 12th ed.; Chapman & Hall: New York, NY, USA, 1994.
27. Fehrenbach, H. Alveolar epithelial type II cell: Defender of the alveolus revisited. *Respir. Res.* **2001**, *2*, 33–46. doi:10.1186/rr36. [CrossRef]
28. Kasper, M.; Barth, K. Potential contribution of alveolar epithelial type I cells to pulmonary fibrosis. *Biosci. Rep.* **2017**, *37*, BSR20171301. doi:10.1042/BSR20171301. [CrossRef]
29. McGrath, J.A.; Lai-Cheong, J.E. Skin and its appendages. In *Anatomy. The Anatomical Basis for Clinical Practice*, 41st ed.; Standring, S., Ed.; Elsevier Limited: Amsterdam, The Netherlands, 2016.
30. Bartels, H.; Oestern, H.J.; Voss-Wermbter, G. Communicating-occluding junction complexes in the alveolar epithelium. *Am. Rev. Respir. Dis.* **1980**, *121*, 1017–1024.
31. Losa, D.; Chanson, M. The lung communication network. *Cell Mol. Life Sci.* **2015**, *72*, 2793–2808. doi:10.1007/s00018-015-1960-9. [CrossRef]
32. Nabhan, A.; Brownfield, D.G.; Harbury, P.B.; Krasnow, M.A.; Desai, T.J. Single-cell Wnt signaling niches

maintain stemness of alveolar type 2 cells. *Science* **2018**, *359*, 1118–1123. doi:10.1126/science.aam6603. [CrossRef]

33. Gehr, P.; Bachofen, M.; Weibel, E.R. The normal human lung: Ultrastructure and morphometric estimation of diffusion capacity. *Respir. Physiol.* **1978**, *32*, 121–140. doi:10.1016/0034-5687(78)90104-4. [CrossRef]
34. Deerinck, T.J.; Bushong, E.A.; Thor, A.; Ellisman, M.H. NCMIR methods for 3D EM: A New Protocol for Preparation Of Biological Specimens for Serial Blockface Scanning Electron Microscopy. 2010. Available online: https://ncmir.ucsd.edu/sbem-protocol (accessed on 21 June 2018).
35. Kremer, J.R.; Mastronarde, D.N.; McIntosh, J.R. Computer visualization of three-dimensional image data using IMOD. *J. Struct. Biol.* **1996**, *116*, 71–76. doi:10.1006/jsbi.1996.0013. [CrossRef] [PubMed]

7

Evidence for Nanoparticle-Induced Lysosomal Dysfunction in Lung Adenocarcinoma (A549) Cells

Arnold Sipos [1,2,*], Kwang-Jin Kim [1,2,3,4,5], Constantinos Sioutas [6] and Edward D. Crandall [1,2,7,8]

1 Will Rogers Institute Pulmonary Research Center and Hastings Center for Pulmonary Research, Keck School of Medicine, University of Southern California, Los Angeles, CA 90033-0906, USA; kjkim@usc.edu (K.-J.K.); edward.crandall@med.usc.edu (E.D.C.)

2 Division of Pulmonary, Critical Care and Sleep Medicine, Department of Medicine, Keck School of Medicine, University of Southern California, Los Angeles, CA 90033-0906, USA

3 Department of Physiology and Neuroscience, Keck School of Medicine, University of Southern California, Los Angeles, CA 90089-9037, USA

4 Department of Pharmacology and Pharmaceutical Sciences, School of Pharmacy, University of Southern California, Los Angeles, CA 90089-9121, USA

5 Department of Biomedical Engineering, Viterbi School of Engineering, University of Southern California, Los Angeles, CA 90089-1111, USA

6 Sonny Astani Department of Civil and Environmental Engineering, Viterbi School of Engineering, University of Southern California, Los Angeles, CA 90089-2531, USA; sioutas@usc.edu

7 Department of Pathology, Keck School of Medicine, University of Southern California, Los Angeles, CA 90033-9092, USA

8 Mork Family Department of Chemical Engineering and Materials Science, Viterbi School of Engineering, University of Southern California, Los Angeles, CA 90089-1211, USA

* Correspondence: asipos@usc.edu

Abstract: Background: Polystyrene nanoparticles (PNP) are taken up by primary rat alveolar epithelial cell monolayers (RAECM) in a time-, dose-, and size-dependent manner without involving endocytosis. Internalized PNP in RAECM activate autophagy, are delivered to lysosomes, and undergo [Ca^{2+}]-dependent exocytosis. In this study, we explored nanoparticle (NP) interactions with A549 cells. Methods: After exposure to PNP or ambient pollution particles (PM0.2), live single A549 cells were studied using confocal laser scanning microscopy. PNP uptake and egress were investigated and activation of autophagy was confirmed by immunolabeling with LC3-II and LC3-GFP transduction/colocalization with PNP. Mitochondrial membrane potential, mitophagy, and lysosomal membrane permeability (LMP) were assessed in the presence/absence of apical nanoparticle (NP) exposure. Results: PNP uptake into A549 cells decreased in the presence of cytochalasin D, an inhibitor of macropinocytosis. PNP egress was not affected by increased cytosolic [Ca^{2+}]. Autophagy activation was indicated by increased LC3 expression and LC3-GFP colocalization with PNP. Increased LMP was observed following PNP or PM0.2 exposure. Mitochondrial membrane potential was unchanged and mitophagy was not detected after NP exposure. Conclusions: Interactions between NP and A549 cells involve complex cellular processes leading to lysosomal dysfunction, which may provide opportunities for improved nanoparticle-based therapeutic approaches to lung cancer management.

Keywords: autophagy; lysosome; lysosomal membrane permeability; mitochondria; pneumocyte

1. Introduction

Nanoparticle (NP) exposure has been reported to induce stress in various cells and tissues [1–4]. The cellular response to NP exposure is dependent on the chemical (e.g., components and surface charge) and physical (e.g., shape and size) characteristics of NP [5–9]. Due to the heterogeneity of the physicochemical properties of NP, it is difficult to generalize their effects in cells. However, it has been reported that NP exposure of cells and tissues affects functions of various intracellular organelles (e.g., mitochondria and endoplasmic reticulum (ER)) [4,10–12]. The involvement of lysosomes in cellular stress (especially in lung alveolar epithelial cells (AEC)) in response to inhaled NP may be especially important in the pathogenesis of chronic lung disease.

Following internalization of foreign materials (e.g., proteins, bacteria, virus and (nano)particles), autophagy is activated as part of cellular defense mechanism(s) [13]. Autophagy is a catabolic process that helps maintain cellular homeostasis by removing excess, harmful, damaged, or foreign cellular components [14,15], although autophagy may play different roles in cancer versus normal cells, leading to either cell survival or death [16–18]. During autophagic processing, autophagosomes are formed to separate the target cytosolic component(s) from the remainder of the cell [19]. The autophagosome then delivers its cargo to the lysosome via autophagosome-lysosome fusion. Intracellular NP have been reported to activate autophagy [20], and NP localized inside (auto)lysosomes were shown to induce alteration(s) in lysosomal function [21]. Inhalation of airborne pollution particles (including those overlapping in size with nanoparticles) may contribute to chronic diseases (e.g., chronic obstructive pulmonary disease and pulmonary fibrosis) [22], although the mechanisms by which this occurs are not well understood [23,24].

A549 is a continuous cell line derived from a human pulmonary adenocarcinoma that is widely used as a model of mammalian lung alveolar epithelial type II cells. Various ultrastructural characteristics of A549 cells are similar to those in type II pneumocytes. Phospholipid composition of the A549 cell line has been shown to be similar to that of primary isolates of type II cells [25].

In this study, ambient air pollution particles (PM0.2, diameter <0.2 μm) and polystyrene nanoparticles (PNP) were used to investigate their intracellular handling/fate and their effects on A549 cells. PM0.2 contain nanoparticles (defined as particles whose size at least in one dimension is ≦100 nm) that may contribute to cellular health effects (including development of chronic lung diseases). PNP are engineered nanoparticles that are relatively nontoxic and non-metabolizable, making them suitable for studies of nanoparticle interactions/kinetics. They are useful especially for live cell imaging by taking advantage of their fluorescent labels. Utilizing NP (i.e., PM0.2 and 20 nm carboxylated PNP) and A549 as a model type II pneumocyte, we investigated in this study the internalization mechanisms, egress characteristics, and intracellular NP fate/handling/effects. We found that apical NP exposure of A549 cells leads to activation of autophagy and increased lysosomal membrane permeability (LMP) without mitochondrial dysfunction.

2. Results

2.1. Live Cell Imaging of Intracellular PNP in A549 Cells

At 24 h of apical PNP exposure of A549 cells, PNP (in red) accumulated in intracellular vesicles (Figure 1), while diffuse cytosolic PNP distribution was also seen. Plasma membranes of A549 cells were labeled by Dylight 488-conjugated tomato lectin (in green).

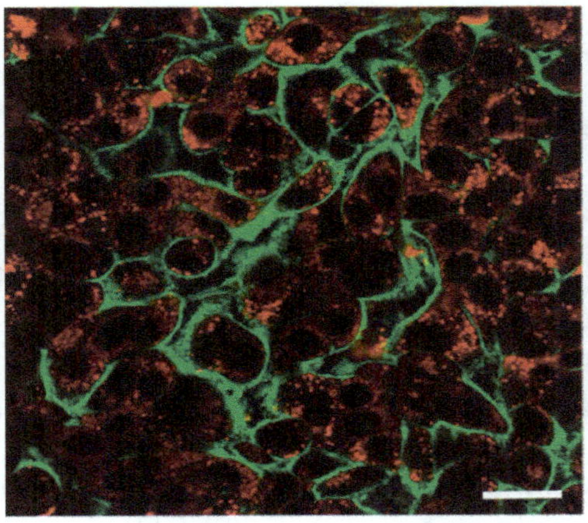

Figure 1. Intracellular accumulation of polystyrene nanoparticles (PNP) in A549 cells. Apical exposure of A549 cells to PNP at 80 µg/mL for 24 h led to accumulation of PNP (red) in intracellular vesicles, while diffuse distribution of PNP in cytosol was also seen. Plasma membranes of A549 cells were labeled by Dylight 488-conjugated tomato lectin (green). Scale bar is 10 µm.

2.2. Mechanism(s) of PNP Entry into A549 Cells

Nocodazole (an inhibitor of microtubule polymerization) decreased intracellular PNP content by 17% and cytochalasin D (CCD) decreased intracellular PNP content by 57%, indicating that macropinocytosis played a role in PNP entry into A549 cells (Figure 2). Clathrin-mediated endocytosis did not appear to be involved in PNP internalization, as monodansylcadaverine (MDC) failed to decrease intracellular PNP content (Figure 2). Further evidence for endocytic internalization of PNP into A549 cells was provided by colocalization of PNP with early endosomes that were pre-transduced with a Rab5-GFP vector (Figure 3).

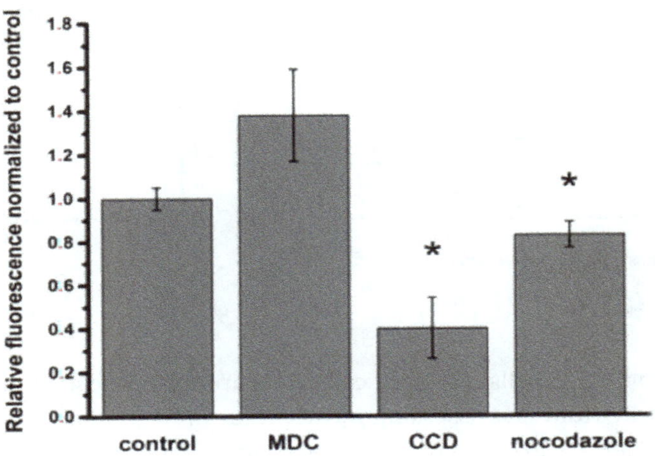

Figure 2. Relative changes in intracellular PNP content in A549 cells in the presence or absence (control) of endocytosis inhibitors after 24 h of apical PNP exposure. Monodansylcadaverine (MDC, an inhibitor of clathrin-mediated endocytosis) failed to decrease intracellular PNP content, whereas cytochalasin D (CCD, an inhibitor of macropinocytosis) and nocodazole (an inhibitor of microtubule polymerization) decreased intracellular PNP content by 60% and 17%, respectively. * $p < 0.05$ compared to control.

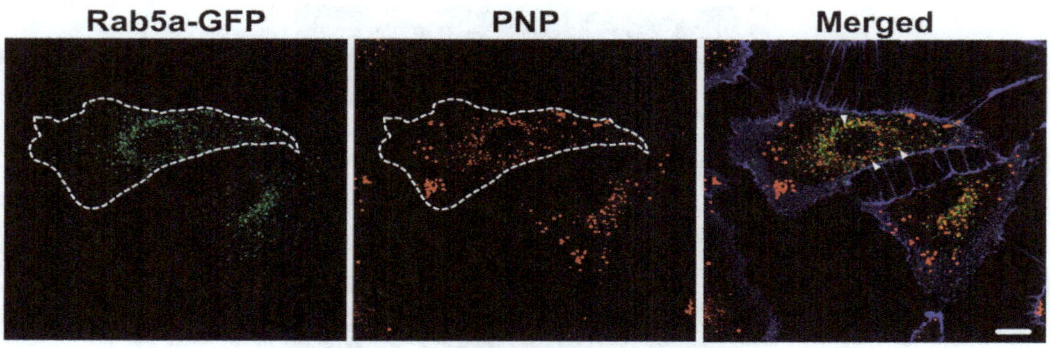

Figure 3. Colocalization of early endosome marker Rab5a-GFP with PNP in A549 cells. A549 cells were transduced for 2 h with an early endosome marker (Rab5a-GFP, green) and apically exposed thereafter to PNP (red) for 24 h. Colocalization (arrowheads, yellow) of PNP with Rab5a-GFP-positive vesicles was observed in some of the vesicles. Contours of cells were added (dotted lines) on the basis of the cell plasma membrane marker Dylight 405-conjugated tomato lectin (blue). Images are representative of 4–5 observations. Scale bar is 10 µm.

2.3. *PNP Egress from A549 Cells*

A549 cells were apically exposed to PNP (80 µg/mL) for 12 h, followed by washing with fresh cell culture fluid. Intracellular PNP content was assessed over time for up to 24 h thereafter. Intracellular PNP content of A549 cells decreased ~90% over 24 h (Figure 4). The egress profile in the continued presence of 10 µM apical ATP was not significantly different from that without ATP (Figure 4a), despite repeated elevations in cytosolic [Ca^{2+}] due to brief (2.5 min) ATP stimulation (Figure 4b).

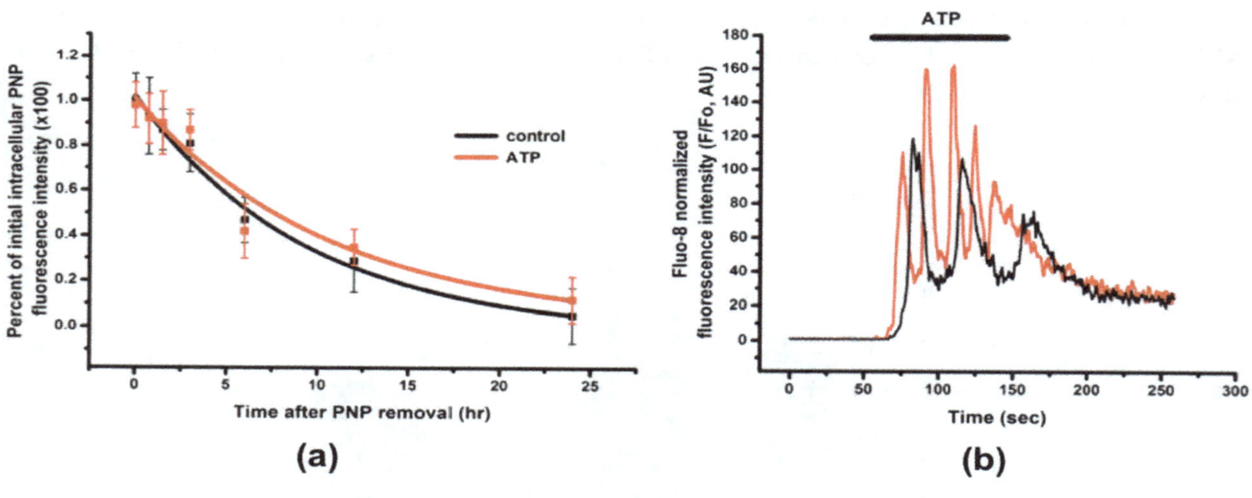

Figure 4. PNP egress from A549 cells. (**a**) A549 cells were apically exposed to PNP for 12 h, followed by washing with fresh culture fluid and assessing intracellular PNP content at designated time points for up to 24 h thereafter. When 10 µM ATP was applied apically to A549 cells at time zero and remained present throughout the entire experiment, no difference in PNP egress kinetics between control (no stimulation) and ATP-treated A549 cells during egress was observed. n = 4–6 for each time point. (**b**) Representative recording of oscillations in intracellular [Ca^{2+}] detected upon 2.5 min presence of 10 µM ATP in the apical bathing fluid of A549 cells. Different colors represent intracellular [Ca^{2+}] observed in two different A549 cells.

2.4. *Intracellular NP Processing in A549 Cells*

We investigated the involvement of autophagy in intracellular processing of NP. A549 cells were preincubated with an inhibitor (e.g., 40 µM chloroquine) of fusion of autophagosomes with lysosomes for 30 min prior to apical NP (PNP at 80 μg/mL or PM0.2 at 1 μg/mL) exposure, followed by exposure to NP (PNP or PM0.2) for 24 h in the continued presence of chloroquine. Immunolabeling for LC3-I/II of NP-exposed and chloroquine-treated A549 cells showed that the intracellular presence of NP led to activation of autophagy (Figure 5). This finding was confirmed in live LC3-GFP-transduced A549 cells (subsequently treated with chloroquine as well), where colocalization of PNP with LC3-GFP-positive intracellular vesicles (i.e., autophagosomes) was found (Figure 6).

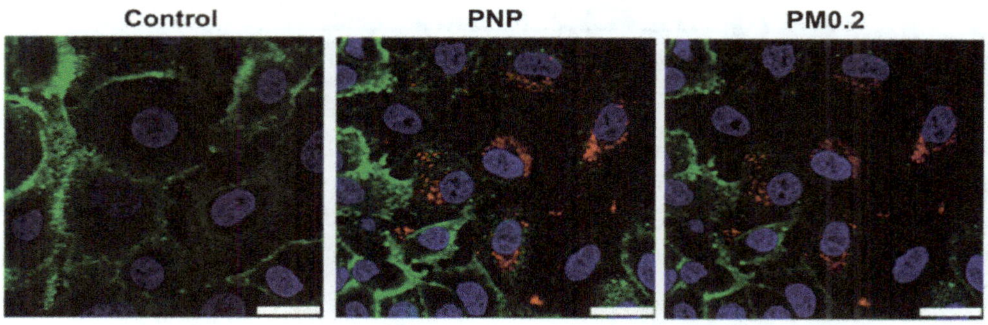

Figure 5. Apical nanoparticle (NP) exposure induced activation of autophagy in A549 cells. A549 cells were preincubated with chloroquine (40 μM, 30 min) and exposed thereafter to NP (PNP or ambient air pollution particles (PM0.2)) for 24 h in the continued presence of chloroquine, followed by assessment of LC3 expression by immunolabeling. LC3 expression (red) was detected in NP-exposed A549 cells. No or very low level of LC3 expression was found in control cells not exposed to NP. Plasma membranes of A549 cells were labeled by Dylight 488-conjugated tomato lectin (green), whereas nuclei were labeled by Hoechst 33342 (blue). Images are representative of 4–5 observations. Scale bars are 25 μm.

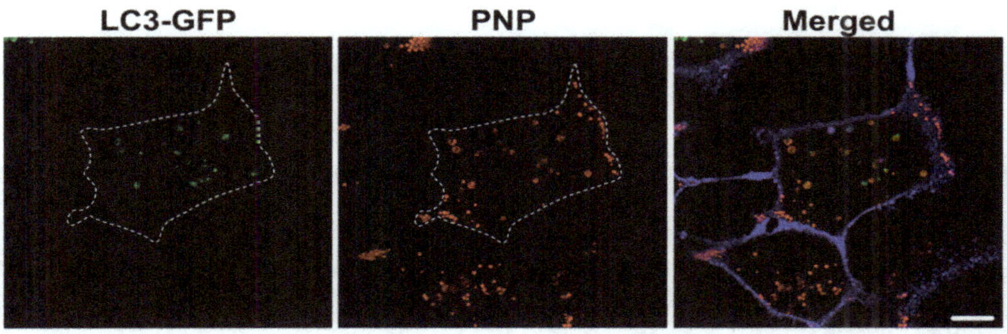

Figure 6. Colocalization of PNP with LC3-GFP in A549 cells. Following transduction of A549 cells with the autophagosome marker LC3-GFP construct for 2 h, cells were preincubated with chloroquine (40 μM) and apically exposed thereafter to PNP for 24 h in the continued presence of chloroquine. Colocalization of PNP (red) with LC3-GFP-positive vesicles (green) was observed. Contour of cell was added (dotted line) on the basis of the cell plasma membrane marker Dylight 405-conjugated tomato lectin (blue). Images are representative of 4–5 observations. Scale bar is 10 μm.

Since autophagic processing of intracellular NP might affect the intracellular content of NP, we assessed intracellular PNP content in A549 cells in the presence of pharmacological inhibitors of autophagy. When autophagosome formation was inhibited by 3-methyladenine (3-MA), intracellular PNP content decreased by 38%, whereas impaired autophagic flux (in the presence of bafilomycin) resulted in a 64% decrease in intracellular PNP content, compared to that in control A549 cells at 24 h post-exposure (Figure 7).

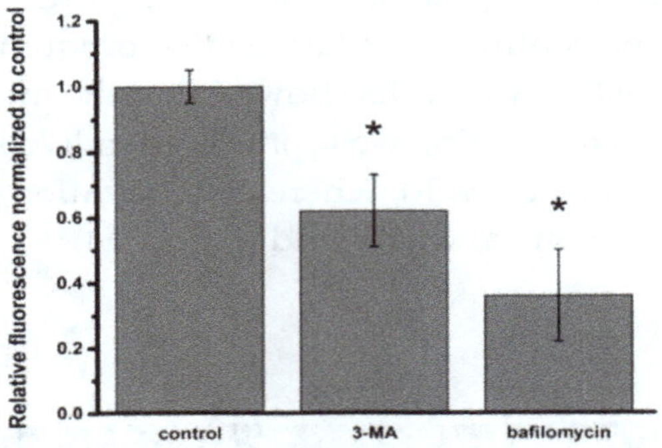

Figure 7. Effects of autophagy inhibitors on intracellular PNP content in A549 cells at 24 h post-exposure to PNP. Intracellular PNP content in A549 cells was reduced by 38% and 64%, respectively, when autophagosome formation was inhibited with 3-methyladenine (3-MA) or autophagosome-lysosome fusion was inhibited with bafilomycin. Data are normalized to control. * $p < 0.05$ compared to control.

2.5. Assessment of NP Exposure-Induced Lysosomal Dysfunction

Colocalization of PNP (red) and lysosomes (green) was observed (Figure 8). PNP were also seen in A549 cells without colocalization with Lysotracker Green. PNP is non-metabolizable and likely to accumulate in lysosomes if intact lysosomal membranes are maintained. Acridine orange (AO) is known to accumulate in lysosomes and can be released upon lysosomal injury (e.g., derangement of lysosomal membrane integrity). When A549 cells were apically exposed to PNP or PM0.2 for 24 h, increased presence of AO in cytosol and nucleus was seen, indicating that LMP was increased (Figure 9).

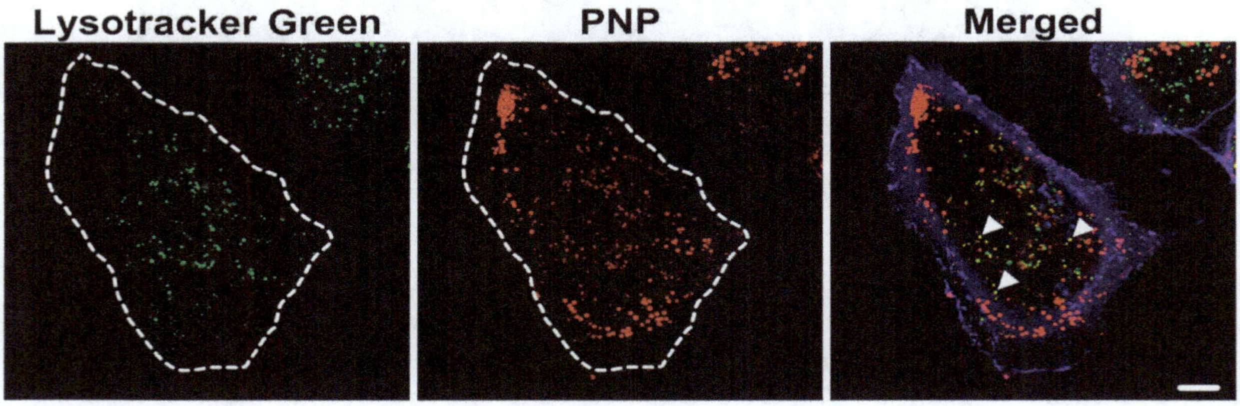

Figure 8. Colocalization of PNP with lysosomes in A549 cells. At 24 h post exposure to PNP, lysosomes in A549 cells were labeled with Lysotracker Green (green). Colocalization (yellow; arrowheads) can be seen between PNP (red) and Lysotracker Green in some of the vesicles in the perinuclear area. Plasma membrane of A549 cells was labeled by Dylight 405-conjugated tomato lectin (blue or shown with dotted line). Images are representative of 4–5 observations. Scale bar is 10 μm.

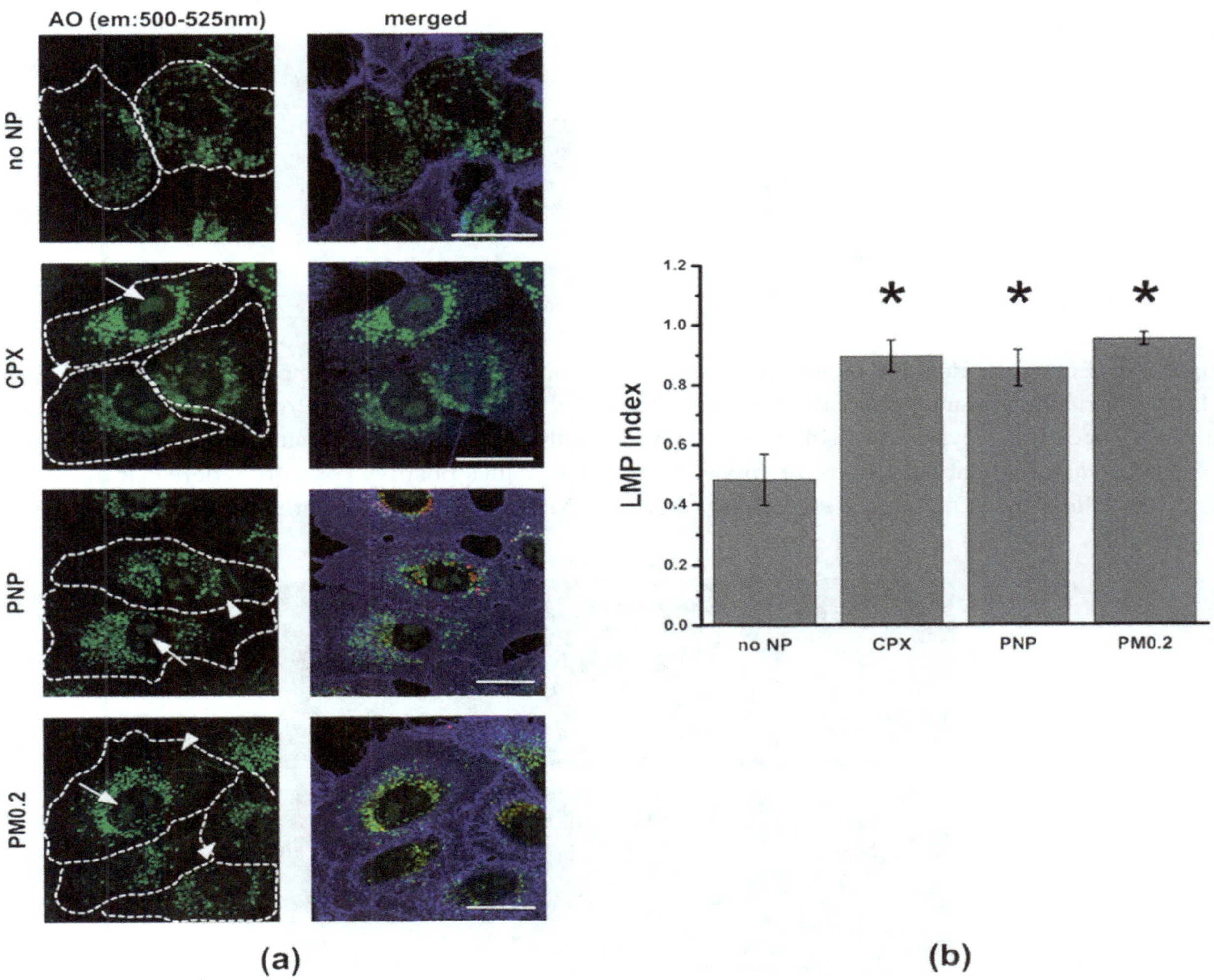

Figure 9. Detection of increased lysosomal membrane permeability (LMP) using acridine orange (AO) in A549 cells. (**a**) Increased LMP was detected when AO (green; ex/em: 488/500–525 nm) intensity in lysosomes was decreased along with increased AO intensity in cytoplasm and nucleus. In "no NP" panels, A549 cells showed virtually no detectable nuclear AO signal. A549 cells pretreated with ciprofloxacin (CPX, 150 μM for 24 h, without NP exposure) as positive control exhibited AO accumulation in both nucleus (arrow) and cytoplasm (arrowhead). NP (PNP or PM0.2) exposure also led to AO accumulation in cytoplasm and nucleus. Contours of cells were added (dotted line) on the basis of the cell plasma membrane marker Dylight 405-conjugated tomato lectin (blue). Scale bars are 20 μm. (**b**) When A549 cells were apically exposed to either PNP or PM0.2 for 24 h, increased LMP index (AO green fluorescence intensity in cytoplasm and nucleus/total cellular AO green fluorescence intensity) was found to be similar to that of positive control (CPX). n = 4–6. * $p < 0.05$ compared to control.

2.6. NP Exposure and Mitochondrial Function in A549 Cells

Mitochondria were labeled with the mitochondrial membrane potential sensitive fluorescent dye tetramethylrhodamine methyl ester (TMRM). When A549 cells were apically exposed to PNP or PM0.2 for 24 h, no change in mitochondrial membrane potential was observed (Figure 10). To confirm these data, we also used the Mtphagy dye, which is capable of staining damaged mitochondria (undergoing mitophagy and being delivered to lysosomes). No colocalization of the Mtphagy dye and LI lysosome marker dye was found, indicating that 24 h of apical exposure of A549 cells to PNP or PM0.2 did not lead to cellular stress involving mitochondrial dysfunction (Figure 11).

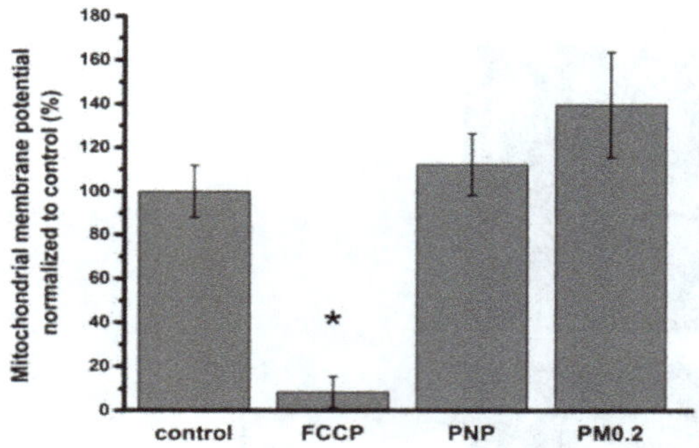

Figure 10. Effect of apical NP exposure for 24 h on mitochondrial membrane potential in A549 cells. Mitochondrial membrane potentials were normalized to the corresponding controls (i.e., not exposed to either NP or carbonyl cyanide 4-(trifluoromethoxy)phenylhydrazone (FCCP)). Mitochondrial membrane potential was nearly abolished in the presence of FCCP (1 μM, positive control), whereas it did not decrease following 24 h of apical exposure to PNP or PM0.2. * $p < 0.05$ compared to control.

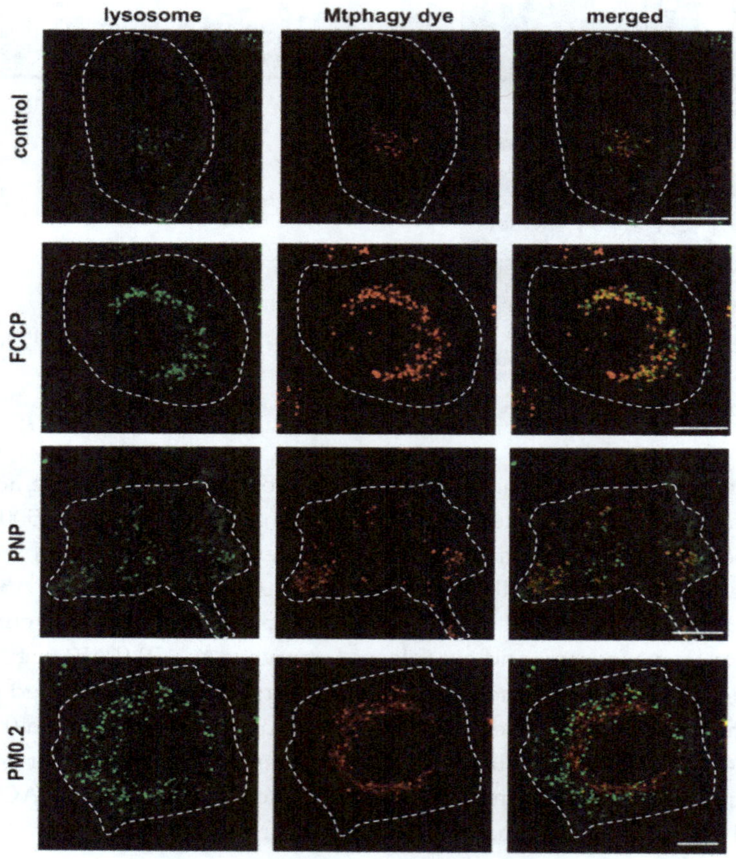

Figure 11. Absence of mitophagy in NP-exposed A549 cells. Mitophagy is detected on the basis of an increase in the fluorescent signal of the Mtphagy dye (in comparison to that of control; red) and colocalization of the Mtphagy dye with lysosomal indicator (LI; green) dye. In control (no exposure to PNP or PM0.2), the Mtphagy dye had weak fluorescence and minimal colocalization with lysosomes. After FCCP exposure (positive control), the Mtphagy dye exhibited strong fluorescence with extensive colocalization with the LI lysosomal marker dye. Exposure of A549 cells to either PNP or PM0.2 yielded weak fluorescence with the Mtphagy dye and showed minimal lysosomal colocalization of the Mtphagy dye, consistent with a low level (or relative absence) of mitophagy. Contours of cells were added (dotted line) on the basis of the cell plasma membrane marker Dylight 405-conjugated tomato lectin. Scale bars (25 μm) are shown in right panels only.

3. Discussion

Using a live cell imaging approach, we demonstrated that PNP are taken up into A549 cells, at least in part by macropinocytosis. Most (>90%) intracellular PNP content is released from A549 cells over 24 h, whereas mobilization of intracellular Ca^{2+} by ATP did not speed up PNP egress from A549 cells. Internalized NP (PNP or PM0.2) activated autophagy, delivering NP to lysosomes. The presence of NP in lysosomes led to increased lysosomal membrane permeability. Mitochondrial membrane potential was not affected and mitophagy was not observed in NP-exposed A549 cells.

3.1. *Uptake of NP into A549 Cells*

We previously reported that primary rat alveolar epithelial cell monolayers (RAECM) do not appear to utilize endocytic process(es) for PNP uptake, which are internalized mainly by diffusion-like entry into RAECM [26]. A549 cells, a lung adenocarcinoma cell line, differ from primary AEC in many ways, including the inability to form a barrier with high transepithelial resistance and utilization of macropinocytosis for NP uptake. PNP internalization that is not inhibited by cytochalasin D may take place via non-endocytic process(es) (e.g., diffusion across and/or poration by PNP of apical cell plasma membranes [27–29]). In addition, clathrin-mediated endocytosis is not involved in PNP uptake into A549 cells (Figure 2). The decrease in PNP uptake in the presence of nocodazole suggests that suppression of vesicle movement on an intracellular microtubular network is insufficient to entirely inhibit endocytosis. When A549 cells were transduced with the early endosome marker Rab5a-GFP, colocalization between early endosomes and PNP was found at 24 h post exposure to PNP, consistent with the presence of PNP endocytosis into A549 cells.

3.2. *Egress of NP from A549 Cells*

Intracellular PNP content decreased 90% over 24 h (Figure 4a) in egress experiments. Intracellular PNP was compartmentalized in A549 cells, as shown in Figure 1, with some PNP diffusely distributed in the cytoplasm. It has been reported that epithelial cells are capable of releasing the content of intracellular vesicles (e.g., lysosomes) [30,31]. For example, release of PNP localized in lysosomes of primary RAECM was dependent on elevations in cytosolic [Ca^{2+}] [26]. By contrast, A549 cells stimulated with ATP led to oscillatory elevations in cytosolic [Ca^{2+}] (Figure 4b) without altering the kinetics of PNP egress over 24 h (Figure 4a). In A549 cells, it is possible that lysosomal PNP leaked into cytosol and may not be available to exit primarily via lysosomal exocytosis.

3.3. *Activation of Autophagy in Intracellular Processing of NP in A549 Cells*

Autophagy is a defense mechanism aiming to maintain cellular homeostasis. The presence of NP in AEC has been reported to activate autophagy in primary RAECM [26]. In order to identify the involvement of autophagy in intracellular fate of internalized NP in A549 cells, we sought to detect the expression of microtubule-associated protein 1A/1B light chain 3B (LC3) protein. LC3 is localized to the phagophore membrane, followed by localization in inner and outer membranes of autophagosomes. Upon fusion of autophagosomes with lysosomes (i.e., autophagic flux), LC3 localized at the inner membrane of (auto)lysosomes is degraded by lysosomal proteolysis. LC3-GFP fusion protein expression is used widely to identify autophagosomes, with the caveat that GFP loses its fluorescence in the lysosomal acidic environment [32,33]. Because the autophagy process is relatively fast [34], there is only a small detection window (before autophagosomes fuse with lysosomes) for observing LC3-GFP, necessitating inhibition of autophagic flux (e.g., with chloroquine or bafilomycin to block the fusion of autophagosomes with lysosomes). In the presence of chloroquine, we observed colocalization of PNP with LC3-GFP after 24 h of apical PNP exposure, indicating that autophagy plays a role in cellular handling of NP in A549 cells (Figure 6). Further evidence for autophagy activation in NP-exposed A549 cells was obtained by immunolabeling of LC3-positive vesicles in NP-exposed A549 cells (Figure 5). PM0.2-exposed primary RAECM exhibited autophagy activation (i.e., expression of LC3) as well.

We observed that interference with autophagy led to decreased intracellular PNP content in A549 cells (Figure 7). When autophagic flux was blocked, autophagosomal content could not be delivered to lysosomes for further processing, as discussed below. Therefore, it is conceivable that the observed lower intracellular PNP content might be related to the decrease in lysosomal PNP localization. It cannot be ruled out that yet-unknown feedback mechanism(s) between autophagy and endocytic process(es) might also play a role. When we performed PNP uptake experiments in primary RAECM in which autophagy was inhibited with 3-MA or bafilomycin, intracellular PNP content was decreased by ~80 and ~50%, respectively [26]. In contrast to primary RAECM, the inhibition in A549 cells of autophagic flux resulted in greater loss in intracellular PNP content (64%) compared to inhibition of autophagosome formation (38%). Although we do not have a clear explanation for this difference between primary RAECM and A549 cells, it may indicate that A549 cell autophagy is regulated differently (especially by 3-MA [35]) from autophagy in primary AEC [36,37]. Lysotracker Green-negative intracellular vesicles that contain PNP may include amphisomes [20,38]. It is possible that the lysosomal dysfunction found in NP-exposed A549 cells (discussed below) also contributed to the difference in intracellular PNP content found in the presence of pharmacological inhibitors of autophagy.

3.4. *Lysosomal Dysfunction in NP-Exposed A549 Cells*

We found relatively low PNP content in lysosomes of A549 cells at 24 h post exposure (Figure 8). Most PNP resided in Lysotracker Green-negative vesicles, indicating that the PNP-filled vesicles were primarily non-lysosomal vesicles. This finding might explain why ATP stimulation failed to speed up the kinetics of PNP egress from A549 cells (Figure 4), as most intracellular PNP are not localized to lysosomes. Acridine orange (AO) is a nucleic acid-sensitive cationic dye often used to label DNA in cells [39,40]. However, when used in nanomolar concentrations, it labels primarily acidic intracellular organelles (e.g., lysosomes) without labeling other intracellular components (e.g., nuclei) (Figure 9a). On the basis of this characteristic, we used 7 nM AO for labeling acidic cellular organelles (mostly lysosomes), followed by detection of increased LMP index in NP-exposed A549 cells (Figure 9b). Apical NP (PNP or PM0.2) exposure caused the release of AO from lysosomes and accumulation in cytosol and nucleus. Interestingly, vesicular staining of AO did not fully disappear following NP exposure of A549 cells, indicating perhaps that the increase in LMP index was not permanent. The magnitude of NP exposure-induced increase in LMP index was comparable to that achieved by the positive control ciprofloxacin (CPX). PNP exposure in HeLa cells has been reported to result in lysosomal dysfunction via the activation of autophagy [41].

3.5. *Absence of Mitochondrial Dysfunction in NP-Exposed A549 Cells*

Mitochondria are often reported as damaged or dysfunctional in the presence of cellular stress (e.g., mild to severe loss in mitochondrial function) following exposure of cells to various NP [42]. One of the most sensitive approaches to test mitochondrial integrity is to monitor changes in fluorescence of the mitochondrial membrane potential sensitive dye TMRM in live cells. We found no appreciable changes in TMRM fluorescence intensity upon apical exposure to NP, although the positive control (i.e., FCCP) lowered TMRM fluorescence intensity by >90%. This finding might suggest that the NP dose we used in this study was too low to induce major mitochondrial impairment and that lysosomes are more sensitive than mitochondria to PNP or PM0.2 exposure at the concentration of NP used to expose A549 cells in this study.

In addition to the mitochondrial membrane potential measurement, we also utilized the novel Mtphagy dye, capable of reporting mitophagy in real time, for assessment of mitochondrial (dys)function. When mitophagy takes place (i.e., damaged mitochondria are delivered to lysosomes), the fluorescence intensity of the Mtphagy dye increases due to acidic lysosomal pH. As a positive control, FCCP treatment of A549 cells led to enhanced fluorescence intensity from the Mtphagy dye with increased colocalization of the Mtphagy dye with the LI lysosomal marker dye. By contrast, NP exposure of A549 cells failed to cause any discernible increase in the Mtphagy dye fluorescence intensity and no measurable colocalization of the Mtphagy dye with the LI lysosome marker dye, indicating no or minimal impairment in mitochondrial function.

3.6. Summary

In summary, we have shown in this study that PNP are taken up in part by macropinocytosis into A549 cells. Egress of PNP from A549 cells is slow and not regulated by increased cytosolic [Ca^{2+}]. Intracellular presence of NP (PNP or PM0.2) activates autophagy, delivering the cargo (i.e., PNP or PM0.2) to lysosomes. Lysosomes become dysfunctional due to the presence of NP in lysosomes. NP exposure of A549 cells induces cellular stress (e.g., increased LMP index) without causing mitochondrial dysfunction(s). Further understanding of the cascade of events in cellular stress caused by NP exposure might help devise approaches to mitigation of cellular/organellar damage and pathogenesis of lung diseases (e.g., pulmonary emphysema and/or fibrosis) caused by chronic intermittent low-level NP exposure. Insights into the differences in the interactions of NP with A549 cells versus those with primary AEC may be useful in devising improved nanoparticle-based therapeutic approaches to lung cancer management.

4. Materials and Methods

4.1. Materials

PNP (20 nm diameter, carboxylated and impregnated with near infrared (NIR) dye) was obtained from Thermo Fischer Scientific, Waltham, WA, USA). Ambient air pollution particles (diameter <0.20 μm (denoted as PM0.2)) were collected from air samples in downtown Los Angeles, CA, USA, per the protocol published elsewhere [43]. Transwell filters of 10.5 mm diameter (with 0.4 μm diameter pores), fetal bovine serum (FBS), and bovine serum albumin (BSA) were purchased from BD Biosciences (Franklin Lakes, NJ, USA). A 1:1 mixture of phenol red-free Dulbecco's modified Eagle's medium and Ham's F-12 medium (DME/F-12), nonessential amino acid solution (NEAA), *N*-(2-hydroxyethyl)piperazine-*N*′-(2-ethanesulfonic acid) hemisodium salt (HEPES), 2-(*N*-morpholino)ethanesulfonic acid sodium salt (MES), monodansylcadaverine (MDC), cytochalasin D (CCD), adenosine triphosphate (ATP), dimethylsulfoxide (DMSO), L-glutamine, 3-methyladenine (3-MA), bafilomycin, nocodazole, carbonyl cyanide 4-(trifluoromethoxy)phenylhydrazone (FCCP), ciprofloxacin, trypsin-EDTA, Triton X-100, paraformaldehyde, chloroquine, and acridine orange (AO) were all obtained from Sigma-Aldrich (St. Louis, MO, USA). Primocin was purchased from InvivoGen (San Diego, CA, USA). 1,2-Bis(2-aminophenoxy)ethane-*N*,*N*,*N*′,*N*′-tetraacetic acid tetrakis(acetoxymethyl ester) (BAPTA-AM) and Hoechst 33342 were obtained from Invitrogen (Carlsbad, CA, USA). Dylight (488 nm)-conjugated tomato lectin was obtained from Vector Laboratories (Burlingame, CA, USA). Some tomato lectin was labeled in-house using Dylight 405 NHS Ester labeling kit (Thermo Fischer Scientific). Fluo-8 AM was purchased from AAT Bioquest (Sunnyvale, CA, USA). BacMam LC3-GFP and Rab5a-GFP constructs, Lysotracker Green, and tetramethylrhodamine methyl ester (TMRM) were bought from Thermo Fischer Scientific. Microtubule-associated protein light chain 3B (LC3B) antibody (that recognizes both LC3B-I and -II) was purchased from Cell Signaling Technology (Danvers, MA, USA). Mitophagy detection kits (including the Mtphagy dye and lysosomal indicator (LI) dye) were obtained from Dojindo Molecular Technologies (Washington, DC, USA). A549 cells were purchased from American Type Culture Collection (Manassas, VA, USA).

4.2. Cell Culture

A549 cells were plated onto Transwell filters at 100,000 cells/0.865 cm^2 and cultured in a defined medium with serum (MDS), composed of 10% FBS and serum-free defined medium (MDSF; DME/F-12 medium supplemented with 1 mM NEAA, 100 U/mL Primocin, 10 mM HEPES, 1.25 mg/mL BSA, and 2 mM L-glutamine). Cells were maintained at 37 °C in a humidified atmosphere of 95% air and 5% CO_2 and fed every other day. Experiments were performed using A549 cells on culture days 2–3.

4.3. Live Cell Imaging

A549 cells cultured on Transwell filters were imaged by confocal microscopy as described elsewhere [26]. Briefly, A549 cells on Transwell filters were mounted in a temperature-controlled chamber (Vestavia Scientific, Vestavia Hills, AL, USA) and bathed with MDS on both sides. In xyz series, intracellular PNP fluorescence intensity was measured stack-by-stack and integrated over the entire volume of a single A549 cell. To demarcate intracellular space at the single cell level, cell plasma membranes were labeled using Dylight (488 or 405 nm)-conjugated tomato lectin. Confocal imaging was at 8 bits, 63× magnification, and 1024 × 1024 resolution with a SP8 confocal microscope system (Leica Microsystems GmbH, Wetzlar, Germany). Gallium nitride (405 nm), argon (488 nm), and helium-neon (633 nm) lasers were utilized for excitation. Image analysis was conducted using Image-J software (NIH, Bethesda, MD, USA) and Leica LAS 3D Process and Quantify Packages.

4.4. Nanoparticle (NP) Exposure of A549 Cells

PM0.2 at 1 μg/mL and near-infrared (NIR) dye-impregnated carboxylated PNP (20 nm diameter with excitation/emission (ex/em) wavelengths of 660/680 nm) at 80 μg/mL were used to apically expose A549 cells for 24 h unless noted otherwise.

4.5. Intracellular PNP Content Assessed after 24 h of Apical PNP Exposure

Incubation of PNP-exposed cells was performed in a humidified atmosphere of 5% CO_2/95% air. At 24 h post exposure, cells were washed with fresh culture medium and intracellular PNP content was estimated using live cell imaging as above.

4.6. Effect of Endocytosis Inhibitors on Intracellular PNP Content

Intracellular PNP content was estimated by live cell imaging in the presence and absence of agents known to interfere with endocytosis pathways, including MDC (inhibiting clathrin-mediated endocytosis; 200 μM), CCD (inhibiting macropinocytosis; 10 μM), and nocodazole (inhibiting microtubule polymerization; 100 nM). A549 cells were exposed both apically and basolaterally to one of these inhibitors, beginning 30 min prior to and during apical PNP exposure of A549 cells, followed by intracellular PNP content assessment. Control represents PNP-exposed A549 cells studied in the absence of endocytosis inhibitors.

4.7. Egress of Intracellular PNP from A549 Cells

A549 cells were apically exposed to 20 nm PNP at 80 μg/mL for 12 h, followed by washing thrice with fresh culture medium. A549 cells were then incubated on both sides with fresh MDS for up to 24 h. Intracellular PNP content of A549 cells at predesignated times was estimated to construct egress time courses.

4.8. Cytosolic Ca^{2+} Mobilization and PNP Exocytosis

The effect of intracellular mobilization of Ca^{2+} on PNP egress was assessed in washed A549 cells (after 12 h of apical PNP exposure as above) stimulated with 10 μM ATP added to both bathing fluids during the egress experiment for up to 24 h. Changes in cytosolic [Ca^{2+}] were detected by Fluo-8 AM (1 μM, 10 min, 25 °C in the presence of 5 mM probenecid to prevent leakage of Fluo-8 from the cells) following a brief presence (for 2.5 min) of apically added 10 μM ATP.

4.9. Nanoparticle Exposure-Induced Activation of Autophagy in A549 Cells

A549 cells were apically exposed to NP (PNP or PM0.2) in the presence or absence of 40 µM chloroquine, which blocks autolysosome formation, that was added to both apical and basolateral bathing fluids 30 min prior to and during NP exposure. After 24 h NP exposure, A549 cells were washed with fresh culture medium thrice and fixed with 4% paraformaldehyde for 10 min at room temperature, followed by immunolabeling of autophagosomes using rabbit LC3B antibody (1:400 dilution, overnight, 4 °C) and Alexa 488-labeled goat anti-rabbit secondary antibody (1:400 dilution, 1 h, 25 °C). Antigen-antibody complexes were detected using confocal microscopy at ex/em of 488/500–550 nm.

4.10. Effects of Inhibitors of Autophagosome or Autolysosome Formation on Intracellular PNP Content

Intracellular PNP content was assessed in the presence of 3-MA (5 mM, an inhibitor of autophagosome formation) or bafilomycin (0.5 µM, an inhibitor of autolysosome formation). A549 cells were pre-incubated with one of these inhibitors in both apical and basolateral fluids 30 min prior to and during apical PNP exposure.

4.11. Assessment of Lysosomal Dysfunction

Lysosomal membrane permeability was assessed in A549 cells labeled with acridine orange (AO, 7 nM, 37 °C and 5% CO_2) for 15 min [40]. Lysosomal dysfunction was detected by release of AO from lysosomes due to increased lysosomal membrane permeability (LMP), followed by accumulation of AO in cytosol and nucleus. In order to quantify LMP, an LMP index was estimated as AO green fluorescence intensity in cytoplasm and nucleus/total cellular AO green fluorescence intensity. Changes in AO fluorescence intensity in A549 cells were monitored using ex/em of 488/500–525 nm. A549 cells treated with ciprofloxacin (150 µM for 24 h) in both apical and basolateral bathing fluids was used as positive control.

4.12. Assessment of Mitochondrial Function

A549 cells were exposed to the mitochondrial membrane potential sensitive fluorescent dye TMRM (1 nM, ex/em: 561/570–630 nm) for 30 min in culture medium at 37 °C and 5% CO_2 prior to live cell imaging. For the detection of mitophagy, A549 cells were apically exposed to Mtphagy dye (100 nM, ex/em: 561/650–800 nm) for 30 min in serum-free culture medium at 37 °C and 5% CO_2. After labeling A549 cells with Mtphagy dye, cells were further apically exposed to NP (PNP or PM0.2), 1 µM FCCP (as a positive control) or DMSO (0.1% as a negative control) for 24 h in MDS. Thirty minutes prior to detection of mitophagy, bathing fluids of A549 cells were changed to MDSF containing LI lysosome marker dye (1 µM, ex/em: 488/490–550 nm). Live cell imaging was performed 30 min later for evidence of mitophagy (i.e., colocalization of the lysosomal marker dye with Mtphagy dye in lysosomes).

4.13. Data Analysis

Data are presented as mean ± standard deviation (n = total number of observations). Student's two-tailed t-tests were used for comparisons of two group means. One-way analysis of variance followed by post-hoc tests based on Tukey procedures was performed using Prism (version 6.07, GraphPad Software, La Jolla, CA, USA) to determine differences among means of ≥3 groups. $p < 0.05$ was considered statistically significant.

Author Contributions: Conceptualization, A.S., K.-J.K., and E.D.C.; methodology, A.S., K.-J.K., and E.D.C.; validation, A.S., K.-J.K., and E.D.C.; formal analysis, A.S., K.-J.K., and E.D.C.; investigation, A.S.; resources, K.-J.K., C.S., and E.D.C.; writing—original draft preparation, A.S. and K.-J.K.; writing—review and editing, A.S., K.-J.K., C.S., and E.D.C.; supervision, K.-J.K. and E.D.C.; project administration, K.-J.K. and E.D.C.; funding acquisition, E.D.C.

Acknowledgments: Many thanks to Yang Chai for generous access to confocal microscopes. Edward D. Crandall is Hastings Professor of Medicine.

Abbreviations

3-MA	3-methyladenine
AEC	Alveolar epithelial cell
AM	Acetoxymethyl ester
ATP	Adenosine triphosphate
CCD	Cytochalasin D
EDTA	Ethylenediaminetetraacetic acid
LMP	Lysosomal membrane permeability
MDC	Monodansylcadaverine
NP	Nanoparticle
LC3	Microtubule-associated proteins 1A/1B light chain 3B
PM0.2	Ambient air pollution particles with a diameter <0.2 μm
PNP	Polystyrene nanoparticle
RAECM	Rat alveolar epithelial cell monolayer

References

1. Buzea, C.; Pacheco, I.I.; Robbie, K. Nanomaterials and nanoparticles: Sources and toxicity. *Biointerphases* **2007**, *2*, 17–71. [CrossRef]
2. Khan, M.I.; Mohammad, A.; Patil, G.; Naqvi, S.A.H.; Chauhan, L.K.S.; Ahmad, I. Induction of ROS, mitochondrial damage and autophagy in lung epithelial cancer cells by iron oxide nanoparticles. *Biomaterials* **2012**, *33*, 1477–1488. [CrossRef] [PubMed]
3. Panariti, A.; Miserocchi, G.; Rivolta, I. The effect of nanoparticle uptake on cellular behavior: Disrupting or enabling functions? *Nanotechnol. Sci. Appl.* **2012**, *5*, 87–100. [PubMed]
4. Cao, Y.; Long, J.; Liu, L.; He, T.; Jiang, L.; Zhao, C.; Li, Z. A review of endoplasmic reticulum (ER) stress and nanoparticle (NP) exposure. *Life Sci.* **2017**, *186*, 33–42. [CrossRef] [PubMed]
5. Andersson, P.O.; Lejon, C.; Ekstrand-Hammarström, B.; Akfur, C.; Ahlinder, L.; Bucht, A.; Österlund, L. Polymorph- and size-dependent uptake and toxicity of TiO_2 nanoparticles in living lung epithelial cells. *Small* **2011**, *7*, 514–523. [CrossRef]
6. Bussy, C.; Pinault, M.; Cambedouzou, J.; Landry, M.J.; Jegou, P.; Mayne-L'hermite, M.; Launois, P.; Boczkowski, J.; Lanone, S. Critical role of surface chemical modifications induced by length shortening on multi-walled carbon nanotubes-induced toxicity. *Part. Fibre Toxicol.* **2012**, *9*, 46. [CrossRef]
7. Gazzano, E.; Ghiazza, M.; Polimeni, M.; Bolis, V.; Fenoglio, I.; Attanasio, A.; Mazzucco, G.; Fubini, B.; Ghigo, D. Physicochemical determinants in the cellular responses to nanostructured amorphous silicas. *Toxicol. Sci.* **2012**, *128*, 158–170. [CrossRef]
8. Chusuei, C.C.; Wu, C.-H.; Mallavarapu, S.; Hou, F.Y.S.; Hsu, C.-M.; Winiarz, J.G.; Aronstam, R.S.; Huang, Y.-W. Cytotoxicity in the age of nano: The role of fourth period transition metal oxide nanoparticle physicochemical properties. *Chem. Biol. Interact.* **2013**, *206*, 319–326. [CrossRef]
9. Kang, S.; Kim, J.-E.; Kim, D.; Woo, C.G.; Pikhitsa, P.V.; Cho, M.-H.; Choi, M. Comparison of cellular toxicity between multi-walled carbon nanotubes and onion-like shell-shaped carbon nanoparticles. *J. Nanopart. Res.* **2015**, *17*, 378. [CrossRef]
10. Yu, K.-N.; Yoon, T.-J.; Minai-Tehrani, A.; Kim, J.-E.; Park, S.J.; Jeong, M.S.; Ha, S.-W.; Lee, J.-K.; Kim, J.S.; Cho, M.-H. Zinc oxide nanoparticle induced autophagic cell death and mitochondrial damage via reactive oxygen species generation. *Toxicol. In Vitro* **2013**, *27*, 1187–1195. [CrossRef]
11. Guo, C.; Wang, J.; Jing, L.; Ma, R.; Liu, X.; Gao, L.; Cao, L.; Duan, J.; Zhou, X.; Li, Y.; et al. Mitochondrial dysfunction, perturbations of mitochondrial dynamics and biogenesis involved in endothelial injury induced by silica nanoparticles. *Environ. Pollut.* **2018**, *236*, 926–936. [CrossRef] [PubMed]

12. Yu, K.-N.; Chang, S.-H.; Park, S.J.; Lim, J.; Lee, J.; Yoon, T.-J.; Kim, J.-S.; Cho, M.-H. Titanium dioxide nanoparticles induce endoplasmic reticulum stress-mediated autophagic cell death via mitochondria-associated endoplasmic reticulum membrane disruption in normal lung cells. *PLoS ONE* **2015**, *10*, e0131208. [CrossRef] [PubMed]
13. Tooze, S.A.; Abada, A.; Elazar, Z. Endocytosis and autophagy: Exploitation or cooperation? *Cold Spring Harb. Perspect. Biol.* **2014**, *6*, a018358. [CrossRef] [PubMed]
14. Glick, D.; Barth, S.; Macleod, K.F. Autophagy: Cellular and molecular mechanisms. *J. Pathol.* **2010**, *221*, 3–12. [CrossRef]
15. Dikic, I.; Elazar, Z. Mechanism and medical implications of mammalian autophagy. *Nat. Rev. Mol. Cell Biol.* **2018**, *19*, 349–364. [CrossRef]
16. Codogno, P.; Meijer, A.J. Autophagy and signaling: Their role in cell survival and cell death. *Cell Death Differ.* **2005**, *12*, 1509–1518. [CrossRef]
17. Das, G.; Shravage, B.V.; Baehrecke, E.H. Regulation and function of autophagy during cell survival and cell death. *Cold Spring Harb. Perspect. Biol.* **2012**, *4*, a008813. [CrossRef]
18. Denton, D.; Kumar, S. Autophagy-dependent cell death. *Cell Death Differ.* **2019**, *26*, 605–616. [CrossRef]
19. Klionsky, D.J. Autophagy: From phenomenology to molecular understanding in less than a decade. *Nat. Rev. Mol. Cell Biol.* **2007**, *8*, 931–937. [CrossRef]
20. Klionsky, D.J.; Eskelinen, E.-L.; Deretic, V. Autophagosomes, phagosomes, autolysosomes, phagolysosomes, autophagolysosomes... wait, I'm confused. *Autophagy* **2014**, *10*, 549–551. [CrossRef]
21. Manshian, B.B.; Pokhrel, S.; Mädler, L.; Soenen, S.J. The impact of nanoparticle-driven lysosomal alkalinization on cellular functionality. *J. Nanobiotechnol.* **2018**, *16*, 85. [CrossRef] [PubMed]
22. Conti, S.; Harari, S.; Caminati, A.; Zanobetti, A.; Schwartz, J.D.; Bertazzi, P.A.; Cesana, G.; Madotto, F. The association between air pollution and the incidence of idiopathic pulmonary fibrosis in Northern Italy. *Eur. Respir. J.* **2018**, *51*, 1700397. [CrossRef] [PubMed]
23. Kurt, O.K.; Zhang, J.; Pinkerton, K.E. Pulmonary health effects of air pollution. *Curr. Opin. Pulm. Med.* **2016**, *22*, 138–143. [CrossRef] [PubMed]
24. Kim, D.; Chen, Z.; Zhou, L.-F.; Huang, S.-X. Air pollutants and early origins of respiratory diseases. *Chronic Dis. Transl. Med.* **2018**, *4*, 75–94. [CrossRef]
25. Nardone, L.L.; Andrews, S.B. Cell line A549 as a model of the type II pneumocyte. *Biochim. Biophys. Acta* **1979**, *573*, 276–295. [CrossRef]
26. Sipos, A.; Kim, K.-J.; Chow, R.H.; Flodby, P.; Borok, Z.; Crandall, E.D. Alveolar epithelial cell processing of nanoparticles activates autophagy and lysosomal exocytosis. *Am. J. Physiol. Lung Cell. Mol. Physiol.* **2018**, *315*, L286–L300. [CrossRef]
27. Contini, C.; Schneemilch, M.; Gaisford, S.; Quirke, N. Nanoparticle—membrane interactions. *J. Exp. Nanosci.* **2018**, *13*, 62–81. [CrossRef]
28. Behzadi, S.; Serpooshan, V.; Tao, W.; Hamaly, M.A.; Alkawareek, M.Y.; Dreaden, E.C.; Brown, D.; Alkilany, A.M.; Farokhzad, O.C.; Mahmoudi, M. Cellular uptake of nanoparticles: Journey inside the cell. *Chem. Soc. Rev.* **2017**, *46*, 4218–4244. [CrossRef]
29. Treuel, L.; Jiang, X.; Nienhaus, G.U. New views on cellular uptake and trafficking of manufactured nanoparticles. *J. R. Soc. Interface* **2013**, *10*, 20120939. [CrossRef]
30. Rodríguez, A.; Webster, P.; Ortego, J.; Andrews, N.W. Lysosomes behave as Ca^{2+}-regulated exocytic vesicles in fibroblasts and epithelial cells. *J. Cell Biol.* **1997**, *137*, 93–104. [CrossRef]
31. Xu, J.; Toops, K.A.; Diaz, F.; Carvajal-Gonzalez, J.M.; Gravotta, D.; Mazzoni, F.; Schreiner, R.; Rodriguez-Boulan, E.; Lakkaraju, A. Mechanism of polarized lysosome exocytosis in epithelial cells. *J. Cell Sci.* **2012**, *125*, 5937–5943. [CrossRef] [PubMed]
32. Kabeya, Y.; Mizushima, N.; Ueno, T.; Yamamoto, A.; Kirisako, T.; Noda, T.; Kominami, E.; Ohsumi, Y.; Yoshimori, T. LC3, a mammalian homologue of yeast Apg8p, is localized in autophagosome membranes after processing. *EMBO J.* **2000**, *19*, 5720–5728. [CrossRef] [PubMed]
33. Kimura, S.; Noda, T.; Yoshimori, T. Dissection of the autophagosome maturation process by a novel reporter protein, tandem fluorescent-tagged LC3. *Autophagy* **2007**, *3*, 452–460. [CrossRef] [PubMed]
34. Antonioli, M.; Di Rienzo, M.; Piacentini, M.; Fimia, G.M. Emerging mechanisms in initiating and terminating autophagy. *Trends Biochem. Sci.* **2017**, *42*, 28–41. [CrossRef] [PubMed]
35. Wu, Y.-T.; Tan, H.-L.; Shui, G.; Bauvy, C.; Huang, Q.; Wenk, M.R.; Ong, C.-N.; Codogno, P.; Shen, H.-M. Dual

role of 3-methyladenine in modulation of autophagy via different temporal patterns of inhibition on class I and III phosphoinositide 3-kinase. *J. Biol. Chem.* **2010**, *285*, 10850–10861. [CrossRef]

36. White, E. The role for autophagy in cancer. *J. Clin. Investig.* **2015**, *125*, 42–46. [CrossRef]
37. Folkerts, H.; Hilgendorf, S.; Vellenga, E.; Bremer, E.; Wiersma, V.R. The multifaceted role of autophagy in cancer and the microenvironment. *Med. Res. Rev.* **2019**, *39*, 517–560. [CrossRef]
38. Zhao, Y.G.; Zhang, H. Autophagosome maturation: An epic journey from the ER to lysosomes. *J. Cell Biol.* **2019**, *218*, 757–770. [CrossRef]
39. Pierzyńska-Mach, A.; Janowski, P.A.; Dobrucki, J.W. Evaluation of acridine orange, LysoTracker Red, and quinacrine as fluorescent probes for long-term tracking of acidic vesicles. *Cytometry A* **2014**, *85*, 729–737. [CrossRef]
40. Repnik, U.; Hafner Česen, M.; Turk, B. Strategies for assaying lysosomal membrane permeabilization. *Cold Spring Harb. Protoc.* **2016**, *2016*. [CrossRef]
41. Song, W.; Popp, L.; Yang, J.; Kumar, A.; Gangoli, V.S.; Segatori, L. The autophagic response to polystyrene nanoparticles is mediated by transcription factor EB and depends on surface charge. *J. Nanobiotechnol.* **2015**, *13*, 87. [CrossRef] [PubMed]
42. Lai, Y.-K.; Lee, W.-C.; Hu, C.-H.; Hammond, G.L. The mitochondria are recognition organelles of cell stress. *J. Surg. Res.* **1996**, *62*, 90–94. [CrossRef] [PubMed]
43. Shirmohammadi, F.; Hasheminassab, S.; Saffari, A.; Schauer, J.J.; Delfino, R.J.; Sioutas, C. Fine and ultrafine particulate organic carbon in the Los Angeles basin: Trends in sources and composition. *Sci. Total Environ.* **2016**, *541*, 1083–1096. [CrossRef] [PubMed]

8

Alveolar Epithelial Type II Cells as Drivers of Lung Fibrosis in Idiopathic Pulmonary Fibrosis

Tanyalak Parimon [1,*], Changfu Yao [1], Barry R Stripp [1,2], Paul W Noble [1] and Peter Chen [1,2]

[1] Division of Pulmonary and Critical Care Medicine, Department of Medicine, Women's Guild Lung Institute, Cedars-Sinai Medical Center, Los Angeles, CA 90048, USA; Changfu.Yao@CSMC.edu (C.Y.); Barry.Stripp@cshs.org (B.R.S.); Paul.Noble@cshs.org (P.W.N.); Peter.Chen@cshs.org (P.C.)

[2] Department of Biomedical Sciences, Cedars-Sinai Medical Center, Los Angeles, CA 90048, USA

* Correspondence: Tanyalak.parimon@cshs.org

Abstract: Alveolar epithelial type II cells (AT2) are a heterogeneous population that have critical secretory and regenerative roles in the alveolus to maintain lung homeostasis. However, impairment to their normal functional capacity and development of a pro-fibrotic phenotype has been demonstrated to contribute to the development of idiopathic pulmonary fibrosis (IPF). A number of factors contribute to AT2 death and dysfunction. As a mucosal surface, AT2 cells are exposed to environmental stresses that can have lasting effects that contribute to fibrogenesis. Genetical risks have also been identified that can cause AT2 impairment and the development of lung fibrosis. Furthermore, aging is a final factor that adds to the pathogenic changes in AT2 cells. Here, we will discuss the homeostatic role of AT2 cells and the studies that have recently defined the heterogeneity of this population of cells. Furthermore, we will review the mechanisms of AT2 death and dysfunction in the context of lung fibrosis.

Keywords: alveolar epithelial cells; pulmonary fibrosis; epithelial cell dysfunction; stem cell exhaustion

---

1. Introduction

Idiopathic Pulmonary Fibrosis (IPF) is a chronic, progressive scarring of the lungs that causes significant healthcare burden due to high morbidity and mortality [1–3]. It is the most common form of idiopathic interstitial pneumonia and exhibits the most severe manifestations carrying the poorest clinical outcomes [4–6]. Recently, two anti-fibrotic medications, Pirfenidone and Nintedanib, have been demonstrated to slow the progression of the disease and are now FDA-approved treatments for IPF [7–15]. Despite the progress made after decades of investigation, there is considerable room for improvement in the treatment of this incurable disease.

Pathological fibrogenesis that occurs in IPF is a dynamic process involving complex interactions between epithelial cells, fibroblasts, immune cells (macrophages, T-cells), and endothelial cells [16,17]. Early theories that chronic inflammation and repetitive damage to the alveolar epithelium promotes fibrogenesis and scar formation in the pathogenesis of lung fibrosis [18] have been largely rejected due to the lack of ongoing inflammation in IPF and the general ineffectiveness of immunosuppressive medications in curbing disease progression. In contrast, a preponderance of more recent evidence suggests that the alveolar epithelium plays a central role. Indeed, honeycombed regions of the lungs have discontinuous epithelium adjacent to hyperplastic alveolar epithelial type II cells (AT2) [19]. Accordingly, the more contemporary paradigm is that chronic injury to distal lung tissue leads to either loss or altered function of epithelial stem cells (i.e., AT2 cells), that promote dysregulated repair and pathogenic activation of fibroblasts.

Both intrinsic (e.g., genetic, aging) and environmental factors have been linked to damage of AT2 cells and contribute to the development of lung fibrosis. Tobacco smoking and viral infections have been associated with IPF [4,20]. IPF is also an age-related disease with a median age of diagnosis of 66 years old [21]. As such, several factors that accumulate with age have been found to contribute to AT2 dysfunction in IPF [22]. However, the most direct evidence supporting a role for AT2 cell dysfunction in the initiation and progression of IPF has come from the characterization of gene defects observed among patients with familial forms of the disease. Two general categories of gene mutations are observed; one category includes genes involved in the regulation of stem cell longevity, the other includes genes whose products contribute to specialized secretory functions of AT2 cells [23].

Altogether, the evidence supports a model in which AT2 injury/dysfunction serves as an early initiating event in IPF that leads to fibroproliferation and progressive loss of lung function [24]. AT2 loss can limit the ability for the repair of the damaged alveolus. Additionally, AT2 cells have maladaptive effects in the IPF lung that can drive fibrosis (Figure 1). Herein, we will review the homeostatic role of the AT2 cell and evidence for both AT2 depletion and dysfunction as contributors to IPF.

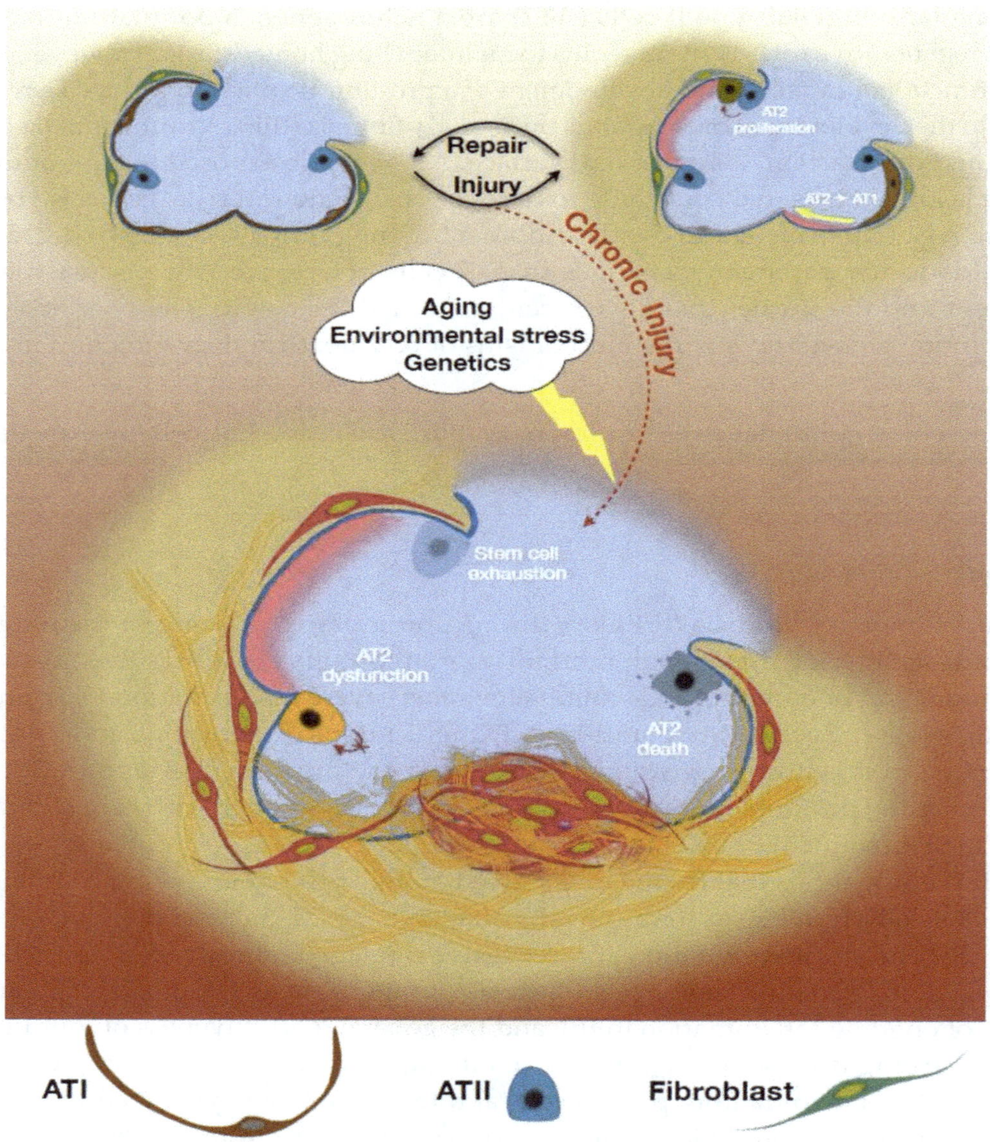

Figure 1. Alveolar epithelial type II cells (AT2) functions in lung fibrosis. An overview schematic illustration described functional roles of AT2 cells to maintain lung homeostasis during injuries and their profibrotic phenotypic changes that promote lung fibrosis upon the presence of risk factors e.g., aging, environmental stress, etc.

2. Alveolar Epithelial Type II Cells (AT2) of the Normal Mammalian Lung

The epithelium lining airspaces of the mammalian lung is maintained by regional stem and progenitor cells that are responsible for replacement of functionally specialized cell types in each compartment during homeostasis and repair [25,26]. In the alveolus, AT2 cells serve as the predominant epithelial progenitor. Lineage tracing experiments in mice show that AT2 cells defined by their expression of surfactant protein C (*Sftpc*/SFTPC) are capable of long-term self-renewal and multipotent differentiation to yield alveolar type I (AT1) cells; two characteristics that suggest either the AT2 population as a whole or a subset of AT2 cells, represent adult tissue stem cells [27]. The observation in this study that a subset of *Sftpc*-lineage positive AT2 cells exhibit greater in vivo clonogenic potential than bulk AT2 cells provides evidence that "stemness" may be a property of a subset of AT2 cells, and by inference, that AT2 cells are functionally heterogeneous. What is not clear from this work is whether AT2 cell heterogeneity is the result of differences in intrinsic potential versus microenvironmental regulation. Recent work defining a Wnt-responsive subset of AT2 cells raises the potential that a Wnt signaling microenvironment may modulate "stemness" of AT2 cells [28,29]; an appealing concept but currently not confirmed by lineage-tracing experiments. However, these data do support the notion that AT2 cells represent a heterogeneous population that includes an abundant pool of facultative progenitors and a more stem-like subset that contributes to homeostatic replacement of specialized alveolar epithelial cells.

Other epithelial stem or progenitor cells have been proposed to contribute to alveolar epithelial renewal and replacement of AT2 cells. So-called bronchio-alveolar stem cells (BASCs) were initially proposed as a multipotent "stem" cell in mouse terminal bronchioles based upon their co-expression of *Sftpc* and *Scgb1a1*, contribution to repair after chemical injury and expansion following induction of activating mutations of the *K-ras* oncogene [30]. Evidence supporting the multipotency and "stemness" of BASCs includes recent studies involving use of dual lineage-tracing strategies demonstrating that *Sftpc/Scgb1a1* dual lineage-labeled cells have potential to contribute to repair following injury to either airways or alveoli [31,32]. However, multipotency of BASCs has currently only been convincingly demonstrated in clonal culture experiments [33], with in vivo confirmation of multipotency confounded by heterogeneity within the lineage-labeled population [32]. Other candidate progenitors for replacement of AT2 cells and the alveolar epithelium include a rare subpopulation of AT1 cells [34] and basal cells that expand to repopulate damaged alveoli following influenza virus infection [35].

3. AT2 Depletion in Idiopathic Pulmonary Fibrosis (IPF)

A prevailing concept is that AT2 depletion potentially through repetitive microinjuries is the underlying cause of lung fibrosis [5]. Indeed, targeted deletion of AT2 cells is sufficient to induce a fibrotic response in the lungs, but it is not sustained [36,37]. Additional data supporting this idea of stem cell exhaustion is that the number of AT2 cells are diminished in IPF lungs [38,39]. However, the depletion of this vital progenitor cell is not only a function of the distorted lung architecture but may also be a precursor to fibrosis [39].

Apoptotic Death of AT2 Cells

Mechanisms of AT2 depletion particularly in the context of early events leading to IPF are not fully elucidated. Clearly, the lung epithelium is under constant stresses as a number of studies have identified increased levels of cells undergoing apoptosis in the lungs from IPF patients, which is not seen in non-fibrotic lungs [40–43]. In fact, TGFβ, a potent pro-fibrotic cytokine, has been demonstrated to mediate its fibroproliferative effects by induction of AT2 apoptosis [44,45]. Apoptosis is a form of programmed cell death that is required as a physiological process for tissue homeostasis but can also be activated in pathological situations [46]. This regulated cell death pathway is tightly controlled at multiple levels, but if the stimulus exceeds a critical threshold, a prescribed pattern of events mediated by caspase cleavage of cellular contents to induce cell death.

In IPF lungs, the Fas-FasL pathway has several components that are upregulated in the alveolar epithelium indicating a preexisting elevation in the signals that induce apoptosis [42,47]. Similar findings were demonstrated in murine models of fibrosis [48]. Global inhibition of apoptosis with captopril or z-VAD also blunts lung fibrosis [49,50]. Additionally, blockade of Fas signaling through various pharmacologic or genetic methods attenuates whereas Fas stimulation augments lung fibrosis in bleomycin-injured mice [51,52]. Many cells that succumb to Fas-mediated death must undergo an amplification loop (type II pathway) that intensifies the death signal by crossing over to the mitochondria through the cleave of BID, a B-cell lymphoma protein-2 (BCL2) family member [53]. Further supporting the importance of the Fas-FasL pathway and apoptosis in general as an important early initiator of lung fibrosis, mice genetically deficient in *Bid* are protected from bleomycin-induced lung fibrosis [45].

4. ER Stress Contributes to AT2 Apoptosis

In addition to receptor-mediated activation of apoptosis, an intrinsic apoptotic pathway can also induce programmed cell death [46]. Various intracellular stresses and damage signals activate pro-apoptotic BCL-2 proteins that permeabilize the mitochondria to release mediators (e.g., cytochrome C) that create a nidus for apoptosome formation and activation of executioner caspases that cause apoptotic death [54].

Endoplasmic reticulum (ER) stress is an important initiator of AT2 apoptosis via the intrinsic pathway that has been linked to IPF [55]. The ER is an important cellular organelle that facilitates the folding and trafficking of proteins to ensure the quality control of proteins required for cellular homeostasis. In situations that overwhelm the protein folding capacity of the ER, the unfolded protein response (UPR) is activated with the aim to restore the physiological activity of the ER. Three transmembrane sensors, specifically inositol-requiring enzyme 1α (IRE1α), pancreatic endoplasmic reticulum kinase (PERK), and activating transcription factor 6 (ATF6), control the UPR [56]. When the UPR is prolonged or severe in nature, proteostasis is lost, and cells become dysfunctional and undergo apoptotic death [55].

Several studies have identified UPR activation in AT2 cells during lung fibrosis [57–59]. Immunohistochemical evaluation of lungs from sporadic and familial IPF demonstrated AT2 co-localization of various ER stress markers and activated caspase-3 [57,58]. Interestingly, AT2 activation of the UPR can be found in histologically normal appearing regions of IPF lungs suggesting ER stress precedes the development of fibrosis. Mice injured with bleomycin also demonstrate ER stress in AT2 cells [59]. More importantly, tunicamycin, an activator of ER stress, augments lung fibrosis [59,60], and specific activation of ER stress in AT2 cells can lead to spontaneous lung fibrosis in transgenic mice [61,62].

Several genetic variants that confer an inherited susceptibility to lung fibrosis can induce ER stress. In particular, pathologic variants of surfactant proteins, which are produced by AT2 cells, have been found to induce ER stress and augment lung fibrosis [23]. In experimental models with transgenic mice that conditionally overexpressed the *SFTPC* mutation (SFTPC^{L188Q}) in AT2 cells, ER stress increased after the induction of the mutant SFTPC^{L188Q} expression [59]. Although these transgenic mice did not develop spontaneous pulmonary fibrosis, they were more susceptible to bleomycin exposure and the resultant injury-induced fibrosis. In contrast, a different *SFTPC* mutation (SFTPC^{C121G}) demonstrated exaggerated ER stress, AT2 apoptosis, and development of spontaneous lung fibrosis after induction of expression in AT2 cells [61].

With aging, the lungs also become more susceptible to ER stress [55]. GRP78 is a chaperone protein that is a central regulator of ER stress by repressing IRE1α, PERK, and ATF6, the three arms that initiate the UPR. A recent study by Borok et al. demonstrated that AT2 expression of GRP78 decreases in both aged mice and in IPF lungs [63]. AT2-specific deletion of *Grp78* induced ER stress, apoptosis and lung fibrosis with an age-dependence on the severity of the effect.

A number of environmental factors that are associated with the development of IPF has also been found to induce ER stress. Smoking, which induces ER stress within the lung epithelium, is associated with an increased risk factor for acquiring IPF [64,65]. Several herpesvirus proteins were identified in AT2 cells that concomitantly showed evidence of UPR activation [20,58]. A recent study also found evidence for increased herpesvirus infections in at-risk subjects for developing interstitial lung disease [66]. Fibrosis can be augmented in mice infected with γherpesvirus [67–70]. Moreover, the viral susceptibility appears be age-related with increased AT2 ER stress and apoptosis, as well as augmented lung fibrosis in old compared to young mice infected with murine γherpesvirus [60,71].

5. Mitochondrial Dysfunction Causes AT2 Death

AT2 cells have the highest number of mitochondria in the lungs due to their high metabolic demands, especially during lung injury and repair [72]. Disturbance and interference of AT2 mitochondrial biogenesis, functions, and homeostasis is a known profibrotic signal [73–75]. The imbalance of mitochondrial dynamic due to impaired mitophagy and accumulation of mtDNA damage or irregularities of protein homeostasis leads to ER stress and program cell death of AT2 cells [74,76]. An accumulation of higher dysmorphic mitochondria (i.e., damaged mitochondria) and ER stress proteins in AT2 cells in IPF compared to control lungs suggests the significance of mitochondria dysfunction in the pathogenesis of lung fibrosis [60,77].

Mitochondrial homeostasis is regulated by integrated pathways primarily for biogenesis and recycling/disposal through mitophagy [78]. Mitofusin 1 and 2 are GTPases required for mitochondrial fusion, and AT2 deletion of either gene augmented lung fibrosis after bleomycin injury [79]. Moreover, combined AT2 deletion of both mitofusin 1 and 2 lead to spontaneous lung fibrosis. Transgenic mice expressing mitochondrial-targeted catalase (MCAT) are also protected from asbestos- and bleomycin-induced lung fibrosis mediated through the inhibition of AT2 cell mtDNA damage and apoptosis [80]. Corroborating with these data, the deficiency of sirtuin 3, a NAD-dependent deacetylase that prevents mtDNA damage, in AT2 cells promoted lung fibrosis by inducing cells apoptosis [81].

PTEN-induced putative kinase 1 (PINK1), a mitochondrial factor that facilitates mitophagy, is depleted during ER stress, with aging, and within fibrotic lungs [60,82,83]. AT2 cells in *Pink1* deficient mice are morphologically similar to AT2 cells in IPF lung, [60]. Furthermore, bleomycin-induced lung fibrosis is augmented in *Pink1* deficient mice and associated with less mitophagy, accumulation of dysmorphic mitochondria, and increased ER stress and AT2 apoptosis [60,77]. Activating transcription factor 3 (*Aft3*), a *Pink1* transcription repressor, has higher expression in fibrotic and aged lungs, suggesting this factor may account for the concomitant depletion of *Pink1* in similar conditions [60,82]. Accordingly, conditional AT2 deletion of *Aft3* protects mice from developing lung fibrosis [82]. Further demonstrating the importance of mitophagy in mediating IPF, a recent finding demonstrated a dysfunctional thyroid axis in IPF, and thyroid hormone administration increased *Pink1* levels, attenuated AT2 apoptosis, and reduced lung fibrosis via a *Pink1*-dependent mechanism [83].

A conflicting finding recently emerged where *Pgam5* deficient mice had decreased mitophagy that improved mitochondrial homeostasis, which had a protective effect during bleomycin-induced lung fibrosis [84]. Because these findings were in global *Pgam5* deficient mice, one possible explanation for the contradictory results is that mitophagy may potentially have profibrotic roles in non-AT2 compartments. Nevertheless, the majority of the evidence suggests mitophagy has a protective effect in AT2 cells and in preventing lung fibrosis [60,77,82,83].

6. AT2 Dysfunction in IPF

Persistent injury to the AT2 compartment not only causes a depletion of these facultative progenitor cells but can also cause irreversible alterations the capacity of these vital cells in carrying out their reparative functions. Indeed, hypertrophic and hyperplastic AT2 cells are found in the fibroblastic foci and have impaired renewal capacity [85]. Furthermore, dysfunctional AT2 cells in the fibrotic lung also produce pro-fibrotic factors that contribute to fibrogenesis [24]. Altogether, AT2 cells are not just simply depleted in the fibrotic lung as collateral damage to ongoing injury, but in addition, these cells have acquired a dysfunctional phenotype that places it as a central driver of fibrosis [37] as depicted in Figure 2.

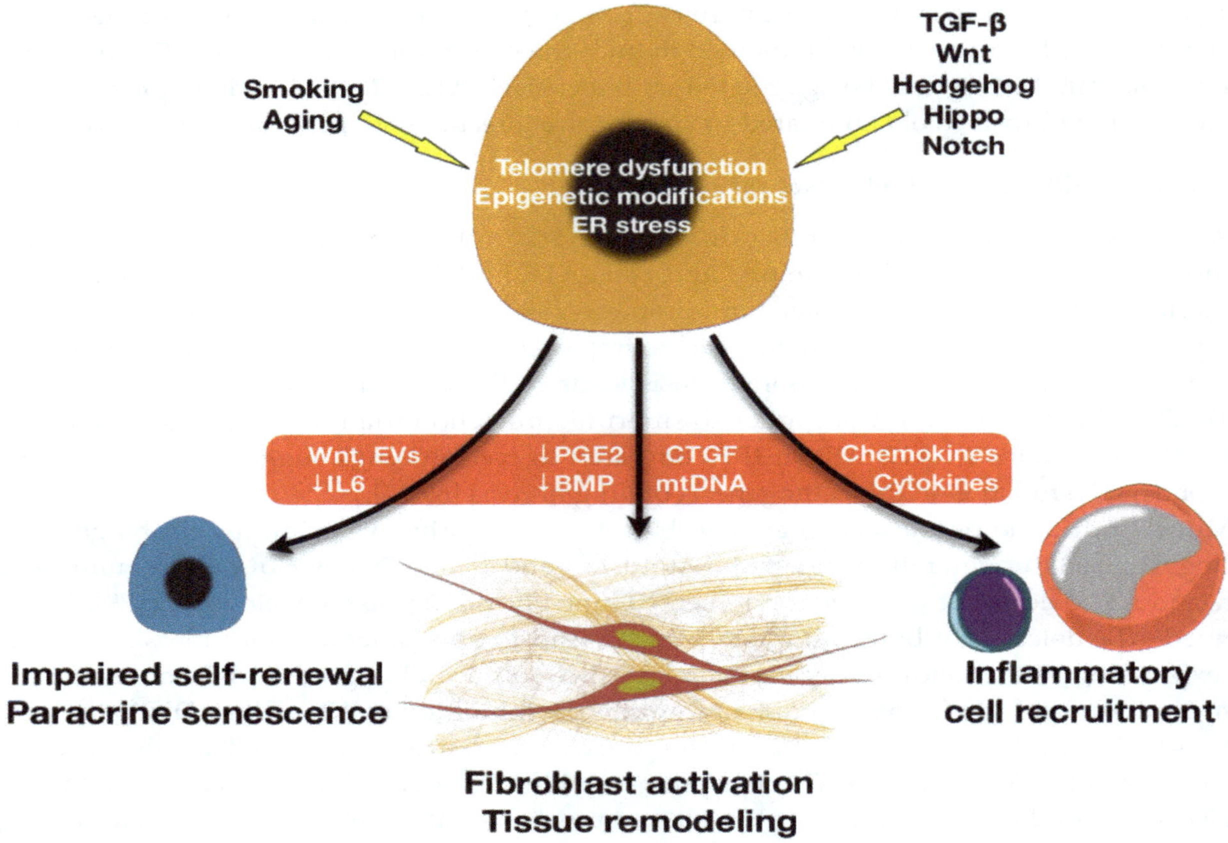

Figure 2. Mechanisms and regulatory signaling of alveolar type II epithelial cells (AT2) dysfunction in lung fibrosis. In lung fibrosis, environmental or intrinsic factors and several signaling regulatory pathways e.g., TGF-β, Wnt, Hedgehog, etc. stimulate AT2 senescence to release senescence-associated secretory phenotype (SASP) and other mediators that can directly activate fibroblasts and tissue remodeling. The indirect effects of SASP include inflammatory cell recruitment and AT2 self-renewal exhaustion through a paracrine effect.

AT2 plasticity has been best demonstrated by the ability of TGFβ to alter their cellular phenotype [86–88]. Although epithelial cells do not directly contribute to the mesenchymal population in IPF [89], what has become evident is that the AT2 cells develop a fundamentally altered state in the IPF lung and acquire a distinctly pro-fibrotic phenotype that promotes expansion of the mesenchymal compartment with myofibroblast activation and matrix deposition [90]. In one respect, the inability of AT2 cells to carry out proper repair of the injured alveolus can lead to scar formation [85]. In fact, AT2 cells play a central role in the activation of TGFβ, which may be self-perpetuating through the rising tension within a fibrotic lung [91]. Additionally, AT2 cells have diminished capacity for transdifferentiation into AT1 cells in the IPF lungs [5]. As such, both ER stress and telomere dysfunction, both of which have the potential to activate a program of cellular senescence, have been found to impair differentiation by stem cells [92–96]. Emerging evidence also demonstrates that induction of AT2 senescence in itself is sufficient to promote lung fibrosis [37].

7. Impaired AT2 Self-Renewal in IPF

Cellular senescence, one of the signature characterizations of the aging process, plays an important role in the pathogenesis of lung fibroproliferative disorders [97–99]. Fibrotic regions of lung tissue from IPF patients show both regional depletion of AT2 cells and the presence of AT2 cells with a senescent-like phenotype [37,38]. As such, AT2 senescence may have a limited reparative capacity that contributes to the fibroproliferation [22,100]. In support of this concept, senolytics show some potential as anti-fibrotics in animal models [101–103]. Moreover, ER stress may not only contribute to IPF through UPR-mediated AT2 death but can also impair the renewal capacity of AT2 cells by inducing cellular senescence [63]. This effect appears to be ubiquitous as the regenerative capacity of multiple types of stem cells is impaired with ER stress [92].

A major contributor to cellular senescence in lung fibrosis is telomere dysfunction [93,104]. Telomeres protect the ends of chromosomes from replicative loss through providing a mechanism for telomerase-dependent repeat expansion, thus maintaining the proliferative potential of stem and progenitor cells [105]. Shortened telomere length has been found in a subset of patients with IPF and correlates with poor survival [66,106,107]. Smoking, a risk factor for IPF, also causes a dose-dependent shortening of telomeres [108]. Similarly, telomere attrition also occurs with aging, another risk for the development of IPF [104].

A number of variants in genes that regulate telomere function has been found in IPF and could be contributing to AT2 senescence and impairment in their renewal capacity [23]. Mutations in *TERC* and *TERT*, telomerase reverse transcriptase family genes that regulate telomere length and functions, are linked to IPF [107,109–112]. A null *TERT* allele conferred a dominant transmission of disease in a familial form of pulmonary fibrosis (FIP) [109]. Risk variants of regulator of telomere elongation helicase 1 (*RTEL1*), a DNA helicase necessary for telomere stability, is also linked to FIP [113–115]. Subsequent studies have also found *TERT* and *RTEL1* mutations to be enriched in patients with IPF [116]. Moreover, a number of other genetic variants in *DKC1* [117], *PARN* [115,116], *NAF1* [118], and *TINF2* [119,120] have been found in FIP and associated with short telomeres. Various animal models have also demonstrated the impact of telomeres in lung fibrosis. Mice with AT2-specific *Tert* deficiency did not develop spontaneous lung fibrosis but upon bleomycin injury had more AT2 senescence and more lung fibrosis [94]. In contrast, conditional AT2 deletion of telomere repeat-binding factor 1 (TRF1), a telomere shelterin protein, caused mice to develop spontaneous lung fibrosis due to an impairment of telomere integrity [95,121].

Several non-cell autonomous factors also contribute to AT2 health and self-renewal capacity [122]. Indeed, the extracellular matrix (ECM) also has a role in the maintenance of AT2 cells [122], and these cell-matrix interactions recently were revealed to be dysfunctional in IPF, diminishing the renewal capacity of these stem cells [39]. Hyaluronan (HA) is a glycosaminoglycan that has increased abundance in the IPF ECM and can promote fibroblast invasiveness to mediate progressive lung fibrosis [123,124]. Interestingly, HA is expressed on the cell surface of normal AT2 cells and promotes stem cell renewal in a Toll-like receptor 4-dependent manner through the release of IL-6 [39]. AT2 cells also have a deficiency in HA signaling during lung fibrosis, leading to IL-6-dependent reductions in their renewal capacity [39]. Furthermore, targeted deletion of hyaluronan synthase 2 in murine AT2 cells leads to loss of progenitor cell functions and increased susceptibility to bleomycin-induced fibrosis [39].

8. Dysregulated Signaling Pathways Causing Intrinsic AT2 Dysfunction in IPF

Advances in single genomics have provided unprecedented opportunities to reveal changes in cellular states during normal development, tissue homeostasis, and disease. As applied to IPF patient samples, these studies have demonstrated reactivation of a series of key developmental pathways (e.g., Wnt, Hippo, Hedgehog, Notch) and the induction of altered cell states (senescence, apoptosis), that provide insights into mechanisms of altered AT2 function [38,125–127]. The Wnt pathway is a particularly prominent signal that is reactivated in fibrotic lungs [125–130]. Although Wnt signaling is necessary for maintaining AT2 self-renewal in development [28,29,131], the aged lung has a maladaptive response where Wnt induces cellular senescence [132,133]. As such, inhibition of Wnt signaling improves lung fibrosis in bleomycin-challenged mice [134–136]. One of the key AT2 functions is to transdifferentiate into AT1 cells. Because of the essential AT1 role in gas exchange,

AT2 self-renewal is an important feature of to provide an endless reparative population that is ready to respond to any injury that damages the alveolar surface [137]. Wnt signaling is a developmental pathway that is activated in adult AT2 cells to drive AT1 transdifferentiation [138]. However, Wnt signaling is largely established as a nefarious event in IPF [128–130]. One possible way to reconcile these divergent observations is that the activated Wnt pathways are a sign of ongoing repair and regeneration of damaged alveoli [139]. Another more likely explanation is that homeostatic signals become maladapted in pathological situations with Wnt signaling causing damaging effects, such as induction of AT2 senescence [132,133].

Hippo signaling, which primarily mediates its signaling via Yes-associated protein (YAP) and transcriptional coactivator with PDZ-binding motif (TAZ), is an evolutionarily conserved pathway that crosses over with Wnt signaling [140,141]. TAZ is expressed by embryonic epithelium and is necessary for branching morphogenesis and alveolarization by promoting AT1 differentiation [142–147]. YAP/TAZ activity is an important transducer of extracellular cues that has important effects in fibrotic lung diseases [148]. In particular, fibroblasts use this mechanosensing pathway to promote a fibrotic phenotype in the fibrotic lung [149–151]. A prediction would be that the epithelium may also alter their phenotype in the IPF as a result of the increased stiffness within their microenvironment. Indeed, Hippo signaling is dysregulated in AT2 cells in the IPF lung to alter cell shape, proliferation, and migration as a possible contributor to lung fibrosis [152].

Notch is another developmental control pathway that regulates cell differentiation and fate through mechanisms involving lateral inhibition [153]. Upon ligand binding, Notch receptors (Notch 1 through 4) are cleaved by γ-secretase, which releases the Notch intracellular domain (NICD) that translocates to the nucleus and induces target gene (e.g., HES, HEY) transcription [154]. Although Notch has distinct roles in distal lung development, AT2 cells also require Notch signaling to coordinate crosstalk with myofibroblasts for proper alveologenesis [155,156]. Reactivation of Notch signaling has been found to be profibrotic in skin, kidney, and cardiac fibrosis [157], and Notch pathways are re-activated in AT2 cells within the IPF lungs [125,158]. Interestingly, alveolar differentiation is inhibited with persistent Notch signaling, which led to a failure to regenerate the damaged alveolus and development of honeycombed cysts that are akin to the pathology found in IPF [159]. Furthermore, Notch activation in AT2 cells induces, whereas Notch inhibition attenuates lung fibrosis [158].

9. Altered AT2-Fibroblast Signaling in IPF

AT2-fibroblast interactions are tightly coordinated in lung development, and this unit works in conjunction after injury to repair a damaged alveolus [29,155,156,160]. This epithelial-mesenchymal crosstalk is clearly disrupted in IPF such that AT2 cells acquire a profibrotic phenotype to aberrantly secrete profibrotic mediators as paracrine factors that stimulate and activate fibroblasts [24]. In fact, TGFβ is predominantly produced by the epithelium where the integrins needed for activation of the latent form is primarily expressed, and abrogation of TGFβ signaling within the lung epithelium can attenuate lung fibrosis [91,161–164]. CTGF is produced by the lung epithelium in response to TGFβ signaling and plays a vital profibrotic role by stimulating collagen deposition by fibroblasts [165–167]. AT2 cells have increased expression of CTGF in bleomycin-induced lung fibrosis, whereas blockade can abrogate fibrosis [167–169]. Hippo signaling (via YAP) also induces activation of target genes such as CTGF and could partially explain how the reactivation of this developmental pathway in IPF contributes to the disease [152]. Release of mtDNA from damaged AT2 cells may also contribute to fibroblast activation in IPF [76].

Hedgehog signaling is a key regulator of the epithelial-mesenchymal interactions during development and fibrosis [127,160,170]. Hedgehog is regulated by the patched surface receptors and upon ligand binding releases smoothened to activate the Gli-family transcription factors [171]. This pathway is active in the alveolar epithelium during alveolarization, after injury, and in tumors as a means to crosstalk with mesenchymal cells and coordinate their activity [152,170]. In the adult lung, hedgehog signaling controls the epithelial-mesenchymal unit by maintaining fibroblast quiescence at homeostasis and during resolution after injury [160]. Pathological reactivation of hedgehog signaling in the alveolar compartment occurs in IPF and in bleomycin-induced lung fibrosis, and pharmacologic and genetic blockade of the hedgehog epithelial-fibroblast crosstalk can attenuate experimental lung fibrosis [127,172–178]. In contrast, it was recently demonstrated that mice deficient in *Gli1* were not protected from lung fibrosis suggesting either *Gli2* or non-canonical hedgehog signaling may be regulating pathological effects in lung fibrosis [179].

The epithelium has defined properties that appear to keep the mesenchymal compartment in check at homeostasis [160,180–183]. Prostaglandin E2 (PGE2) levels are suppressed in IPF and have been identified as an important epithelial factor that suppresses fibroblast proliferation and activation [183–185]. Recently, bone morphogenic protein (BMP) was also identified to mediate a similar inhibitory effect on fibroblasts [186]. Thus, AT2 cells not only promote fibrosis through release of profibrotic mediators, but the loss of negative reinforcement factors such as PGE2 and BMP can contribute to fibroproliferation.

10. The Senescence-associated Secretory Phenotype Has Pro-fibrotic Effects

AT2 senescence plays a prominent role in lung fibrosis through the acquisition of a senescence-associated secretory phenotype (SASP) and is a feature of senescent cells that result in the release of a myriad of factors with inflammatory and fibrogenic properties [187]. AT2 cells within the lungs of IPF patients and bleomycin-injured mice gain features consistent with a SASP [37,38,93,125,126]. Indeed, a number of secreted inflammatory and profibrotic factors are released from AT2 cells within the fibrotic lung that can have autocrine and paracrine actions within the fibrotic microenvironment to promote lung fibrosis [24].

Several genetic variants have been found to be associated with lung fibrosis and could be mediating fibrosis through the development of the SASP in AT2 cells. Telomere-mediated senescence causes the SASP [93], and it is plausible that the various telomerase mutations associated with lung fibrosis mediate their pro-fibrotic effects by inducing a SASP in AT2 cells [107,109–112]. Hermansky–Pudlak syndrome (HPS) is an autosomal recessive disease that causes oculocutaneous albinism, bleeding diathesis, and lung fibrosis [188]. AT2 produced excessive monocyte chemotactic protein-1 (MCP-1, also known as C-C motif ligand 2 (CCL2)) that in turn promoted macrophage recruitments and TGFβ production leading to lung fibrosis [189]. This finding is consistent with the acquisition of a SASP. A *SFTPC* genetic variant associated with IPF (*SFPTC*^{I73T}) also induces AT2 secretion of several chemokines, which are consistent with a SASP, to recruit Ly6C^{hi}CD64^{-} monocytes [62]. Although not evaluated, this constellation of findings suggests a SASP may also be regulating the development of the spontaneous fibrosis found in this murine model.

Interestingly, a "bystander effect" is found with cellular senescence in which paracrine factors can induce neighboring cells to undergo cellular senescence [190–192]. Notch signaling can also promote the transfer of the senescent phenotype, which makes one posit if Notch activation in IPF may be perpetuating cell senescence in neighboring cells [193–195]. Extracellular vesicles (EVs) are released from cells and carry a number of factors including proteins, nucleic acids, and lipids as cargo that can be delivered to distal cells as a means of intercellular communication [196]. EVs not only change quantity and quality with cell senescence but can also play a role in causing senescence through a variety of cargo [197]. Recent evidence demonstrates increased EV production in IPF lungs could potentially be produced by senescent cells; Moreover, these EVs carry cargo such as interferon-induced transmembrane protein 3 to promote paracrine senescence [198]. EV quantify increases in the IPF lungs, and EVs isolated from fibrotic lungs can augment fibroproliferation in bleomycin-injured mice [126,199]. Wnt5a, which can induce senescence, is found on EVs from IPF lungs [132,199]. Furthermore, several microRNA cargos within EVs from IPF lungs have been found to regulate cellular senescence [126]. With the ability of EVs to carry a number of cargos that can functionally regulate distal cell phenotype, they are poised to facilitate cellular dysfunction in lung fibrosis and understanding how EVs mediate the pathological effects of the SASP could lead to interesting targets for therapeutic intervention.

11. Epigenetic Changes in the AT2 Promote Lung Fibrosis

The accumulation of environmental and age-related stresses over time can permanently reshape the cellular response through epigenetic changes [200]. Epigenetics refers to hereditable changes in gene expression that occur in the absence of DNA sequence alterations. Specifically, DNA methylation, histone modifications, chromatin high-order structure and remodeling, and noncoding RNAs regulate genetic accessibility to the transcriptional machinery and post-transcriptional regulation of protein translation [201]. Distinctly different patterns of DNA methylation are found in IPF patients, and multiple histone modifications have been associated with alterations in key pro-fibrotic pathways [200,202–204].

IPF tends to occur in older adults, and aging is an inherent risk in accumulating epigenetic changes [24,205–207]. IPF is more prevalent in smokers [4], and several lines of evidence have demonstrated tobacco smoke to induce long-lasting changes in gene expression, which are largely attributed to epigenetic modification of the lung epithelium [208–212]. Moreover, differential patterns in DNA methylation patterns can be determined by gender, which may also contribute to the increased incidence of IPF in males [213–216]. Several lines of evidence support the ability of epigenetic modulators to alter the course of lung fibrosis. Changes to the methylation state and Histone deacetylase (HDAC) inhibition by pharmacological treatment or with genetically-modified mice can blunt lung fibrosis [37,217–222]. Several noncoding RNAs have also been demonstrated to regulate lung fibrosis [200,223].

Noncoding RNAs operate through suppress of protein translation, and although without controversy, is generally considered epigenetic modifiers [201]. Moreover, multiple lines of evidence support a crossover of traditional mechanisms of epigenetic modification with microRNA expression. For example, HDAC3 controls expression of the miR-17-92 family to regulate TGFβ expression, which controls alveolar sacculation [224]. The miR-17-92 family has decreased expression in IPF and after bleomycin-induced fibrosis, whereas augmented expression after 5′-aza-2′-deoxycytidine treatment attenuated lung fibrosis [217]. The Dlk-Dio3 domain is an imprinted region that contains clusters of miRNAs and genes [225]. Methylation of the paternal intergenic germline-derived differentially methylated region (IG-DMR) represses miRNA expression from this allele such that only the miRNAs on the maternally inherited allele are transcribed [226]. Expression changes of miRNAs within the Dlk-Dio3 regions alters WNT signaling and has been associated with lung fibrosis [227,228]. Similar to the miR-17-92 family, HDAC3 controls the expression of the microRNAs within the Dlk-Dio3 region [224]. Moreover, microRNAs in the Dlk-Dio3 region have decreased expression in fibrotic conditions and can target TGFβ expression and signaling [180,224]. In particular, miR-323a-3p, which is located in the Dlk-Dio3 region, has been demonstrated to attenuate lung fibrosis in bleomycin-injured mice [180].

12. Conclusions

AT2 cells as a driver of IPF is an established concept supported by an abundance of evidence that demonstrates their loss and dysfunction to have a central role in fibroproliferation. Recent delineation of AT2 subsets has improved the understanding of the way these cells participate in lung development and repair after injury. What remains to be determined is how this cellular heterogeneity may have differential AT2 responses to the various environmental exposures, genetics, and age-associated changes that contribute to injury and culminate over time in a dysfunctional phenotype that shifts from reparative programs to pathogenic fibrogenesis.

Abbreviations

IPF	Idiopathic Pulmonary Fibrosis
FDA	U.S. Food and Drug Administration

U.S. The United States of America

AT2 Alveolar Epithelial Type II Cells

References

1. Ley, B.; Collard, H.R.; King, T.E., Jr. Clinical course and prediction of survival in idiopathic pulmonary fibrosis. *Am. J. Respir. Crit. Care Med.* **2011**, *183*, 431–440. [CrossRef]
2. Hutchinson, J.; Fogarty, A.; Hubbard, R.; McKeever, T. Global incidence and mortality of idiopathic pulmonary fibrosis: A systematic review. *Eur. Respir. J.* **2015**, *46*, 795–806. [CrossRef] [PubMed]
3. Hutchinson, J.P.; McKeever, T.M.; Fogarty, A.W.; Navaratnam, V.; Hubbard, R.B. Increasing Global Mortality from Idiopathic Pulmonary Fibrosis in the Twenty-First Century. *Ann. ATS* **2014**, *11*, 1176–1185. [CrossRef] [PubMed]
4. Martinez, F.J.; Collard, H.R.; Pardo, A.; Raghu, G.; Richeldi, L.; Selman, M.; Swigris, J.J.; Taniguchi, H.; Wells, A.U. Idiopathic pulmonary fibrosis. *Nat. Rev. Dis. Primers* **2017**, *3*, 17074. [CrossRef] [PubMed]
5. Noble, P.W.; Barkauskas, C.E.; Jiang, D. Pulmonary fibrosis: Patterns and perpetrators. *J. Clin. Investig.* **2012**, *122*, 2756–2762. [CrossRef] [PubMed]
6. Robbie, H.; Daccord, C.; Chua, F.; Devaraj, A. Evaluating disease severity in idiopathic pulmonary fibrosis. *Eur. Respir. Rev.* **2017**, *26*, 170051. [CrossRef]
7. Karimi-Shah, B.A.; Chowdhury, B.A. Forced vital capacity in idiopathic pulmonary fibrosis—FDA review of pirfenidone and nintedanib. *N. Engl. J. Med.* **2015**, *372*, 1189–1191. [CrossRef]
8. Noble, P.W.; Albera, C.; Bradford, W.Z.; Costabel, U.; Glassberg, M.K.; Kardatzke, D.; King, T.E., Jr.; Lancaster, L.; Sahn, S.A.; Szwarcberg, J.; et al. Pirfenidone in patients with idiopathic pulmonary fibrosis (CAPACITY): Two randomised trials. *Lancet* **2011**, *377*, 1760–1769. [CrossRef]
9. King, T.E., Jr.; Bradford, W.Z.; Castro-Bernardini, S.; Fagan, E.A.; Glaspole, I.; Glassberg, M.K.; Gorina, E.; Hopkins, P.M.; Kardatzke, D.; Lancaster, L.; et al. A phase 3 trial of pirfenidone in patients with idiopathic pulmonary fibrosis. *N. Engl. J. Med.* **2014**, *370*, 2083–2092. [CrossRef]
10. Noble, P.W.; Albera, C.; Bradford, W.Z.; Costabel, U.; Du Bois, R.M.; Fagan, E.A.; Fishman, R.S.; Glaspole, I.; Glassberg, M.K.; Lancaster, L.; et al. Pirfenidone for idiopathic pulmonary fibrosis: Analysis of pooled data from three multinational phase 3 trials. *Eur. Respir. J.* **2016**, *47*, 243–253. [CrossRef]
11. Richeldi, L.; Costabel, U.; Selman, M.; Kim, D.S.; Hansell, D.M.; Nicholson, A.G.; Brown, K.K.; Flaherty, K.R.; Noble, P.W.; Raghu, G.; et al. Efficacy of a tyrosine kinase inhibitor in idiopathic pulmonary fibrosis. *N. Engl. J. Med.* **2011**, *365*, 1079–1087. [CrossRef] [PubMed]
12. Richeldi, L.; Du Bois, R.M.; Raghu, G.; Azuma, A.; Brown, K.K.; Costabel, U.; Cottin, V.; Flaherty, K.R.; Hansell, D.M.; Inoue, Y.; et al. Efficacy and safety of nintedanib in idiopathic pulmonary fibrosis. *N. Engl. J. Med.* **2014**, *370*, 2071–2082. [CrossRef] [PubMed]
13. Azuma, A.; Nukiwa, T.; Tsuboi, E.; Suga, M.; Abe, S.; Nakata, K.; Taguchi, Y.; Nagai, S.; Itoh, H.; Ohi, M.; et al. Double-blind, placebo-controlled trial of pirfenidone in patients with idiopathic pulmonary fibrosis. *Am. J. Respir. Crit. Care Med.* **2005**, *171*, 1040–1047. [CrossRef] [PubMed]
14. Corte, T.; Bonella, F.; Crestani, B.; Demedts, M.G.; Richeldi, L.; Coeck, C.; Pelling, K.; Quaresma, M.; Lasky, J.A. Safety, tolerability and appropriate use of nintedanib in idiopathic pulmonary fibrosis. *Respir. Res.* **2015**, *16*, 116. [CrossRef] [PubMed]
15. Costabel, U.; Inoue, Y.; Richeldi, L.; Collard, H.R.; Tschoepe, I.; Stowasser, S.; Azuma, A. Efficacy of Nintedanib in Idiopathic Pulmonary Fibrosis across Prespecified Subgroups in INPULSIS. *Am. J. Respir. Crit. Care Med.* **2016**, *193*, 178–185. [CrossRef] [PubMed]
16. Wynn, T.A. Integrating mechanisms of pulmonary fibrosis. *J. Exp. Med.* **2011**, *208*, 1339–1350. [CrossRef] [PubMed]
17. Barkauskas, C.E.; Noble, P.W. Cellular mechanisms of tissue fibrosis. 7. New insights into the cellular mechanisms of pulmonary fibrosis. *Am. J. Physiol. Cell Physiol.* **2014**, *306*, C987–C996. [CrossRef]
18. Selman, M.; Pardo, A. Role of epithelial cells in idiopathic pulmonary fibrosis: From innocent targets to serial killers. *Proc. Am. Thorac. Soc.* **2006**, *3*, 364–372. [CrossRef]
19. Pardo, A.; Selman, M. Molecular mechanisms of pulmonary fibrosis. *Front. Biosci.* **2002**, *7*, d1743–d1761. [CrossRef]

20. Tang, Y.W.; Johnson, J.E.; Browning, P.J.; Cruz-Gervis, R.A.; Davis, A.; Graham, B.S.; Brigham, K.L.; Oates, J.A., Jr.; Loyd, J.E.; Stecenko, A.A. Herpesvirus DNA is consistently detected in lungs of patients with idiopathic pulmonary fibrosis. *J. Clin. Microbiol.* **2003**, *41*, 2633–2640. [CrossRef]
21. King, T.E., Jr.; Pardo, A.; Selman, M. Idiopathic pulmonary fibrosis. *Lancet* **2011**, *378*, 1949–1961. [CrossRef]
22. Meiners, S.; Eickelberg, O.; Konigshoff, M. Hallmarks of the ageing lung. *Eur. Respir. J.* **2015**, *45*, 807–827. [CrossRef] [PubMed]
23. Garcia, C.K. Insights from human genetic studies of lung and organ fibrosis. *J. Clin. Investig.* **2018**, *128*, 36–44. [CrossRef] [PubMed]
24. Selman, M.; Pardo, A. The leading role of epithelial cells in the pathogenesis of idiopathic pulmonary fibrosis. *Cell Signal.* **2019**, *66*, 109482. [CrossRef] [PubMed]
25. Hogan, B.L.; Barkauskas, C.E.; Chapman, H.A.; Epstein, J.A.; Jain, R.; Hsia, C.C.; Niklason, L.; Calle, E.; Le, A.; Randell, S.H.; et al. Repair and regeneration of the respiratory system: Complexity, plasticity, and mechanisms of lung stem cell function. *Cell Stem Cell* **2014**, *15*, 123–138. [CrossRef]
26. Rackley, C.R.; Stripp, B.R. Building and maintaining the epithelium of the lung. *J. Clin. Investig.* **2012**, *122*, 2724–2730. [CrossRef]
27. Barkauskas, C.E.; Cronce, M.J.; Rackley, C.R.; Bowie, E.J.; Keene, D.R.; Stripp, B.R.; Randell, S.H.; Noble, P.W.; Hogan, B.L. Type 2 alveolar cells are stem cells in adult lung. *J. Clin. Investig.* **2013**, *123*, 3025–3036. [CrossRef]
28. Zacharias, W.J.; Frank, D.B.; Zepp, J.A.; Morley, M.P.; Alkhaleel, F.A.; Kong, J.; Zhou, S.; Cantu, E.; Morrisey, E.E. Regeneration of the lung alveolus by an evolutionarily conserved epithelial progenitor. *Nature* **2018**, *555*, 251–255. [CrossRef]
29. Nabhan, A.N.; Brownfield, D.G.; Harbury, P.B.; Krasnow, M.A.; Desai, T.J. Single-cell Wnt signaling niches maintain stemness of alveolar type 2 cells. *Science* **2018**, *359*, 1118–1123. [CrossRef]
30. Kim, C.F.; Jackson, E.L.; Woolfenden, A.E.; Lawrence, S.; Babar, I.; Vogel, S.; Crowley, D.; Bronson, R.T.; Jacks, T. Identification of bronchioalveolar stem cells in normal lung and lung cancer. *Cell* **2005**, *121*, 823–835. [CrossRef]
31. Salwig, I.; Spitznagel, B.; Vazquez-Armendariz, A.I.; Khalooghi, K.; Guenther, S.; Herold, S.; Szibor, M.; Braun, T. Bronchioalveolar stem cells are a main source for regeneration of distal lung epithelia in vivo. *EMBO J.* **2019**, *38*. [CrossRef] [PubMed]
32. Liu, Q.; Liu, K.; Cui, G.; Huang, X.; Yao, S.; Guo, W.; Qin, Z.; Li, Y.; Yang, R.; Pu, W.; et al. Lung regeneration by multipotent stem cells residing at the bronchioalveolar-duct junction. *Nat. Genet.* **2019**, *51*, 728–738. [CrossRef] [PubMed]
33. Lee, J.H.; Bhang, D.H.; Beede, A.; Huang, T.L.; Stripp, B.R.; Bloch, K.D.; Wagers, A.J.; Tseng, Y.H.; Ryeom, S.; Kim, C.F. Lung stem cell differentiation in mice directed by endothelial cells via a BMP4-NFATc1-thrombospondin-1 axis. *Cell* **2014**, *156*, 440–455. [CrossRef] [PubMed]
34. Jain, R.; Barkauskas, C.E.; Takeda, N.; Bowie, E.J.; Aghajanian, H.; Wang, Q.; Padmanabhan, A.; Manderfield, L.J.; Gupta, M.; Li, D.; et al. Plasticity of Hopx(+) type I alveolar cells to regenerate type II cells in the lung. *Nat. Commun.* **2015**, *6*, 6727. [CrossRef] [PubMed]
35. Kumar, P.A.; Hu, Y.; Yamamoto, Y.; Hoe, N.B.; Wei, T.S.; Mu, D.; Sun, Y.; Joo, L.S.; Dagher, R.; Zielonka, E.M.; et al. Distal airway stem cells yield alveoli in vitro and during lung regeneration following H1N1 influenza infection. *Cell* **2011**, *147*, 525–538. [CrossRef] [PubMed]
36. Sisson, T.H.; Mendez, M.; Choi, K.; Subbotina, N.; Courey, A.; Cunningham, A.; Dave, A.; Engelhardt, J.F.; Liu, X.; White, E.S.; et al. Targeted injury of type II alveolar epithelial cells induces pulmonary fibrosis. *Am. J. Respir. Crit. Care Med.* **2010**, *181*, 254–263. [CrossRef] [PubMed]
37. Yao, C.; Guan, X.; Carraro, G.; Parimon, T.; Liu, X.; Huang, G.; Soukiasian, H.J.; David, G.; Weigt, S.S.; Belperio, J.A.; et al. Senescence of alveolar stem cells drives progressive pulmonary fibrosis. *Cell Stem Cell* **2019**, *59*, 00545. [CrossRef]
38. Xu, Y.; Mizuno, T.; Sridharan, A.; Du, Y.; Guo, M.; Tang, J.; Wikenheiser-Brokamp, K.A.; Perl, A.-K.T.; Funari, V.A.; Gokey, J.J.; et al. Single-cell RNA sequencing identifies diverse roles of epithelial cells in idiopathic pulmonary fibrosis. *JCI Insight* **2016**, *1*, e90558. [CrossRef] [PubMed]
39. Liang, J.; Zhang, Y.; Xie, T.; Liu, N.; Chen, H.; Geng, Y.; Kurkciyan, A.; Mena, J.M.; Stripp, B.R.; Jiang, D.; et al. Hyaluronan and TLR4 promote surfactant-protein-C-positive alveolar progenitor cell renewal and prevent severe pulmonary fibrosis in mice. *Nat. Med.* **2016**, *22*, 1285–1293. [CrossRef]

40. Uhal, B.D.; Joshi, I.; Hughes, W.F.; Ramos, C.; Pardo, A.; Selman, M. Alveolar epithelial cell death adjacent to underlying myofibroblasts in advanced fibrotic human lung. *Am. J. Physiol.* **1998**, *275*, L1192–L1199. [CrossRef]
41. Barbas-Filho, J.V.; Ferreira, M.A.; Sesso, A.; Kairalla, R.A.; Carvalho, C.R.; Capelozzi, V.L. Evidence of type II pneumocyte apoptosis in the pathogenesis of idiopathic pulmonary fibrosis (IFP)/usual interstitial pneumonia (UIP). *J. Clin. Pathol.* **2001**, *54*, 132–138. [CrossRef] [PubMed]
42. Maeyama, T.; Kuwano, K.; Kawasaki, M.; Kunitake, R.; Hagimoto, N.; Matsuba, T.; Yoshimi, M.; Inoshima, I.; Yoshida, K.; Hara, N. Upregulation of Fas-signalling molecules in lung epithelial cells from patients with idiopathic pulmonary fibrosis. *Eur. Respir. J.* **2001**, *17*, 180–189. [CrossRef] [PubMed]
43. Plataki, M.; Koutsopoulos, A.V.; Darivianaki, K.; Delides, G.; Siafakas, N.M.; Bouros, D. Expression of apoptotic and antiapoptotic markers in epithelial cells in idiopathic pulmonary fibrosis. *Chest* **2005**, *127*, 266–274. [CrossRef] [PubMed]
44. Lee, C.G.; Cho, S.J.; Kang, M.J.; Chapoval, S.P.; Lee, P.J.; Noble, P.W.; Yehualaeshet, T.; Lu, B.; Flavell, R.A.; Milbrandt, J.; et al. Early growth response gene 1-mediated apoptosis is essential for transforming growth factor beta1-induced pulmonary fibrosis. *J. Exp. Med.* **2004**, *200*, 377–389. [CrossRef] [PubMed]
45. Budinger, G.R.; Mutlu, G.M.; Eisenbart, J.; Fuller, A.C.; Bellmeyer, A.A.; Baker, C.M.; Wilson, M.; Ridge, K.; Barrett, T.A.; Lee, V.Y.; et al. Proapoptotic Bid is required for pulmonary fibrosis. *Proc. Natl. Acad. Sci. USA* **2006**, *103*, 4604–4609. [CrossRef]
46. Galluzzi, L.; Vitale, I.; Aaronson, S.A.; Abrams, J.M.; Adam, D.; Agostinis, P.; Alnemri, E.S.; Altucci, L.; Amelio, I.; Andrews, D.W.; et al. Molecular mechanisms of cell death: Recommendations of the Nomenclature Committee on Cell Death 2018. *Cell Death Differ.* **2018**, *25*, 486–541. [CrossRef]
47. Kuwano, K.; Miyazaki, H.; Hagimoto, N.; Kawasaki, M.; Fujita, M.; Kunitake, R.; Kaneko, Y.; Hara, N. The involvement of Fas-Fas ligand pathway in fibrosing lung diseases. *Am. J. Respir. Cell Mol. Biol.* **1999**, *20*, 53–60. [CrossRef]
48. Hagimoto, N.; Kuwano, K.; Nomoto, Y.; Kunitake, R.; Hara, N. Apoptosis and expression of Fas/Fas ligand mRNA in bleomycin-induced pulmonary fibrosis in mice. *Am. J. Respir. Cell Mol. Biol.* **1997**, *16*, 91–101. [CrossRef]
49. Wang, R.; Ibarra-Sunga, O.; Verlinski, L.; Pick, R.; Uhal, B.D. Abrogation of bleomycin-induced epithelial apoptosis and lung fibrosis by captopril or by a caspase inhibitor. *Am. J. Physiol. Lung Cell Mol. Physiol.* **2000**, *279*, L143–L151. [CrossRef]
50. Kuwano, K.; Kunitake, R.; Maeyama, T.; Hagimoto, N.; Kawasaki, M.; Matsuba, T.; Yoshimi, M.; Inoshima, I.; Yoshida, K.; Hara, N. Attenuation of bleomycin-induced pneumopathy in mice by a caspase inhibitor. *Am. J. Physiol. Lung Cell Mol. Physiol.* **2001**, *280*, L316–L325. [CrossRef]
51. Kuwano, K.; Hagimoto, N.; Kawasaki, M.; Yatomi, T.; Nakamura, N.; Nagata, S.; Suda, T.; Kunitake, R.; Maeyama, T.; Miyazaki, H.; et al. Essential roles of the Fas-Fas ligand pathway in the development of pulmonary fibrosis. *J. Clin. Investig.* **1999**, *104*, 13–19. [CrossRef] [PubMed]
52. Hagimoto, N.; Kuwano, K.; Miyazaki, H.; Kunitake, R.; Fujita, M.; Kawasaki, M.; Kaneko, Y.; Hara, N. Induction of apoptosis and pulmonary fibrosis in mice in response to ligation of Fas antigen. *Am. J. Respir. Cell Mol. Biol.* **1997**, *17*, 272–278. [CrossRef] [PubMed]
53. Schutze, S.; Tchikov, V.; Schneider-Brachert, W. Regulation of TNFR1 and CD95 signalling by receptor compartmentalization. *Nat. Rev. Mol. Cell Biol.* **2008**, *9*, 655–662. [CrossRef] [PubMed]
54. Fuchs, Y.; Steller, H. Live to die another way: Modes of programmed cell death and the signals emanating from dying cells. *Nat. Rev. Mol. Cell Biol.* **2015**, *16*, 329–344. [CrossRef] [PubMed]
55. Kropski, J.A.; Blackwell, T.S. Endoplasmic reticulum stress in the pathogenesis of fibrotic disease. *J. Clin. Investig.* **2018**, *128*, 64–73. [CrossRef] [PubMed]
56. Hipp, M.S.; Kasturi, P.; Hartl, F.U. The proteostasis network and its decline in ageing. *Nat. Rev. Mol. Cell Biol.* **2019**, *20*, 421–435. [CrossRef]
57. Korfei, M.; Ruppert, C.; Mahavadi, P.; Henneke, I.; Markart, P.; Koch, M.; Lang, G.; Fink, L.; Bohle, R.M.; Seeger, W.; et al. Epithelial endoplasmic reticulum stress and apoptosis in sporadic idiopathic pulmonary fibrosis. *Am. J. Respir. Crit. Care Med.* **2008**, *178*, 838–846. [CrossRef]
58. Lawson, W.E.; Crossno, P.F.; Polosukhin, V.V.; Roldan, J.; Cheng, D.S.; Lane, K.B.; Blackwell, T.R.; Xu, C.; Markin, C.; Ware, L.B.; et al. Endoplasmic reticulum stress in alveolar epithelial cells is prominent in IPF: Association with altered surfactant protein processing and herpesvirus infection. *Am. J. Physiol. Lung Cell

Mol. Physiol. **2008**, *294*, L1119–L1126. [CrossRef]

59. Lawson, W.E.; Cheng, D.S.; Degryse, A.L.; Tanjore, H.; Polosukhin, V.V.; Xu, X.C.; Newcomb, D.C.; Jones, B.R.; Roldan, J.; Lane, K.B.; et al. Endoplasmic reticulum stress enhances fibrotic remodeling in the lungs. *Proc. Natl. Acad. Sci. USA* **2011**, *108*, 10562–10567. [CrossRef]
60. Bueno, M.; Lai, Y.C.; Romero, Y.; Brands, J.; St Croix, C.M.; Kamga, C.; Corey, C.; Herazo-Maya, J.D.; Sembrat, J.; Lee, J.S.; et al. PINK1 deficiency impairs mitochondrial homeostasis and promotes lung fibrosis. *J. Clin. Investig.* **2015**, *125*, 521–538. [CrossRef]
61. Katzen, J.; Wagner, B.D.; Venosa, A.; Kopp, M.; Tomer, Y.; Russo, S.J.; Headen, A.C.; Basil, M.C.; Stark, J.M.; Mulugeta, S.; et al. An SFTPC BRICHOS mutant links epithelial ER stress and spontaneous lung fibrosis. *JCI Insight* **2019**, *4*. [CrossRef] [PubMed]
62. Nureki, S.I.; Tomer, Y.; Venosa, A.; Katzen, J.; Russo, S.J.; Jamil, S.; Barrett, M.; Nguyen, V.; Kopp, M.; Mulugeta, S.; et al. Expression of mutant Sftpc in murine alveolar epithelia drives spontaneous lung fibrosis. *J. Clin. Investig.* **2018**, *128*, 4008–4024. [CrossRef] [PubMed]
63. Borok, Z.; Horie, M.; Flodby, P.; Wang, H.; Liu, Y.; Ganesh, S.; Ryan Firth, A.L.; Minoo, P.; Li, C.; Beers, M.F.; et al. Grp78 Loss in Epithelial Progenitors Reveals an Age-Linked Role for ER Stress in Pulmonary Fibrosis. *Am. J. Respir. Crit. Care Med.* **2019**. [CrossRef]
64. Baumgartner, K.B.; Samet, J.M.; Stidley, C.A.; Colby, T.V.; Waldron, J.A. Cigarette smoking: A risk factor for idiopathic pulmonary fibrosis. *Am. J. Respir. Crit. Care Med.* **1997**, *155*, 242–248. [CrossRef]
65. Jorgensen, E.; Stinson, A.; Shan, L.; Yang, J.; Gietl, D.; Albino, A.P. Cigarette smoke induces endoplasmic reticulum stress and the unfolded protein response in normal and malignant human lung cells. *BMC Cancer* **2008**, *8*, 229. [CrossRef]
66. Kropski, J.A.; Pritchett, J.M.; Zoz, D.F.; Crossno, P.F.; Markin, C.; Garnett, E.T.; Degryse, A.L.; Mitchell, D.B.; Polosukhin, V.V.; Rickman, O.B.; et al. Extensive phenotyping of individuals at risk for familial interstitial pneumonia reveals clues to the pathogenesis of interstitial lung disease. *Am. J. Respir. Crit. Care Med.* **2015**, *191*, 417–426. [CrossRef]
67. McMillan, T.R.; Moore, B.B.; Weinberg, J.B.; Vannella, K.M.; Fields, W.B.; Christensen, P.J.; Van Dyk, L.F.; Toews, G.B. Exacerbation of established pulmonary fibrosis in a murine model by gammaherpesvirus. *Am. J. Respir. Crit. Care Med.* **2008**, *177*, 771–780. [CrossRef]
68. Vannella, K.M.; Luckhardt, T.R.; Wilke, C.A.; Van Dyk, L.F.; Toews, G.B.; Moore, B.B. Latent herpesvirus infection augments experimental pulmonary fibrosis. *Am. J. Respir. Crit. Care Med.* **2010**, *181*, 465–477. [CrossRef]
69. Mora, A.L.; Woods, C.R.; Garcia, A.; Xu, J.; Rojas, M.; Speck, S.H.; Roman, J.; Brigham, K.L.; Stecenko, A.A. Lung infection with gamma-herpesvirus induces progressive pulmonary fibrosis in Th2-biased mice. *Am. J. Physiol. Lung Cell Mol. Physiol.* **2005**, *289*, L711–L721. [CrossRef]
70. Lok, S.S.; Haider, Y.; Howell, D.; Stewart, J.P.; Hasleton, P.S.; Egan, J.J. Murine gammaherpes virus as a cofactor in the development of pulmonary fibrosis in bleomycin resistant mice. *Eur. Respir. J.* **2002**, *20*, 1228–1232. [CrossRef]
71. Torres-Gonzalez, E.; Bueno, M.; Tanaka, A.; Krug, L.T.; Cheng, D.S.; Polosukhin, V.V.; Sorescu, D.; Lawson, W.E.; Blackwell, T.S.; Rojas, M.; et al. Role of endoplasmic reticulum stress in age-related susceptibility to lung fibrosis. *Am. J. Respir. Cell Mol. Biol.* **2012**, *46*, 748–756. [CrossRef] [PubMed]
72. Piantadosi, C.A.; Suliman, H.B. Mitochondrial Dysfunction in Lung Pathogenesis. *Annu. Rev. Physiol.* **2017**, *79*, 495–515. [CrossRef] [PubMed]
73. Cloonan, S.M.; Choi, A.M. Mitochondria in lung disease. *J. Clin. Investig.* **2016**, *126*, 809–820. [CrossRef] [PubMed]
74. Mora, A.L.; Bueno, M.; Rojas, M. Mitochondria in the spotlight of aging and idiopathic pulmonary fibrosis. *J. Clin. Investig.* **2017**, *127*, 405–414. [CrossRef]
75. Rangarajan, S.; Bernard, K.; Thannickal, V.J. Mitochondrial Dysfunction in Pulmonary Fibrosis. *Ann. Am. Thorac. Soc.* **2017**, *14*, S383–S388. [CrossRef]
76. Bueno, M.; Zank, D.; Buendia-Roldan, I.; Fiedler, K.; Mays, B.G.; Alvarez, D.; Sembrat, J.; Kimball, B.; Bullock, J.K.; Martin, J.L.; et al. PINK1 attenuates mtDNA release in alveolar epithelial cells and TLR9 mediated profibrotic responses. *PLoS ONE* **2019**, *14*, e0218003. [CrossRef]
77. Patel, A.S.; Song, J.W.; Chu, S.G.; Mizumura, K.; Osorio, J.C.; Shi, Y.; El-Chemaly, S.; Lee, C.G.; Rosas, I.O.; Elias, J.A.; et al. Epithelial cell mitochondrial dysfunction and PINK1 are induced by transforming growth factor-beta1 in pulmonary fibrosis. *PLoS ONE* **2015**, *10*, e0121246. [CrossRef]

78. Dorn, G.W., 2nd. Evolving Concepts of Mitochondrial Dynamics. *Annu. Rev. Physiol.* **2019**, *81*, 1–17. [CrossRef]
79. Chung, K.-P.; Hsu, C.-L.; Fan, L.-C.; Huang, Z.; Bhatia, D.; Chen, Y.-J.; Hisata, S.; Cho, S.J.; Nakahira, K.; Imamura, M.; et al. Mitofusins regulate lipid metabolism to mediate the development of lung fibrosis. *Nat. Commun.* **2019**, *10*, 3390. [CrossRef]
80. Kim, S.-J.; Cheresh, P.; Jablonski, R.P.; Morales-Nebreda, L.; Cheng, Y.; Hogan, E.; Yeldandi, A.; Chi, M.; Piseaux, R.; Ridge, K.; et al. Mitochondrial catalase overexpressed transgenic mice are protected against lung fibrosis in part via preventing alveolar epithelial cell mitochondrial DNA damage. *Free Radic. Biol. Med.* **2016**, *101*, 482–490. [CrossRef]
81. Jablonski, R.P.; Kim, S.-J.; Cheresh, P.; Williams, D.B.; Morales-Nebreda, L.; Cheng, Y.; Yeldandi, A.; Bhorade, S.; Pardo, A.; Selman, M.; et al. SIRT3 deficiency promotes lung fibrosis by augmenting alveolar epithelial cell mitochondrial DNA damage and apoptosis. *FASEB J.* **2017**, *31*, 2520–2532. [CrossRef] [PubMed]
82. Bueno, M.; Brands, J.; Voltz, L.; Fiedler, K.; Mays, B.; St Croix, C.; Sembrat, J.; Mallampalli, R.K.; Rojas, M.; Mora, A.L. ATF3 represses PINK1 gene transcription in lung epithelial cells to control mitochondrial homeostasis. *Aging Cell* **2018**, *17*. [CrossRef] [PubMed]
83. Yu, G.; Tzouvelekis, A.; Wang, R.; Herazo-Maya, J.D.; Ibarra, G.H.; Srivastava, A.; De Castro, J.P.W.; DeIuliis, G.; Ahangari, F.; Woolard, T.; et al. Thyroid hormone inhibits lung fibrosis in mice by improving epithelial mitochondrial function. *Nat. Med.* **2018**, *24*, 39–49. [CrossRef] [PubMed]
84. Ganzleben, I.; He, G.W.; Gunther, C.; Prigge, E.S.; Richter, K.; Rieker, R.J.; Mougiakakos, D.; Neurath, M.F.; Becker, C. PGAM5 is a key driver of mitochondrial dysfunction in experimental lung fibrosis. *Cell Mol. Life Sci.* **2019**. [CrossRef]
85. Kulkarni, T.; De Andrade, J.; Zhou, Y.; Luckhardt, T.; Thannickal, V.J. Alveolar epithelial disintegrity in pulmonary fibrosis. *Am. J. Physiol. Lung Cell Mol. Physiol.* **2016**, *311*, L185–L191. [CrossRef]
86. Kim, K.K.; Kugler, M.C.; Wolters, P.J.; Robillard, L.; Galvez, M.G.; Brumwell, A.N.; Sheppard, D.; Chapman, H.A. Alveolar epithelial cell mesenchymal transition develops in vivo during pulmonary fibrosis and is regulated by the extracellular matrix. *Proc. Natl. Acad. Sci. USA* **2006**, *103*, 13180–13185. [CrossRef]
87. Kim, K.K.; Wei, Y.; Szekeres, C.; Kugler, M.C.; Wolters, P.J.; Hill, M.L.; Frank, J.A.; Brumwell, A.N.; Wheeler, S.E.; Kreidberg, J.A.; et al. Epithelial cell alpha3beta1 integrin links beta-catenin and Smad signaling to promote myofibroblast formation and pulmonary fibrosis. *J. Clin. Investig.* **2009**, *119*, 213–224. [CrossRef]
88. Kim, Y.; Kugler, M.C.; Wei, Y.; Kim, K.K.; Li, X.; Brumwell, A.N.; Chapman, H.A. Integrin alpha3beta1-dependent beta-catenin phosphorylation links epithelial Smad signaling to cell contacts. *J. Cell Biol.* **2009**, *184*, 309–322. [CrossRef]
89. Rock, J.R.; Barkauskas, C.E.; Cronce, M.J.; Xue, Y.; Harris, J.R.; Liang, J.; Noble, P.W.; Hogan, B.L. Multiple stromal populations contribute to pulmonary fibrosis without evidence for epithelial to mesenchymal transition. *Proc. Natl. Acad. Sci. USA* **2011**, *108*, E1475–E1483. [CrossRef]
90. Borok, Z.; Whitsett, J.A.; Bitterman, P.B.; Thannickal, V.J.; Kotton, D.N.; Reynolds, S.D.; Krasnow, M.A.; Bianchi, D.W.; Morrisey, E.E.; Hogan, B.L.; et al. Cell plasticity in lung injury and repair: Report from an NHLBI workshop, April 19–20, 2010. *Proc. Am. Thorac. Soc.* **2011**, *8*, 215–222. [CrossRef]
91. Wu, H.; Yu, Y.; Huang, H.; Hu, Y.; Fu, S.; Wang, Z.; Shi, M.; Zhao, X.; Yuan, J.; Li, J.; et al. Progressive Pulmonary Fibrosis Is Caused by Elevated Mechanical Tension on Alveolar Stem Cells. *Cell* **2019**, *180*, 107–121. [CrossRef] [PubMed]
92. Yang, Y.; Cheung, H.H.; Tu, J.; Miu, K.K.; Chan, W.Y. New insights into the unfolded protein response in stem cells. *Oncotarget* **2016**, *7*, 54010–54027. [CrossRef] [PubMed]
93. Alder, J.K.; Barkauskas, C.E.; Limjunyawong, N.; Stanley, S.E.; Kembou, F.; Tuder, R.M.; Hogan, B.L.; Mitzner, W.; Armanios, M. Telomere dysfunction causes alveolar stem cell failure. *Proc. Natl. Acad. Sci. USA* **2015**, *112*, 5099–5104. [CrossRef] [PubMed]
94. Liu, T.; Gonzalez De Los Santos, F.; Zhao, Y.; Wu, Z.; Rinke, A.E.; Kim, K.K.; Phan, S.H. Telomerase reverse transcriptase ameliorates lung fibrosis by protecting alveolar epithelial cells against senescence. *J. Biol. Chem.* **2019**, *294*, 8861–8871. [CrossRef]
95. Naikawadi, R.P.; Disayabutr, S.; Mallavia, B.; Donne, M.L.; Green, G.; La, J.L.; Rock, J.R.; Looney, M.R.; Wolters, P.J. Telomere dysfunction in alveolar epithelial cells causes lung remodeling and fibrosis. *JCI Insight* **2016**, *1*, e86704. [CrossRef]

96. Povedano, J.M.; Martinez, P.; Serrano, R.; Tejera, A.; Gomez-Lopez, G.; Bobadilla, M.; Flores, J.M.; Bosch, F.; Blasco, M.A. Therapeutic effects of telomerase in mice with pulmonary fibrosis induced by damage to the lungs and short telomeres. *Elife* **2018**, *7*. [CrossRef] [PubMed]
97. Gulati, S.; Thannickal, V.J. The Aging Lung and Idiopathic Pulmonary Fibrosis. *Am. J. Med. Sci.* **2019**, *357*, 384–389. [CrossRef]
98. Selman, M.; Buendia-Roldan, I.; Pardo, A. Aging and Pulmonary Fibrosis. *Rev. Investig. Clin.* **2016**, *68*, 75–83.
99. Thannickal, V.J. Mechanistic links between aging and lung fibrosis. *Biogerontology* **2013**, *14*, 609–615. [CrossRef]
100. Chilosi, M.; Carloni, A.; Rossi, A.; Poletti, V. Premature lung aging and cellular senescence in the pathogenesis of idiopathic pulmonary fibrosis and COPD/emphysema. *Transl. Res.* **2013**, *162*, 156–173. [CrossRef] [PubMed]
101. Lehmann, M.; Korfei, M.; Mutze, K.; Klee, S.; Skronska-Wasek, W.; Alsafadi, H.N.; Ota, C.; Costa, R.; Schiller, H.B.; Lindner, M.; et al. Senolytic drugs target alveolar epithelial cell function and attenuate experimental lung fibrosis ex vivo. *Eur. Respir. J.* **2017**, *50*. [CrossRef] [PubMed]
102. Justice, J.N.; Nambiar, A.M.; Tchkonia, T.; LeBrasseur, N.K.; Pascual, R.; Hashmi, S.K.; Prata, L.; Masternak, M.M.; Kritchevsky, S.B.; Musi, N.; et al. Senolytics in idiopathic pulmonary fibrosis: Results from a first-in-human, open-label, pilot study. *EBioMedicine* **2019**, *40*, 554–563. [CrossRef]
103. Schafer, M.J.; White, T.A.; Iijima, K.; Haak, A.J.; Ligresti, G.; Atkinson, E.J.; Oberg, A.L.; Birch, J.; Salmonowicz, H.; Zhu, Y.; et al. Cellular senescence mediates fibrotic pulmonary disease. *Nat. Commun.* **2017**, *8*, 14532. [CrossRef]
104. Arish, N.; Petukhov, D.; Wallach-Dayan, S.B. The Role of Telomerase and Telomeres in Interstitial Lung Diseases: From Molecules to Clinical Implications. *Int. J. Mol. Sci.* **2019**, *20*. [CrossRef] [PubMed]
105. Shay, J.W.; Wright, W.E. Telomeres and telomerase: Three decades of progress. *Nat. Rev. Genet.* **2019**, *20*, 299–309. [CrossRef] [PubMed]
106. Snetselaar, R.; Van Batenburg, A.A.; Van Oosterhout, M.F.M.; Kazemier, K.M.; Roothaan, S.M.; Peeters, T.; Van der Vis, J.J.; Goldschmeding, R.; Grutters, J.C.; Van Moorsel, C.H.M. Short telomere length in IPF lung associates with fibrotic lesions and predicts survival. *PLoS ONE* **2017**, *12*, e0189467. [CrossRef] [PubMed]
107. Alder, J.K.; Chen, J.J.; Lancaster, L.; Danoff, S.; Su, S.C.; Cogan, J.D.; Vulto, I.; Xie, M.; Qi, X.; Tuder, R.M.; et al. Short telomeres are a risk factor for idiopathic pulmonary fibrosis. *Proc. Natl. Acad. Sci. USA* **2008**, *105*, 13051–13056. [CrossRef]
108. Morla, M.; Busquets, X.; Pons, J.; Sauleda, J.; MacNee, W.; Agusti, A.G. Telomere shortening in smokers with and without COPD. *Eur. Respir. J.* **2006**, *27*, 525–528. [CrossRef]
109. Armanios, M.Y.; Chen, J.J.; Cogan, J.D.; Alder, J.K.; Ingersoll, R.G.; Markin, C.; Lawson, W.E.; Xie, M.; Vulto, I.; Phillips, J.A., 3rd; et al. Telomerase mutations in families with idiopathic pulmonary fibrosis. *N. Engl. J. Med.* **2007**, *356*, 1317–1326. [CrossRef]
110. Cronkhite, J.T.; Xing, C.; Raghu, G.; Chin, K.M.; Torres, F.; Rosenblatt, R.L.; Garcia, C.K. Telomere shortening in familial and sporadic pulmonary fibrosis. *Am. J. Respir. Crit. Care Med.* **2008**, *178*, 729–737. [CrossRef]
111. Tsakiri, K.D.; Cronkhite, J.T.; Kuan, P.J.; Xing, C.; Raghu, G.; Weissler, J.C.; Rosenblatt, R.L.; Shay, J.W.; Garcia, C.K. Adult-onset pulmonary fibrosis caused by mutations in telomerase. *Proc. Natl. Acad. Sci. USA* **2007**, *104*, 7552–7557. [CrossRef] [PubMed]
112. Diaz de Leon, A.; Cronkhite, J.T.; Katzenstein, A.L.; Godwin, J.D.; Raghu, G.; Glazer, C.S.; Rosenblatt, R.L.; Girod, C.E.; Garrity, E.R.; Xing, C.; et al. Telomere lengths, pulmonary fibrosis and telomerase (TERT) mutations. *PLoS ONE* **2010**, *5*, e10680. [CrossRef] [PubMed]
113. Kannengiesser, C.; Borie, R.; Menard, C.; Reocreux, M.; Nitschke, P.; Gazal, S.; Mal, H.; Taille, C.; Cadranel, J.; Nunes, H.; et al. Heterozygous RTEL1 mutations are associated with familial pulmonary fibrosis. *Eur. Respir. J.* **2015**, *46*, 474–485. [CrossRef] [PubMed]
114. Cogan, J.D.; Kropski, J.A.; Zhao, M.; Mitchell, D.B.; Rives, L.; Markin, C.; Garnett, E.T.; Montgomery, K.H.; Mason, W.R.; McKean, D.F.; et al. Rare variants in RTEL1 are associated with familial interstitial pneumonia. *Am. J. Respir. Crit. Care Med.* **2015**, *191*, 646–655. [CrossRef]
115. Stuart, B.D.; Choi, J.; Zaidi, S.; Xing, C.; Holohan, B.; Chen, R.; Choi, M.; Dharwadkar, P.; Torres, F.; Girod, C.E.; et al. Exome sequencing links mutations in PARN and RTEL1 with familial pulmonary fibrosis and telomere shortening. *Nat. Genet.* **2015**, *47*, 512–517. [CrossRef]
116. Petrovski, S.; Todd, J.L.; Durheim, M.T.; Wang, Q.; Chien, J.W.; Kelly, F.L.; Frankel, C.; Mebane, C.M.; Ren, Z.; Bridgers, J.; et al. An Exome Sequencing Study to Assess the Role of Rare Genetic Variation in Pulmonary Fibrosis. *Am. J. Respir. Crit. Care Med.* **2017** *196*, 82–93. [CrossRef]

117. Kropski, J.A.; Mitchell, D.B.; Markin, C.; Polosukhin, V.V.; Choi, L.; Johnson, J.E.; Lawson, W.E.; Phillips, J.A., 3rd; Cogan, J.D.; Blackwell, T.S.; et al. A novel dyskerin (DKC1) mutation is associated with familial interstitial pneumonia. *Chest* **2014**, *146*, e1–e7. [CrossRef]
118. Stanley, S.E.; Gable, D.L.; Wagner, C.L.; Carlile, T.M.; Hanumanthu, V.S.; Podlevsky, J.D.; Khalil, S.E.; DeZern, A.E.; Rojas-Duran, M.F.; Applegate, C.D.; et al. Loss-of-function mutations in the RNA biogenesis factor NAF1 predispose to pulmonary fibrosis-emphysema. *Sci. Transl. Med.* **2016**, *8*, 351ra107. [CrossRef]
119. Alder, J.K.; Stanley, S.E.; Wagner, C.L.; Hamilton, M.; Hanumanthu, V.S.; Armanios, M. Exome sequencing identifies mutant TINF2 in a family with pulmonary fibrosis. *Chest* **2015**, *147*, 1361–1368. [CrossRef]
120. Hoffman, T.W.; Van der Vis, J.J.; Van Oosterhout, M.F.; Van Es, H.W.; Van Kessel, D.A.; Grutters, J.C.; Van Moorsel, C.H. TINF2 Gene Mutation in a Patient with Pulmonary Fibrosis. *Case Rep. Pulmonol.* **2016**, *2016*, 1310862. [CrossRef]
121. Povedano, J.M.; Martinez, P.; Flores, J.M.; Mulero, F.; Blasco, M.A. Mice with Pulmonary Fibrosis Driven by Telomere Dysfunction. *Cell Rep.* **2015**, *12*, 286–299. [CrossRef] [PubMed]
122. Adamson, I.Y.; King, G.M.; Young, L. Influence of extracellular matrix and collagen components on alveolar type 2 cell morphology and function. *In Vitro Cell Dev. Biol.* **1989**, *25*, 494–502. [CrossRef] [PubMed]
123. Li, Y.; Jiang, D.; Liang, J.; Meltzer, E.B.; Gray, A.; Miura, R.; Wogensen, L.; Yamaguchi, Y.; Noble, P.W. Severe lung fibrosis requires an invasive fibroblast phenotype regulated by hyaluronan and CD44. *J. Exp. Med.* **2011**, *208*, 1459–1471. [CrossRef] [PubMed]
124. Bjermer, L.; Lundgren, R.; Hallgren, R. Hyaluronan and type III procollagen peptide concentrations in bronchoalveolar lavage fluid in idiopathic pulmonary fibrosis. *Thorax* **1989**, *44*, 126–131. [CrossRef] [PubMed]
125. Reyfman, P.A.; Walter, J.M.; Joshi, N.; Anekalla, K.R.; McQuattie-Pimentel, A.C.; Chiu, S.; Fernandez, R.; Akbarpour, M.; Chen, C.I.; Ren, Z.; et al. Single-Cell Transcriptomic Analysis of Human Lung Provides Insights into the Pathobiology of Pulmonary Fibrosis. *Am. J. Respir. Crit. Care Med.* **2019**, *199*, 1517–1536. [CrossRef]
126. Parimon, T.; Yao, C.; Habiel, D.M.; Ge, L.; Bora, S.A.; Brauer, R.; Evans, C.M.; Xie, T.; Alonso-Valenteen, F.; Medina-Kauwe, L.K.; et al. Syndecan-1 promotes lung fibrosis by regulating epithelial reprogramming through extracellular vesicles. *JCI Insight* **2019**, *5*. [CrossRef]
127. Raredon, M.S.B.; Adams, T.S.; Suhail, Y.; Schupp, J.C.; Poli, S.; Neumark, N.; Leiby, K.L.; Greaney, A.M.; Yuan, Y.; Horien, C.; et al. Single-cell connectomic analysis of adult mammalian lungs. *Sci. Adv.* **2019**, *5*, eaaw3851. [CrossRef]
128. Konigshoff, M.; Kramer, M.; Balsara, N.; Wilhelm, J.; Amarie, O.V.; Jahn, A.; Rose, F.; Fink, L.; Seeger, W.; Schaefer, L.; et al. WNT1-inducible signaling protein-1 mediates pulmonary fibrosis in mice and is upregulated in humans with idiopathic pulmonary fibrosis. *J. Clin. Investig.* **2009**, *119*, 772–787. [CrossRef]
129. Konigshoff, M.; Balsara, N.; Pfaff, E.M.; Kramer, M.; Chrobak, I.; Seeger, W.; Eickelberg, O. Functional Wnt signaling is increased in idiopathic pulmonary fibrosis. *PLoS ONE* **2008**, *3*, e2142. [CrossRef]
130. Chilosi, M.; Poletti, V.; Zamo, A.; Lestani, M.; Montagna, L.; Piccoli, P.; Pedron, S.; Bertaso, M.; Scarpa, A.; Murer, B.; et al. Aberrant Wnt/beta-catenin pathway activation in idiopathic pulmonary fibrosis. *Am. J. Pathol.* **2003**, *162*, 1495–1502. [CrossRef]
131. Frank, D.B.; Peng, T.; Zepp, J.A.; Snitow, M.; Vincent, T.L.; Penkala, I.J.; Cui, Z.; Herriges, M.J.; Morley, M.P.; Zhou, S.; et al. Emergence of a Wave of Wnt Signaling that Regulates Lung Alveologenesis by Controlling Epithelial Self-Renewal and Differentiation. *Cell Rep.* **2016**, *17*, 2312–2325. [CrossRef] [PubMed]
132. Liu, H.; Fergusson, M.M.; Castilho, R.M.; Liu, J.; Cao, L.; Chen, J.; Malide, D.; Rovira, I.I.; Schimel, D.; Kuo, C.J.; et al. Augmented Wnt signaling in a mammalian model of accelerated aging. *Science* **2007**, *317*, 803–806. [CrossRef] [PubMed]
133. Kovacs, T.; Csongei, V.; Feller, D.; Ernszt, D.; Smuk, G.; Sarosi, V.; Jakab, L.; Kvell, K.; Bartis, D.; Pongracz, J.E. Alteration in the Wnt microenvironment directly regulates molecular events leading to pulmonary senescence. *Aging Cell* **2014**, *13*, 838–849. [CrossRef] [PubMed]
134. Lam, A.P.; Herazo-Maya, J.D.; Sennello, J.A.; Flozak, A.S.; Russell, S.; Mutlu, G.M.; Budinger, G.R.; DasGupta, R.; Varga, J.; Kaminski, N.; et al. Wnt coreceptor Lrp5 is a driver of idiopathic pulmonary fibrosis. *Am. J. Respir. Crit. Care Med.* **2014**, *190*, 185–195. [CrossRef]
135. Henderson, W.R., Jr.; Chi, E.Y.; Ye, X.; Nguyen, C.; Tien, Y.T.; Zhou, B.; Borok, Z.; Knight, D.A.; Kahn, M. Inhibition of Wnt/beta-catenin/CREB binding protein (CBP) signaling reverses pulmonary fibrosis. *Proc. Natl. Acad. Sci. USA* **2010**, *107*, 14309–14314. [CrossRef]

136. Ulsamer, A.; Wei, Y.; Kim, K.K.; Tan, K.; Wheeler, S.; Xi, Y.; Thies, R.S.; Chapman, H.A. Axin pathway activity regulates in vivo pY654-beta-catenin accumulation and pulmonary fibrosis. *J. Biol. Chem.* **2012**, *287*, 5164–5172. [CrossRef]
137. Olajuyin, A.M.; Zhang, X.; Ji, H.L. Alveolar type 2 progenitor cells for lung injury repair. *Cell Death Discov.* **2019**, *5*, 63. [CrossRef]
138. Mutze, K.; Vierkotten, S.; Milosevic, J.; Eickelberg, O.; Konigshoff, M. Enolase 1 (ENO1) and protein disulfide-isomerase associated 3 (PDIA3) regulate Wnt/beta-catenin-driven trans-differentiation of murine alveolar epithelial cells. *Dis. Model. Mech.* **2015**, *8*, 877–890. [CrossRef]
139. Konigshoff, M.; Eickelberg, O. WNT signaling in lung disease: A failure or a regeneration signal? *Am. J. Respir. Cell Mol. Biol.* **2010**, *42*, 21–31. [CrossRef]
140. Azzolin, L.; Panciera, T.; Soligo, S.; Enzo, E.; Bicciato, S.; Dupont, S.; Bresolin, S.; Frasson, C.; Basso, G.; Guzzardo, V.; et al. YAP/TAZ incorporation in the beta-catenin destruction complex orchestrates the Wnt response. *Cell* **2014**, *158*, 157–170. [CrossRef]
141. Azzolin, L.; Zanconato, F.; Bresolin, S.; Forcato, M.; Basso, G.; Bicciato, S.; Cordenonsi, M.; Piccolo, S. Role of TAZ as mediator of Wnt signaling. *Cell* **2012**, *151*, 1443–1456. [CrossRef] [PubMed]
142. Mitani, A.; Nagase, T.; Fukuchi, K.; Aburatani, H.; Makita, R.; Kurihara, H. Transcriptional coactivator with PDZ-binding motif is essential for normal alveolarization in mice. *Am. J. Respir. Crit. Care Med.* **2009**, *180*, 326–338. [CrossRef] [PubMed]
143. Park, K.S.; Whitsett, J.A.; Di Palma, T.; Hong, J.H.; Yaffe, M.B.; Zannini, M. TAZ interacts with TTF-1 and regulates expression of surfactant protein-C. *J. Biol. Chem.* **2004**, *279*, 17384–17390. [CrossRef] [PubMed]
144. Makita, R.; Uchijima, Y.; Nishiyama, K.; Amano, T.; Chen, Q.; Takeuchi, T.; Mitani, A.; Nagase, T.; Yatomi, Y.; Aburatani, H.; et al. Multiple renal cysts, urinary concentration defects, and pulmonary emphysematous changes in mice lacking TAZ. *Am. J. Physiol. Ren. Physiol.* **2008**, *294*, F542–F553. [CrossRef]
145. Lin, C.; Yao, E.; Zhang, K.; Jiang, X.; Croll, S.; Thompson-Peer, K.; Chuang, P.T. YAP is essential for mechanical force production and epithelial cell proliferation during lung branching morphogenesis. *Elife* **2017**, *6*. [CrossRef]
146. Liu, Z.; Wu, H.; Jiang, K.; Wang, Y.; Zhang, W.; Chu, Q.; Li, J.; Huang, H.; Cai, T.; Ji, H.; et al. MAPK-Mediated YAP Activation Controls Mechanical-Tension-Induced Pulmonary Alveolar Regeneration. *Cell Rep.* **2016**, *16*, 1810–1819. [CrossRef]
147. Sun, T.; Huang, Z.; Zhang, H.; Posner, C.; Jia, G.; Ramalingam, T.R.; Xu, M.; Brightbill, H.; Egen, J.G.; Dey, A.; et al. TAZ is required for lung alveolar epithelial cell differentiation after injury. *JCI Insight* **2019**, *5*. [CrossRef]
148. Tschumperlin, D.J.; Ligresti, G.; Hilscher, M.B.; Shah, V.H. Mechanosensing and fibrosis. *J. Clin. Investig.* **2018**, *128*, 74–84. [CrossRef]
149. Liu, F.; Lagares, D.; Choi, K.M.; Stopfer, L.; Marinkovic, A.; Vrbanac, V.; Probst, C.K.; Hiemer, S.E.; Sisson, T.H.; Horowitz, J.C.; et al. Mechanosignaling through YAP and TAZ drives fibroblast activation and fibrosis. *Am. J. Physiol. Lung Cell Mol. Physiol.* **2015**, *308*, L344–L357. [CrossRef]
150. Piersma, B.; Bank, R.A. Keeping fibroblasts in suspense: TAZ-mediated signaling activates a context-dependent profibrotic phenotype. Focus on "TAZ activation drives fibroblast spheroid growth, expression of profibrotic paracrine signals, and context-dependent ECM gene expression". *Am. J. Physiol. Cell Physiol.* **2017**, *312*, C274–C276. [CrossRef]
151. Noguchi, S.; Saito, A.; Mikami, Y.; Urushiyama, H.; Horie, M.; Matsuzaki, H.; Takeshima, H.; Makita, K.; Miyashita, N.; Mitani, A.; et al. TAZ contributes to pulmonary fibrosis by activating profibrotic functions of lung fibroblasts. *Sci. Rep.* **2017**, *7*, 42595. [CrossRef]
152. Gokey, J.J.; Sridharan, A.; Xu, Y.; Green, J.; Carraro, G.; Stripp, B.R.; Perl, A.-K.T.; Whitsett, J.A. Active epithelial Hippo signaling in idiopathic pulmonary fibrosis. *JCI Insight* **2018**, *3*, e98738. [CrossRef]
153. Hussain, M.; Xu, C.; Ahmad, M.; Yang, Y.; Lu, M.; Wu, X.; Tang, L.; Wu, X. Notch Signaling: Linking Embryonic Lung Development and Asthmatic Airway Remodeling. *Mol. Pharmacol.* **2017**, *92*, 676–693. [CrossRef]
154. Bray, S.J. Notch signalling in context. *Nat. Rev. Mol. Cell Biol.* **2016**, *17*, 722–735. [CrossRef]

155. Tsao, P.N.; Matsuoka, C.; Wei, S.C.; Sato, A.; Sato, S.; Hasegawa, K.; Chen, H.K.; Ling, T.Y.; Mori, M.; Cardoso, W.V.; et al. Epithelial Notch signaling regulates lung alveolar morphogenesis and airway epithelial integrity. *Proc. Natl. Acad. Sci. USA* **2016**, *113*, 8242–8247. [CrossRef]
156. Xu, K.; Nieuwenhuis, E.; Cohen, B.L.; Wang, W.; Canty, A.J.; Danska, J.S.; Coultas, L.; Rossant, J.; Wu, M.Y.; Piscione, T.D.; et al. Lunatic Fringe-mediated Notch signaling is required for lung alveogenesis. *Am. J. Physiol. Lung Cell Mol. Physiol.* **2010**, *298*, L45–L56. [CrossRef]
157. Kavian, N.; Servettaz, A.; Weill, B.; Batteux, F. New insights into the mechanism of notch signalling in fibrosis. *Open Rheumatol. J.* **2012**, *6*, 96–102. [CrossRef]
158. Wasnick, R.M.; Korfei, M.; Piskulak, K.; Henneke, I.; Wilhelm, J.; Mahavadi, P.; Von der Beck, D.; Koch, M.; Shalashova, I.; Klymenko, O.; et al. Restored alveolar epithelial differentiation and reversed human lung fibrosis upon Notch inhibition. *BioRxiv* **2019**, 580498. [CrossRef]
159. Vaughan, A.E.; Brumwell, A.N.; Xi, Y.; Gotts, J.E.; Brownfield, D.G.; Treutlein, B.; Tan, K.; Tan, V.; Liu, F.C.; Looney, M.R.; et al. Lineage-negative progenitors mobilize to regenerate lung epithelium after major injury. *Nature* **2015**, *517*, 621–625. [CrossRef]
160. Peng, T.; Frank, D.B.; Kadzik, R.S.; Morley, M.P.; Rathi, K.S.; Wang, T.; Zhou, S.; Cheng, L.; Lu, M.M.; Morrisey, E.E. Hedgehog actively maintains adult lung quiescence and regulates repair and regeneration. *Nature* **2015**, *526*, 578–582. [CrossRef]
161. Li, M.; Krishnaveni, M.S.; Li, C.; Zhou, B.; Xing, Y.; Banfalvi, A.; Li, A.; Lombardi, V.; Akbari, O.; Borok, Z.; et al. Epithelium-specific deletion of TGF-beta receptor type II protects mice from bleomycin-induced pulmonary fibrosis. *J. Clin. Investig.* **2011**, *121*, 277–287. [CrossRef]
162. Coker, R.K.; Laurent, G.J.; Jeffery, P.K.; Du Bois, R.M.; Black, C.M.; McAnulty, R.J. Localisation of transforming growth factor beta1 and beta3 mRNA transcripts in normal and fibrotic human lung. *Thorax* **2001**, *56*, 549–556. [CrossRef]
163. Mu, D.; Cambier, S.; Fjellbirkeland, L.; Baron, J.L.; Munger, J.S.; Kawakatsu, H.; Sheppard, D.; Broaddus, V.C.; Nishimura, S.L. The integrin alpha(v)beta8 mediates epithelial homeostasis through MT1-MMP-dependent activation of TGF-beta1. *J. Cell Biol.* **2002**, *157*, 493–507. [CrossRef]
164. Munger, J.S.; Huang, X.; Kawakatsu, H.; Griffiths, M.J.; Dalton, S.L.; Wu, J.; Pittet, J.F.; Kaminski, N.; Garat, C.; Matthay, M.A.; et al. The integrin alpha v beta 6 binds and activates latent TGF beta 1: A mechanism for regulating pulmonary inflammation and fibrosis. *Cell* **1999**, *96*, 319–328. [CrossRef]
165. Bonniaud, P.; Martin, G.; Margetts, P.J.; Ask, K.; Robertson, J.; Gauldie, J.; Kolb, M. Connective tissue growth factor is crucial to inducing a profibrotic environment in "fibrosis-resistant" BALB/c mouse lungs. *Am. J. Respir. Cell Mol. Biol.* **2004**, *31*. 510–516. [CrossRef]
166. Bonniaud, P.; Margetts, P.J.; Kolb, M.; Haberberger, T.; Kelly, M.; Robertson, J.; Gauldie, J. Adenoviral gene transfer of connective tissue growth factor in the lung induces transient fibrosis. *Am. J. Respir. Crit. Care Med.* **2003**, *168*, 770–778. [CrossRef]
167. Watts, K.L.; Spiteri, M.A. Connective tissue growth factor expression and induction by transforming growth factor-beta is abrogated by simvastatin via a Rho signaling mechanism. *Am. J. Physiol. Lung Cell Mol. Physiol.* **2004**, *287*, L1323–L1332. [CrossRef]
168. Lasky, J.A.; Ortiz, L.A.; Tonthat, B.; Hoyle, G.W.; Corti, M.; Athas, G.; Lungarella, G.; Brody, A.; Friedman, M. Connective tissue growth factor mRNA expression is upregulated in bleomycin-induced lung fibrosis. *Am. J. Physiol.* **1998**, *275*, L365–L371. [CrossRef]
169. Pan, L.H.; Yamauchi, K.; Uzuki, M.; Nakanishi, T.; Takigawa, M.; Inoue, H.; Sawai, T. Type II alveolar epithelial cells and interstitial fibroblasts express connective tissue growth factor in IPF. *Eur. Respir. J.* **2001**, *17*, 1220–1227. [CrossRef] [PubMed]
170. Wang, C.; Cassandras, M.; Peng, T. The Role of Hedgehog Signaling in Adult Lung Regeneration and Maintenance. *J. Dev. Biol.* **2019**, *7*. [CrossRef]
171. Kugler, M.C.; Joyner, A.L.; Loomis, C.A.; Munger, J.S. Sonic hedgehog signaling in the lung. From development to disease. *Am. J. Respir. Cell Mol. Biol.* **2015**, *52*, 1–13. [CrossRef] [PubMed]
172. Hu, B.; Liu, J.; Wu, Z.; Liu, T.; Ullenbruch, M.R.; Ding, L.; Henke, C.A.; Bitterman, P.B.; Phan, S.H. Reemergence of hedgehog mediates epithelial-mesenchymal crosstalk in pulmonary fibrosis. *Am. J. Respir. Cell Mol. Biol.* **2015**, *52*, 418–428. [CrossRef] [PubMed]
173. Bolanos, A.L.; Milla, C.M.; Lira, J.C.; Ramirez, R.; Checa, M.; Barrera, L.; Garcia-Alvarez, J.; Carbajal, V.; Becerril, C.; Gaxiola, M.; et al. Role of Sonic Hedgehog in idiopathic pulmonary fibrosis. *Am. J. Physiol. Lung

Cell Mol. Physiol. **2012**, *303*, L978–L990. [CrossRef] [PubMed]

174. Stewart, G.A.; Hoyne, G.F.; Ahmad, S.A.; Jarman, E.; Wallace, W.A.; Harrison, D.J.; Haslett, C.; Lamb, J.R.; Howie, S.E. Expression of the developmental Sonic hedgehog (Shh) signalling pathway is up-regulated in chronic lung fibrosis and the Shh receptor patched 1 is present in circulating T lymphocytes. *J. Pathol.* **2003**, *199*, 488–495. [CrossRef] [PubMed]
175. Coon, D.R.; Roberts, D.J.; Loscertales, M.; Kradin, R. Differential epithelial expression of SHH and FOXF1 in usual and nonspecific interstitial pneumonia. *Exp. Mol. Pathol.* **2006**, *80*, 119–123. [CrossRef]
176. Fitch, P.M.; Howie, S.E.; Wallace, W.A. Oxidative damage and TGF-beta differentially induce lung epithelial cell sonic hedgehog and tenascin-C expression: Implications for the regulation of lung remodelling in idiopathic interstitial lung disease. *Int. J. Exp. Pathol.* **2011**, *92*, 8–17. [CrossRef]
177. Moshai, E.F.; Wemeau-Stervinou, L.; Cigna, N.; Brayer, S.; Somme, J.M.; Crestani, B.; Mailleux, A.A. Targeting the hedgehog-glioma-associated oncogene homolog pathway inhibits bleomycin-induced lung fibrosis in mice. *Am. J. Respir. Cell Mol. Biol.* **2014**, *51*, 11–25. [CrossRef]
178. Liu, L.; Kugler, M.C.; Loomis, C.A.; Samdani, R.; Zhao, Z.; Chen, G.J.; Brandt, J.P.; Brownell, I.; Joyner, A.L.; Rom, W.N.; et al. Hedgehog signaling in neonatal and adult lung. *Am. J. Respir. Cell Mol. Biol.* **2013**, *48*, 703–710. [CrossRef]
179. Kugler, M.C.; Yie, T.A.; Cai, Y.; Berger, J.Z.; Loomis, C.A.; Munger, J.S. The Hedgehog target Gli1 is not required for bleomycin-induced lung fibrosis. *Exp. Lung Res.* **2019**, *45*, 22–29. [CrossRef]
180. Ge, L.; Habiel, D.M.; Hansbro, P.M.; Kim, R.Y.; Gharib, S.A.; Edelman, J.D.; Konigshoff, M.; Parimon, T.; Brauer, R.; Huang, Y.; et al. miR-323a-3p regulates lung fibrosis by targeting multiple profibrotic pathways. *JCI Insight* **2016**, *1*, e90301. [CrossRef]
181. Pan, T.; Mason, R.J.; Westcott, J.Y.; Shannon, J.M. Rat alveolar type II cells inhibit lung fibroblast proliferation in vitro. *Am. J. Respir. Cell Mol. Biol.* **2001**, *25*, 353–361. [CrossRef] [PubMed]
182. Portnoy, J.; Pan, T.; Dinarello, C.A.; Shannon, J.M.; Westcott, J.Y.; Zhang, L.; Mason, R.J. Alveolar type II cells inhibit fibroblast proliferation: Role of IL-1alpha. *Am. J. Physiol. Lung Cell Mol. Physiol.* **2006**, *290*, L307–L316. [CrossRef] [PubMed]
183. Moore, B.B.; Peters-Golden, M.; Christensen, P.J.; Lama, V.; Kuziel, W.A.; Paine, R., 3rd; Toews, G.B. Alveolar epithelial cell inhibition of fibroblast proliferation is regulated by MCP-1/CCR2 and mediated by PGE2. *Am. J. Physiol. Lung Cell Mol. Physiol.* **2003**, *284*, L342–L349. [CrossRef] [PubMed]
184. Borok, Z.; Gillissen, A.; Buhl, R.; Hoyt, R.F.; Hubbard, R.C.; Ozaki, T.; Rennard, S.I.; Crystal, R.G. Augmentation of functional prostaglandin E levels on the respiratory epithelial surface by aerosol administration of prostaglandin E. *Am. Rev. Respir. Dis.* **1991**, *144*, 1080–1084. [CrossRef]
185. Lama, V.; Moore, B.B.; Christensen, P.; Toews, G.B.; Peters-Golden, M. Prostaglandin E2 synthesis and suppression of fibroblast proliferation by alveolar epithelial cells is cyclooxygenase-2-dependent. *Am. J. Respir. Cell Mol. Biol.* **2002**, *27*, 752–758. [CrossRef]
186. Tan, Q.; Ma, X.Y.; Liu, W.; Meridew, J.A.; Jones, D.L.; Haak, A.J.; Sicard, D.; Ligresti, G.; Tschumperlin, D.J. Nascent Lung Organoids Reveal Epithelium- and Bone Morphogenetic Protein-mediated Suppression of Fibroblast Activation. *Am. J. Respir. Cell Mol. Biol.* **2019**, *61*, 607–619. [CrossRef]
187. Munoz-Espin, D.; Serrano, M. Cellular senescence: From physiology to pathology. *Nat. Rev. Mol. Cell Biol.* **2014**, *15*, 482–496. [CrossRef]
188. Gahl, W.A.; Brantly, M.; Kaiser-Kupfer, M.I.; Iwata, F.; Hazelwood, S.; Shotelersuk, V.; Duffy, L.F.; Kuehl, E.M.; Troendle, J.; Bernardini, I. Genetic defects and clinical characteristics of patients with a form of oculocutaneous albinism (Hermansky-Pudlak syndrome). *N. Engl. J. Med.* **1998**, *338*, 1258–1264. [CrossRef]
189. Young, L.R.; Gulleman, P.M.; Short, C.W.; Tanjore, H.; Sherrill, T.; Qi, A.; McBride, A.P.; Zaynagetdinov, R.; Benjamin, J.T.; Lawson, W.E.; et al. Epithelial-macrophage interactions determine pulmonary fibrosis susceptibility in Hermansky-Pudlak syndrome. *JCI Insight* **2016**, *1*, e88947. [CrossRef]
190. Acosta, J.C.; Banito, A.; Wuestefeld, T.; Georgilis, A.; Janich, P.; Morton, J.P.; Athineos, D.; Kang, T.W.; Lasitschka, F.; Andrulis, M.; et al. A complex secretory program orchestrated by the inflammasome controls paracrine senescence. *Nat. Cell Biol.* **2013**, *15*, 978–990. [CrossRef]
191. Nelson, G.; Wordsworth, J.; Wang, C.; Jurk, D.; Lawless, C.; Martin-Ruiz, C.; Von Zglinicki, T. A senescent cell bystander effect: Senescence-induced senescence. *Aging Cell* **2012**, *11*, 345–349. [CrossRef] [PubMed]
192. Hubackova, S.; Krejcikova, K.; Bartek, J.; Hodny, Z. IL1- and TGFbeta-Nox4 signaling, oxidative stress and DNA damage response are shared features of replicative, oncogene-induced, and drug-induced paracrine

'bystander senescence'. *Aging (Albany N.Y.)* **2012**, *4*, 932–951. [CrossRef]

193. Hoare, M.; Narita, M. Notch and Senescence. *Adv. Exp. Med. Biol.* **2018**, *1066*, 299–318. [CrossRef] [PubMed]
194. Hoare, M.; Narita, M. NOTCH and the 2 SASPs of senescence. *Cell Cycle* **2017**, *16*, 239–240. [CrossRef]
195. Hoare, M.; Ito, Y.; Kang, T.W.; Weekes, M.P.; Matheson, N.J.; Patten, D.A.; Shetty, S.; Parry, A.J.; Menon, S.; Salama, R.; et al. NOTCH1 mediates a switch between two distinct secretomes during senescence. *Nat. Cell Biol.* **2016**, *18*, 979–992. [CrossRef]
196. Van Niel, G.; D'Angelo, G.; Raposo, G. Shedding light on the cell biology of extracellular vesicles. *Nat. Rev. Mol. Cell Biol.* **2018**, *19*, 213–228. [CrossRef]
197. Takasugi, M. Emerging roles of extracellular vesicles in cellular senescence and aging. *Aging Cell* **2018**, *17*. [CrossRef]
198. Borghesan, M.; Fafian-Labora, J.; Eleftheriadou, O.; Carpintero-Fernandez, P.; Paez-Ribes, M.; Vizcay-Barrena, G.; Swisa, A.; Kolodkin-Gal, D.; Ximenez-Embun, P.; Lowe, R.; et al. Small Extracellular Vesicles Are Key Regulators of Non-cell Autonomous Intercellular Communication in Senescence via the Interferon Protein IFITM3. *Cell Rep.* **2019**, *27*, 3956–3971. [CrossRef]
199. Martin-Medina, A.; Lehmann, M.; Burgy, O.; Hermann, S.; Baarsma, H.A.; Wagner, D.E.; De Santis, M.M.; Ciolek, F.; Hofer, T.P.; Frankenberger, M.; et al. Increased Extracellular Vesicles Mediate WNT-5A Signaling in Idiopathic Pulmonary Fibrosis. *Am. J. Respir. Crit. Care Med.* **2018**. [CrossRef]
200. Yang, I.V.; Schwartz, D.A. Epigenetics of idiopathic pulmonary fibrosis. *Transl. Res.* **2015**, *165*, 48–60. [CrossRef]
201. Chen, Z.; Li, S.; Subramaniam, S.; Shyy, J.Y.; Chien, S. Epigenetic Regulation: A New Frontier for Biomedical Engineers. *Annu. Rev. Biomed. Eng.* **2017**, *19*, 195–219. [CrossRef] [PubMed]
202. Yang, I.V.; Pedersen, B.S.; Rabinovich, E.; Hennessy, C.E.; Davidson, E.J.; Murphy, E.; Guardela, B.J.; Tedrow, J.R.; Zhang, Y.; Singh, M.K.; et al. Relationship of DNA methylation and gene expression in idiopathic pulmonary fibrosis. *Am. J. Respir. Crit. Care Med.* **2014**, *190*, 1263–1272. [CrossRef] [PubMed]
203. Sanders, Y.Y.; Ambalavanan, N.; Halloran, B.; Zhang, X.; Liu, H.; Crossman, D.K.; Bray, M.; Zhang, K.; Thannickal, V.J.; Hagood, J.S. Altered DNA methylation profile in idiopathic pulmonary fibrosis. *Am. J. Respir. Crit. Care Med.* **2012**, *186*, 525–535. [CrossRef]
204. Rabinovich, E.I.; Kapetanaki, M.G.; Steinfeld, I.; Gibson, K.F.; Pandit, K.V.; Yu, G.; Yakhini, Z.; Kaminski, N. Global methylation patterns in idiopathic pulmonary fibrosis. *PLoS ONE* **2012**, *7*, e33770. [CrossRef]
205. Fraga, M.F.; Ballestar, E.; Paz, M.F.; Ropero, S.; Setien, F.; Ballestar, M.L.; Heine-Suner, D.; Cigudosa, J.C.; Urioste, M.; Benitez, J.; et al. Epigenetic differences arise during the lifetime of monozygotic twins. *Proc. Natl. Acad. Sci. USA* **2005**, *102*, 10604–10609. [CrossRef] [PubMed]
206. Heyn, H.; Li, N.; Ferreira, H.J.; Moran, S.; Pisano, D.G.; Gomez, A.; Diez, J.; Sanchez-Mut, J.V.; Setien, F.; Carmona, F.J.; et al. Distinct DNA methylomes of newborns and centenarians. *Proc. Natl. Acad. Sci. USA* **2012**, *109*, 10522–10527. [CrossRef] [PubMed]
207. Issa, J.P. Aging and epigenetic drift: A vicious cycle. *J. Clin. Investig.* **2014**, *124*, 24–29. [CrossRef] [PubMed]
208. Silvestri, G.A.; Vachani, A.; Whitney, D.; Elashoff, M.; Porta Smith, K.; Ferguson, J.S.; Parsons, E.; Mitra, N.; Brody, J.; Lenburg, M.E.; et al. A Bronchial Genomic Classifier for the Diagnostic Evaluation of Lung Cancer. *N. Engl. J. Med.* **2015**, *373*, 243–251. [CrossRef]
209. Steiling, K.; Kadar, A.Y.; Bergerat, A.; Flanigon, J.; Sridhar, S.; Shah, V.; Ahmad, Q.R.; Brody, J.S.; Lenburg, M.E.; Steffen, M.; et al. Comparison of proteomic and transcriptomic profiles in the bronchial airway epithelium of current and never smokers. *PLoS ONE* **2009**, *4*, e5043. [CrossRef]
210. Sridhar, S.; Schembri, F.; Zeskind, J.; Shah, V.; Gustafson, A.M.; Steiling, K.; Liu, G.; Dumas, Y.M.; Zhang, X.; Brody, J.S.; et al. Smoking-induced gene expression changes in the bronchial airway are reflected in nasal and buccal epithelium. *BMC Genom.* **2008**, *9*, 259. [CrossRef]
211. Shah, V.; Sridhar, S.; Beane, J.; Brody, J.S.; Spira, A. SIEGE: Smoking Induced Epithelial Gene Expression Database. *Nucleic Acids Res.* **2005**, *33*, D573–D579. [CrossRef] [PubMed]
212. Buro-Auriemma, L.J.; Salit, J.; Hackett, N.R.; Walters, M.S.; Strulovici-Barel, Y.; Staudt, M.R.; Fuller, J.; Mahmoud, M.; Stevenson, C.S.; Hilton, H.; et al. Cigarette smoking induces small airway epithelial epigenetic changes with corresponding modulation of gene expression. *Hum. Mol. Genet.* **2013**, *22*, 4726–4738. [CrossRef] [PubMed]
213. Cotton, A.M.; Lam, L.; Affleck, J.G.; Wilson, I.M.; Penaherrera, M.S.; McFadden, D.E.; Kobor, M.S.; Lam, W.L.; Robinson, W.P.; Brown, C.J. Chromosome-wide DNA methylation analysis predicts human tissue-specific X

inactivation. *Hum. Genet.* **2011**, *130*, 187–201. [CrossRef] [PubMed]
214. Boks, M.P.; Derks, E.M.; Weisenberger, D.J.; Strengman, E.; Janson, E.; Sommer, I.E.; Kahn, R.S.; Ophoff, R.A. The relationship of DNA methylation with age, gender and genotype in twins and healthy controls. *PLoS ONE* **2009**, *4*, e6767. [CrossRef] [PubMed]
215. Sarter, B.; Long, T.I.; Tsong, W.H.; Koh, W.P.; Yu, M.C.; Laird, P.W. Sex differential in methylation patterns of selected genes in Singapore Chinese. *Hum. Genet.* **2005**, *117*, 402–403. [CrossRef]
216. El-Maarri, O.; Becker, T.; Junen, J.; Manzoor, S.S.; Diaz-Lacava, A.; Schwaab, R.; Wienker, T.; Oldenburg, J. Gender specific differences in levels of DNA methylation at selected loci from human total blood: A tendency toward higher methylation levels in males. *Hum. Genet.* **2007**, *122*, 505–514. [CrossRef] [PubMed]
217. Dakhlallah, D.; Batte, K.; Wang, Y.; Cantemir-Stone, C.Z.; Yan, P.; Nuovo, G.; Mikhail, A.; Hitchcock, C.L.; Wright, V.P.; Nana-Sinkam, S.P.; et al. Epigenetic regulation of miR-17~92 contributes to the pathogenesis of pulmonary fibrosis. *Am. J. Respir. Crit. Care Med.* **2013**, *187*, 397–405. [CrossRef] [PubMed]
218. Rubio, K.; Singh, I.; Dobersch, S.; Sarvari, P.; Gunther, S.; Cordero, J.; Mehta, A.; Wujak, L.; Cabrera-Fuentes, H.; Chao, C.M.; et al. Inactivation of nuclear histone deacetylases by EP300 disrupts the MiCEE complex in idiopathic pulmonary fibrosis. *Nat. Commun.* **2019**, *10*, 2229. [CrossRef] [PubMed]
219. Korfei, M.; Skwarna, S.; Henneke, I.; MacKenzie, B.; Klymenko, O.; Saito, S.; Ruppert, C.; Von der Beck, D.; Mahavadi, P.; Klepetko, W.; et al. Aberrant expression and activity of histone deacetylases in sporadic idiopathic pulmonary fibrosis. *Thorax* **2015**, *70*, 1022–1032. [CrossRef]
220. Sanders, Y.Y.; Hagood, J.S.; Liu, H.; Zhang, W.; Ambalavanan, N.; Thannickal, V.J. Histone deacetylase inhibition promotes fibroblast apoptosis and ameliorates pulmonary fibrosis in mice. *Eur. Respir. J.* **2014**, *43*, 1448–1458. [CrossRef]
221. Conforti, F.; Davies, E.R.; Calderwood, C.J.; Thatcher, T.H.; Jones, M.G.; Smart, D.E.; Mahajan, S.; Alzetani, A.; Havelock, T.; Maher, T.M.; et al. The histone deacetylase inhibitor, romidepsin, as a potential treatment for pulmonary fibrosis. *Oncotarget* **2017**, *8*, 48737–48754. [CrossRef] [PubMed]
222. Tang, X.; Peng, R.; Phillips, J.E.; Deguzman, J.; Ren, Y.; Apparsundaram, S.; Luo, Q.; Bauer, C.M.; Fuentes, M.E.; DeMartino, J.A.; et al. Assessment of Brd4 inhibition in idiopathic pulmonary fibrosis lung fibroblasts and in vivo models of lung fibrosis. *Am. J. Pathol.* **2013**, *183*, 470–479. [CrossRef] [PubMed]
223. Miao, C.; Xiong, Y.; Zhang, G.; Chang, J. MicroRNAs in idiopathic pulmonary fibrosis, new research progress and their pathophysiological implication. *Exp. Lung Res.* **2018**, *44*, 178–190. [CrossRef]
224. Wang, Y.; Frank, D.B.; Morley, M.P.; Zhou, S.; Wang, X.; Lu, M.M.; Lazar, M.A.; Morrisey, E.E. HDAC3-Dependent Epigenetic Pathway Controls Lung Alveolar Epithelial Cell Remodeling and Spreading via miR-17-92 and TGF-beta Signaling Regulation. *Dev. Cell* **2016**, *36*, 303–315. [CrossRef] [PubMed]
225. Da Rocha, S.T.; Edwards, C.A.; Ito, M.; Ogata, T.; Ferguson-Smith, A.C. Genomic imprinting at the mammalian Dlk1-Dio3 domain. *Trends Genet.* **2008**, *24*, 306–316. [CrossRef] [PubMed]
226. Seitz, H.; Royo, H.; Bortolin, M.L.; Lin, S.P.; Ferguson-Smith, A.C.; Cavaille, J. A large imprinted microRNA gene cluster at the mouse Dlk1-Gtl2 domain. *Genome Res.* **2004**, *14*, 1741–1748. [CrossRef]
227. Snyder, C.M.; Rice, A.L.; Estrella, N.L.; Held, A.; Kandarian, S.C.; Naya, F.J. MEF2A regulates the Gtl2-Dio3 microRNA mega-cluster to modulate WNT signaling in skeletal muscle regeneration. *Development* **2013**, *140*, 31–42. [CrossRef]
228. Milosevic, J.; Pandit, K.; Magister, M.; Rabinovich, E.; Ellwanger, D.C.; Yu, G.; Vuga, L.J.; Weksler, B.; Benos, P.V.; Gibson, K.F.; et al. Profibrotic role of miR-154 in pulmonary fibrosis. *Am. J. Respir. Cell Mol. Biol.* **2012**, *47*, 879–887. [CrossRef]

9

P2X7 Receptor Indirectly Regulates the JAM-A Protein Content via Modulation of GSK-3β

Karl-Philipp Wesslau, Anabel Stein, Michael Kasper and Kathrin Barth *

Institute of Anatomy, Dresden University of Technology, D-01307 Dresden, Germany; karl-philipp@wesslau.de (K-P.W.); bella.stein@yahoo.de (A.S.); michael.kasper@tu-dresden.de (M.K.)

* Correspondence: kathrin.barth@tu-dresden.de

Abstract: The alveolar epithelial cells represent an important part of the alveolar barrier, which is maintained by tight junction proteins, particularly JAM-A, occludin, and claudin-18, which regulate paracellular permeability. In this study, we report on a strong increase in epithelial JAM-A expression in P2X7 receptor knockout mice when compared to the wildtype. Precision-cut lung slices of wildtype and knockout lungs and immortal epithelial lung E10 cells were treated with bleomycin, the P2X7 receptor inhibitor oxATP, and the agonist BzATP, respectively, to evaluate early changes in JAM-A expression. Biochemical and immunohistochemical data showed evidence for P2X7 receptor-dependent JAM-A expression in vitro. Inhibition of the P2X7 receptor using oxATP increased JAM-A, whereas activation of the receptor decreased the JAM-A protein level. In order to examine the role of GSK-3β in the expression of JAM-A in alveolar epithelial cells, we used lithium chloride for GSK-3β inhibiting experiments, which showed a modulating effect on bleomycin-induced alterations in JAM-A levels. Our data suggest that an increased constitutive JAM-A protein level in P2X7 receptor knockout mice may have a protective effect against bleomycin-induced lung injury. Bleomycin-treated precision-cut lung slices from P2X7 receptor knockout mice responded with a lower increase in mRNA expression of JAM-A than bleomycin-treated precision-cut lung slices from wildtype mice.

Keywords: JAM-A; P2X7 receptor; mouse lung; alveolar epithelium; bleomycin-induced lung injury; GSK-3β

---

1. Introduction

Alveolar epithelial cells (AEC) represent the most vulnerable cells of the distal lung parenchyma and consist of flat AECI type I and cuboidal AECII type II cells in most vertebrates, including humans. Under normal physiological conditions, both cell types are involved in gas exchange and fluid homeostasis [1] and participate in alveolar barrier functions and wound repair processes after lung injury [2]. To maintain cellular polarity and barrier functions of AEC, several types of intercellular junctions exist such as tight junctions (TJ), adherens junctions (AJ), gap junctions, and desmosomes. TJ proteins are particularly important in the regulation of the transcellular permeability of AEC.

Besides their completely different morphological appearance, AECI and AECII specifically differ in their protein pattern, which allows, to a certain degree, their distinction from each other [3]. Knockout of AECI-specific proteins lead to the early death of the animals (T1α knockout, [4], or the lungs exhibit a pathologic phenotype (e.g., caveolin-1 [5], RAGE [6], and aquaporin-5 [7] knockouts). One exception is the P2X7 receptor deficient mouse, which does not exhibit a single sign of histomorphological alterations during its lifetime [8]. The P2X7 receptor (P2X7R) is a ligand-gated ion channel activated by extracellular ATP. In the most distal part of lung, P2X7R is selectively present in AECI [9] and in alveolar macrophages [10]. The intracellular pathways activated by the receptor influence pulmonary inflammation (reviewed in Reference [11]) and the P2X7R knockout (P2X7$^{-/-}$) lung show altered tight junction protein expression [12].

In experimental studies, $P2X7^{-/-}$ deficient mice have presented dramatically reduced lung inflammation with reduced fibrosis markers in the bleomycin (BLM) model [13]. Deletion of P2X7R has a protective effect and the receptor is a therapeutic target for the amelioration of hyperoxia-induced lung injury [14]. $P2X7^{-/-}$ animals showed no significant effect of LPS on lung function, alveolar collapse, or fiber deposition in lung parenchyma when compared with wildtype (WT) mice [15].

Treatment with BLM, an anti-cancer agent, is often used as an experimental model of lung injury and pulmonary fibrosis. Molecular changes after BLM exposure include genes encoding growth factors, signaling molecules, and structural proteins, for example, caveolin-1 and diverse junctional proteins. BLM causes an increase in reactive oxygen species and thus induces apoptosis in epithelial and other cells of the lung, leading to disruption of the alveolar barrier. Recently, it was shown that bleomycin-induced lung injury was attenuated in $P2X7^{-/-}$ mice [13].

The TJ and AJ are collectively referred to as the apical junctional complex (AJC) and constitute apical intercellular contacts. The AJC contains the key transmembrane proteins occludin, the claudin protein family, and junctional adhesion molecules (JAM) localized to the TJ, as well as E-cadherin in the AJ. JAMs are expressed by a variety of different cells, mainly epithelial cells, endothelial cells, and cells of the immune system, e.g., leukocytes. The importance of JAM-A in regulating barrier function is shown for JAM-A in epithelial and endothelial cells where siRNA mediated loss of JAM-A expression results in enhanced permeability, as determined by transepithelial resistance (TER) [16]. A complex series of poorly understood signaling events establish epithelial barrier function culminating in the formation of mature TJs, whereby JAM-A seems to be important in early events required for TJ assembly. Adhesion complexes are not formed at low Ca^{2+} concentration in epithelial cells.

In earlier work, we have shown that high intracellular Ca^{2+} content through activation of P2X7R after BLM treatment leads to increased protein kinase (PKC)-β1 in alveolar epithelial cells [17]. The comparison of lung tissues from WT and $P2X7^{-/-}$ mice revealed decreased protein and mRNA levels of PKC-β1 and calmodulin (CaM). We demonstrated that the inhibition of P2X7R after BLM treatment also leads to decreased CaM and PKC-β1 content. This indicates that in the BLM model, P2X7R is involved in the regulation of intracellular calcium content and that the PKC-β1 acts downstream of the P2X7R. By stimulating and inhibiting various isoforms, the conventional PKCs, including the isoforms α, β1, β2, and γ are activated by calcium and diacylglycerol. Both factors have been described as triggers of TJ dissolution [18]. In addition to modified TJ protein levels in the $P2X7^{-/-}$, we also found an increased inactivation of the glycogen synthase kinase (GSK)-3β in the $P2X7^{-/-}$ compared to the WT mice [12]. In vitro experiments demonstrated that GSK-3β phosphorylation mediated by PKC enhanced GSK-3β activity. It has also been reported that in vitro GSK-3β is inactivated in the same manner by particular forms of PKCs [19]. The physiological importance of GSK-3β activity in the regulation of the normal epithelial barrier was shown by Severson et al. [20], which implicates the active role of GSK-3β in controlling the expression of the AJC proteins occludin, claudin-1, and E-cadherin.

The aim of this study was to investigate the expression of the tight junction molecule JAM-A in WT and $P2X7^{-/-}$ mice and to investigate the involvement of GSK-3β, which has previously been shown to be increased in $P2X7^{-/-}$ mice [12]. We further studied the influence of BLM on JAM-A in precision-cut lung slices (PCLS) of WT and $P2X7^{-/-}$ mice and in immortal AECI-like E10 cells and whether the GSK-3β(Ser9) phosphorylation changed after BLM treatment. The influence of the inhibition of P2X7R under BLM treatment was studied using the P2X7R inhibitor oxATP. We also investigated whether inactivation of P2X7R led to changes in the phosphorylation of GSK-3β at Ser9 and if this subsequently had an impact on JAM-A protein content.

2. Results

2.1. *P2X7$^{-/-}$ Mice Show Strongly Enhanced JAM-A Protein Level in the Lung Parenchyma*

We analyzed the mRNA expression and total protein content of JAM-A in lung tissue homogenates of WT and P2X7$^{-/-}$ mice (Figure 1).

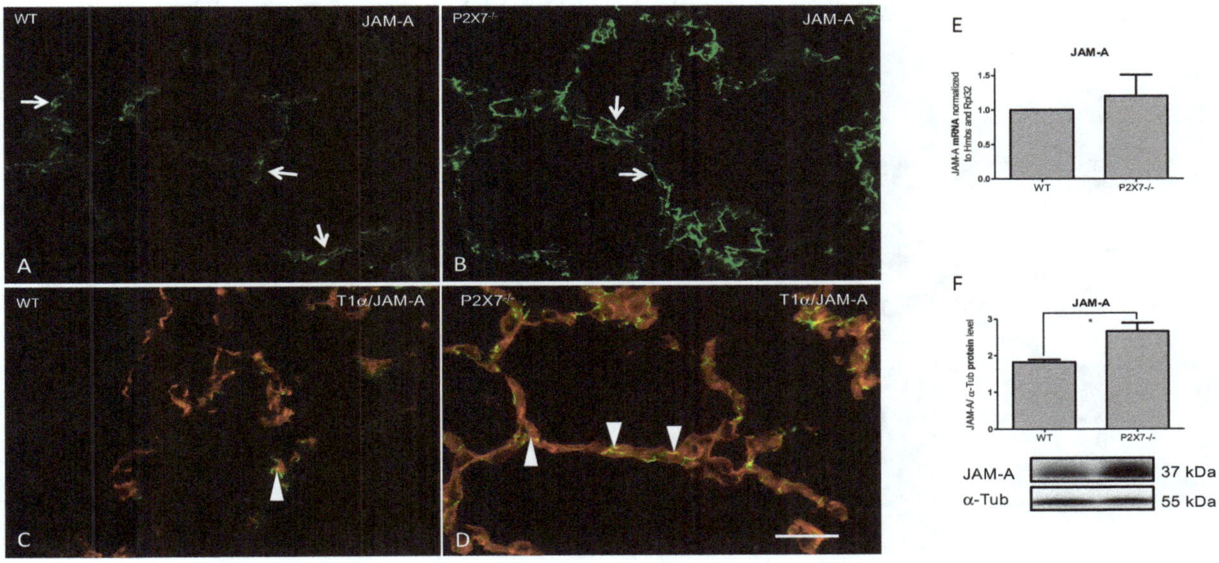

Figure 1. Frozen sections of mouse lung tissue. Immunofluorescence demonstration of JAM-A in WT and P2X7$^{-/-}$ mice (**A**–**D**). Note the increase in immunoreactivity of JAM-A in P2X7$^{-/-}$ mice (**B**,**D**). (**C**,**D**) Double immunofluorescence with the AECI marker T1α (TexasRed). Arrows show the linear pattern of JAM-A. Arrowheads depict examples of epithelial junctions. Bar = 100 μm. Corresponding mRNA (**E**) (Wildtype (WT) normalized to 1; $n = 3$; p-value 0.5737) and protein (**F**) ($n = 3$, p-value 0.0357) levels in lung homogenates. * $p < 0.05$.

A significant increase in JAM-A protein content was found in the P2X7$^{-/-}$ mice. The total mRNA level of JAM-A was also found to be increased.

Immunofluorescence staining confirmed the change in JAM-A expression. WT mice showed a predominantly linear staining pattern of localization for JAM-A. This pattern of immunoreactivity did not change in the P2X7$^{-/-}$ mice. Only quantitative alterations were observable. There were no signs of disrupted junctions. Double immunofluorescence experiments with AECI specific T1α revealed a prominent JAM-A localization related to the AECI-AECI and AECI-AECII border.

2.2. *Influence of BLM Treatment on mRNA Expression of JAM-A and Localization in the Lung Tissue of P2X7$^{-/-}$ Mice in Comparison to the WT*

To investigate whether the BLM treatment in the lung tissue of P2X7$^{-/-}$ led to an altered expression of JAM-A in comparison to the WT animals, the PCLS of wildtype and P2X7$^{-/-}$ mice were prepared and treated with BLM for 24 h and 48 h (Figure 2). Using quantitative RT-PCR, we were able to demonstrate a marked increase in JAM-A expression in the PCLS of BLM-treated WT mice compared to BLM-treated PCLS of P2X7$^{-/-}$ mice (Figure 2, inset in A and E).

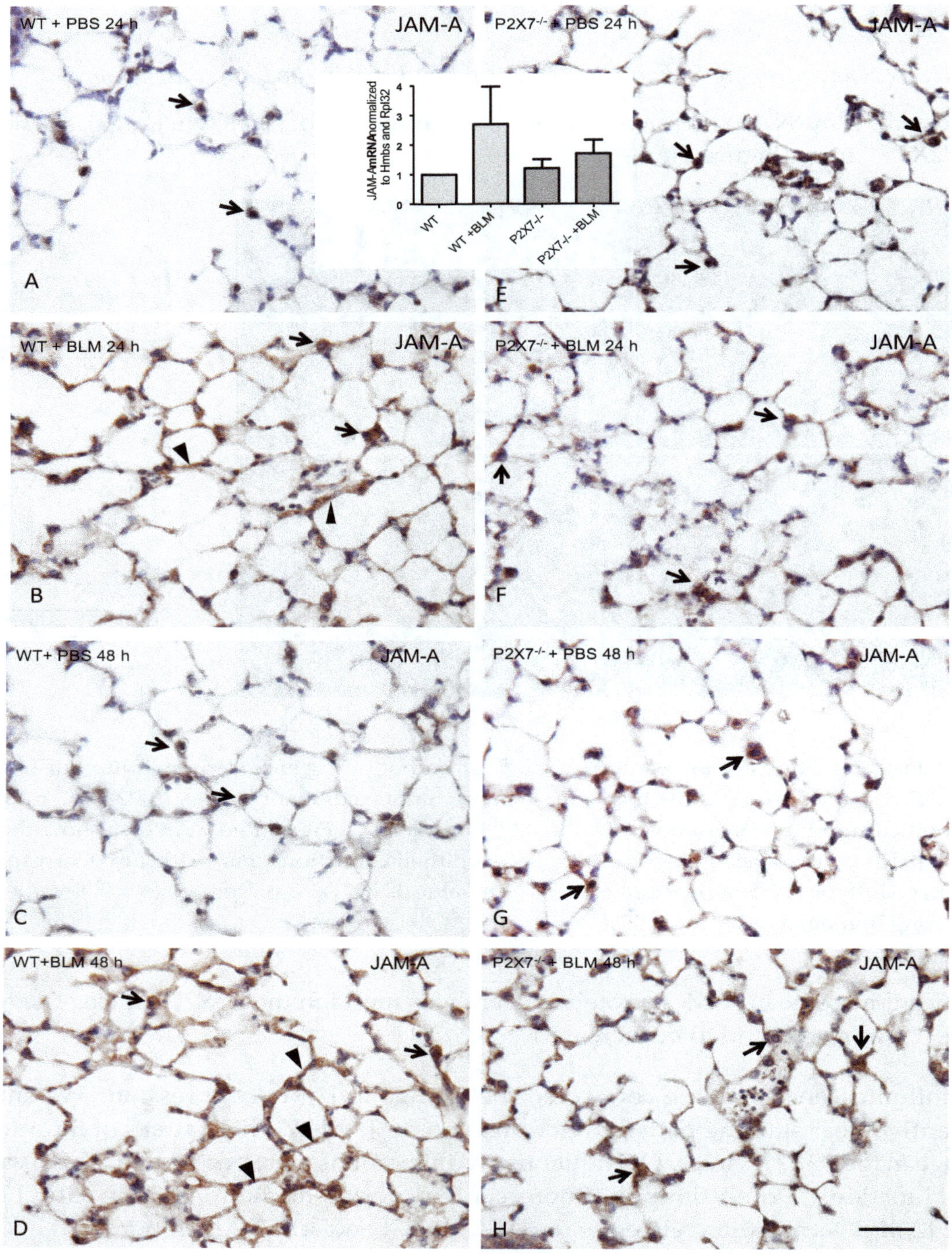

Figure 2. Paraffin sections from embedded PCLS after 300 mU/mL BLM exposure for 24 h (**A**,**B**,**E**,**F**) and 48 h (**C**,**D**,**G**,**H**). Immunoperoxidase demonstration of JAM-A in WT (**A**–**D**) and P2X7$^{-/-}$ (**E**–**H**) mice. Note the preferable immunostaining of AECII in untreated WT (arrows in **A**,**C**), a weak increase in P2X7$^{-/-}$ mice (**E**,**G**), and the strongest immunostaining of the AECs in the BLM-treated WT mice (**B**,**D**). Arrowheads depict the alveolar lining of JAM-A immunoreactivity. Bar = 100 μm. Inset over (**A**) and (**E**): Analysis of mRNA content in paraffin sections of PCLS from WT and P2X7$^{-/-}$ mice after 24 h. mRNA content of *JAM-A* was analyzed by quantitative real time RT-PCR using *Hmbs* and *Rpl32* as housekeeping genes. Charts are represented as mean ± SEM (WT normalized to 1; n = 3; p-value 0.4550).

Immunoperoxidase staining for JAM-A in the PCLS of WT lungs exhibited prominent staining at the AECI/II border and some additional cytoplasmic AECII staining, with increased immunoreactivity in the PCLS of P2X7$^{-/-}$. The entire JAM-A immunoreactivity, as seen in frozen sections (compared to Figure 1), could not be reproduced in the paraffin sections, since fixation and paraffin embedding impaired the immunoreactivity and the structural conciseness of immunolocalization. The 24 h treatment with BLM led to a strongly enhanced immunoreactivity of the entire alveolar lining layer in the WT, but to a lesser extent in the P2X7$^{-/-}$ (Figure 2). This effect was stronger after 48 h of BLM treatment (Figure 2).

Some additional endothelial JAM-A immunostaining could not be excluded, since double staining with endothelial markers could not be performed in the present study due to the lack of suitable antibodies.

2.3. *The Inhibition of GSK-3β Leads to the Reduction of the Protein Content of JAM-A under BLM Treatment*

In the following experiment, different influences on JAM-A were evaluated. Based on the findings in the P2X7$^{-/-}$ mice where the inactivated form of GSK-3β, the GSK-3β(Ser9), was upregulated compared to WT [12], the GSK-3β(Ser9) protein level was investigated after BLM treatment in the alveolar epithelial E10 cells. In order to examine the role of GSK-3β in the expression of JAM-A, we used lithium chloride (LiCl), an inhibitor of GSK-3β, to treat the undamaged cells. Additionally, inactivation of GSK-3β under BLM treatment was performed to investigate the effects of inactivated GSK-3β on JAM-A under these conditions. After 24 h and 48 h of treatment with BLM, BLM + LiCl, or LiCl alone, the expression of the total GSK-3β was unchanged under all conditions when compared with the untreated E10 cells (Figure 3A).

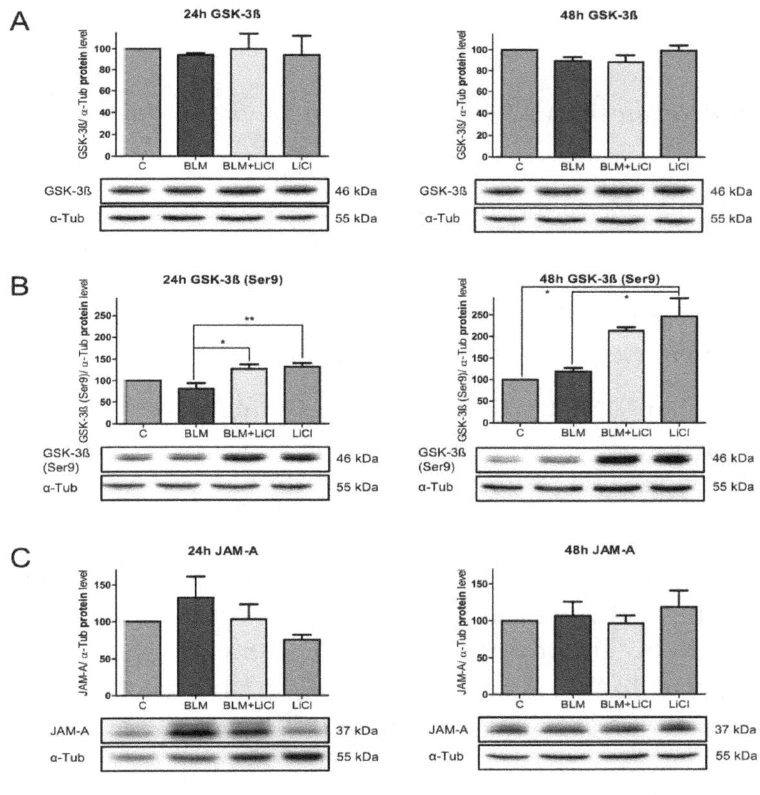

Figure 3. Expression of total GSK-3β (**A**), GSK-3β(Ser9) (**B**), and JAM-A (**C**) were analyzed by Western blot after 24 h and 48 h treatment with 100 mU/mL BLM, 100 mU/mL BLM, and 10 mM LiCl or 10 mM LiCl alone. Equal protein amounts of cell lysates were used in SDS-PAGE and analyzed by Western blot. α-Tub served as the loading control. Untreated cells were used as the control and normalized to 100%. Representative blots from three independent experiments are shown. Charts presented as mean ± SEM (n = 3) of GSK-3β /α-Tub, GSK-3β(Ser9)/α-Tub, and JAM-A/α-Tub. P-values: 24 h GSK-3β 0.9447; 48 h GSK-3β 0.0625; 24 h GSK-3β(Ser9) 0.0046; 48 h GSK-3β(Ser9) 0.0066; 24 h JAM-A 0.186; and 48 h JAM-A 0.6123. * $p < 0.05$, ** $p < 0.01$.

After 24 h of BLM treatment, no increase in GSK-3β(Ser9) was seen (Figure 3B). The addition of LiCl to BLM or LiCl alone increased the expression of GSK-3β(Ser9) only slightly (Figure 3B), but significantly in comparison to the BLM-treated cells.

As shown in Figure 3C, 24 h of BLM treatment of the E10 cells induced an increase of 132.3% in JAM-A. Inhibition of GSK-3β with LiCl in combination with BLM reduced the increase of JAM-A, indicating that the inactivation of the GSK-3β under BLM treatment had consequences for the expression of JAM-A (Figure 3C). Treatment of E10 cells with LiCl alone also downregulated the protein content of JAM-A to 75.6% compared to the untreated control cells.

After 48 h of BLM treatment, no increase in GSK-3β(Ser9) was also seen (Figure 3B). The addition of LiCl after 48 h of BLM treatment resulted in a strong increase in the protein content of the inactive form GSK-3β(Ser9) to 178.5% compared to the BLM-treated cells (Figure 3B). Likewise, treatment with LiCl alone led to a dramatic increase in GSK-3β(Ser9).

After 48 h of BLM treatment, the early increase in JAM-A returned to the level seen in the control cells (Figure 3C) The strong upregulation of GSK-3β(Ser9) under BLM treatment or by sole LiCl treatment in the control cells did not lead to any changes in the JAM-A protein.

In summary, early BLM treatment (24 h) in alveolar epithelial cells induced an increase in JAM-A. The BLM treatment did not inactivate GSK-3β within a period of 48 h. The early rise of JAM-A after BLM exposure could be reduced to the protein level of the control cells by inactivation of GSK-3β. This means that the upregulation of the inactive form of GSK-3β prevents the rise of JAM-A under BLM treatment.

2.4. The P2X7R Indirectly Regulates JAM-A Protein Content by the Modulation of GSK-3β(Ser9)

The aim of the following experiment in the E10 cells was to investigate how the inhibition of P2X7R under BLM treatment (24 h) affected the inactive form of GSK-3β and whether subsequent changes in JAM-A occurred. The increase in the protein content of P2X7R after BLM treatment in the E10 cells has already been shown in one of our previous studies [17]. Additionally, the increase in JAM-A after BLM treatment was confirmed (Figure 3) and there was no inactivation of GSK-3β at this time when compared to the untreated control cells (Figure 3).

To test the hypothesis that P2X7R could indirectly modulate JAM-A following BLM treatment by regulating the inactive form of GSK-3β, we studied the GSK-3β(Ser9) and JAM-A protein contents after inhibition of P2X7R by oxATP (Figure 4).

The inhibition of P2X7R under BLM treatment led to a strong decrease in the GSK-3β(Ser9) protein content in the alveolar epithelial cells in comparison to the untreated or BLM-treated cells. The significant reduction in GSK-3β(Ser9) protein content compared to BLM-treated cells resulted in a re-upregulation of JAM-A. Treatment with oxATP alone led to significant downregulation of GSK-3β(Ser9) when compared to the untreated cells. The inhibition of P2X7R under these conditions also produced an increase in JAM-A when compared to the untreated cells.

2.5. Localization of JAM-A in Alveolar Epithelial Cells after BLM Treatment and the Influence of oxATP

Confluent E10 cells were incubated with 100 mU/mL BLM to study the effect of BLM on the distribution of JAM-A. Immunofluorescence revealed a regular localization of JAM-A to TJ at sites of cell–cell contact in the control cells (Figure 4). BLM exposure for 24 h (Figure 4B) or oxATP alone (Figure 4C) did not change JAM-A immunoreactivity and its cellular localization, but the cell size increased after BLM exposure. oxATP and BLM together normalized the BLM induced cell swelling (Figure 4D).

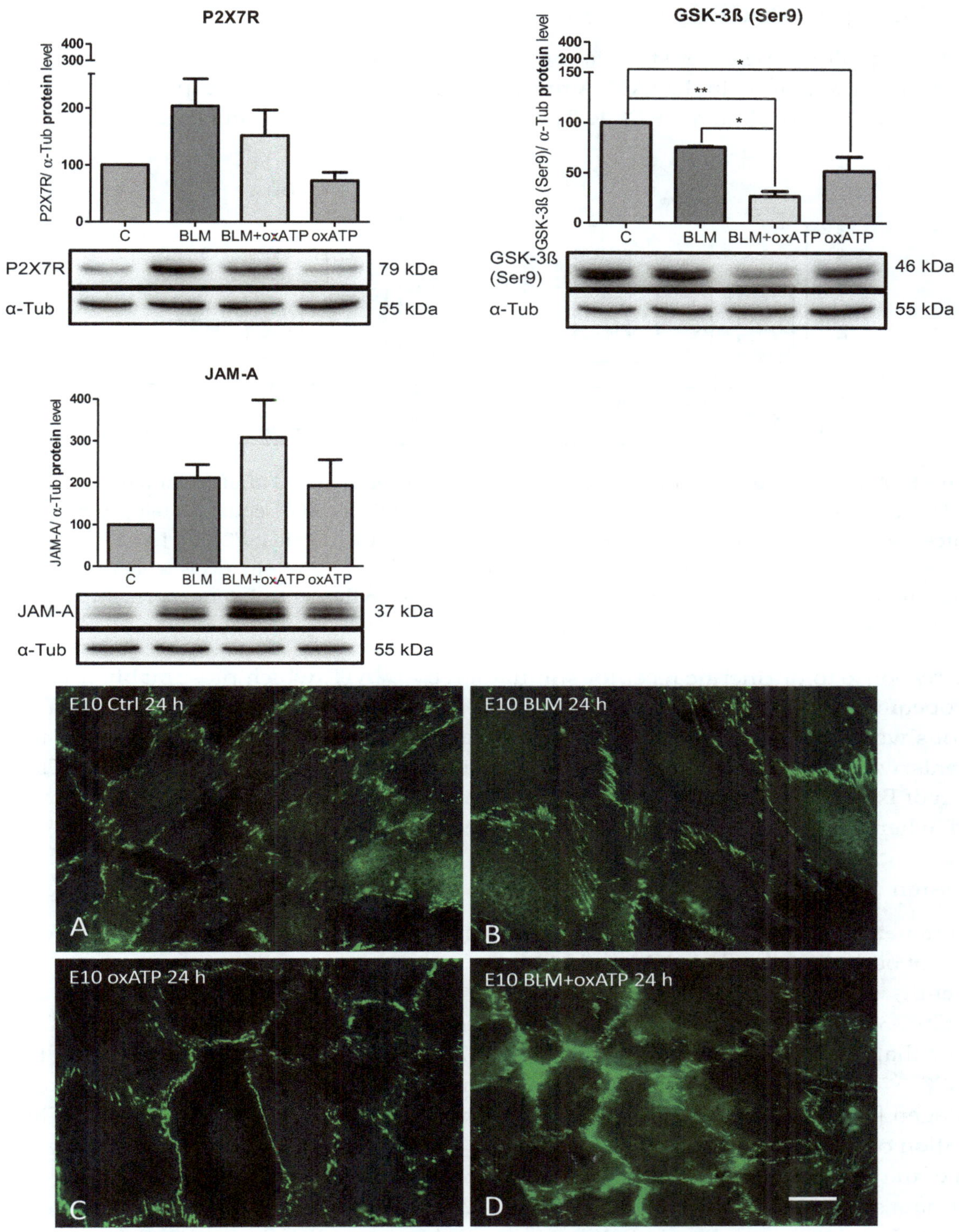

Figure 4. Effects of P2X7R inhibition by 150 μM oxATP, which was added 2 h prior to 100 mU/mL BLM treatment. Equal protein amounts of cell lysates were used in SDS-PAGE and analyzed by Western blot. α-Tub served as the loading control. Untreated cells were used as the control and normalized to 100%. Representative blots from three independent experiments are shown. Charts are presented as the mean ± SEM (n = 3) of P2X7R/ α-Tub, GSK-3β(Ser9)/ α-Tub and JAM-A/ α-Tub. P-values: P2X7R 0.0338; GSK-3β(Ser9) 0.002; and JAM-A 0.05. Immunofluorescence demonstration of JAM-A in untreated (**A**), BLM (**B**), or oxATP (**C**) treated E10 cells. Note the increased cell size after BLM exposure (**B**), which was ameliorated after oxATP (**D**). Representative images of multiple experiments (n = 3) are shown. Bar = 20 μm. * $p < 0.05$, ** $p < 0.01$.

2.6. The P2X7R Agonist BzATP Affects the JAM-A Protein Content

Next, we explored whether stimulation of P2X7R in alveolar epithelial E10 cells with BzATP would induce a modulation in the JAM-A protein content. E10 cells were exposed to 100 μM BzATP for one and two days to stimulate P2X7R. The Western blots are shown in Figure 5.

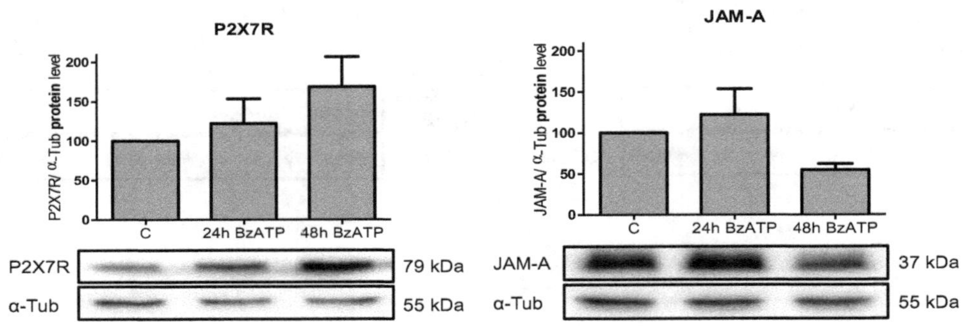

Figure 5. Analysis of protein levels in alveolar epithelial cell line E10 after treatment with 150 μM BzATP. Cells were treated with BzATP for 24 h and 48 h. For SDS-PAGE, equal protein amounts of cell lysates were used and analyzed by Western blot with antibodies against P2X7R, JAM-A, and α-Tub. Untreated cells were used as the control and normalized to 100%. Protein levels were normalized to α-Tub and are shown as the mean ± SEM (n = 3) in relation to the control. One representative blot is pictured. P-values: P2X7R 0.1667 and JAM-A 0.1048.

The response to purinergic receptor stimulation by BzATP, which presumably involves a Ca^{2+} channel opening, resulted in an increase in Ca^{2+} [17]. As an indication for this, we were able to show in previous work that the CaM content was increased after BzATP treatment [17]. In the present experiments, we demonstrated that the JAM-A protein content was influenced by the BzATP treatment. After 24 h of BzATP treatment in E10 cells, a minimal increase in the JAM-A protein concentration occurred, whereas a stronger decrease was seen after 48 h (Figure 5).

3. Discussion

Maintenance of the integrity of the alveolar barrier is realized by TJ among neighboring AECs consisting of occludin, claudins, ZOs, and JAM-A.

Recently, we have demonstrated that in $P2X7^{-/-}$ mice, claudin-18 is upregulated and the inactive form of GSK-3β, GSK-3β(Ser9), is also upregulated in comparison to WT mice [12]. Our current data show that another TJ protein, JAM-A, in $P2X7^{-/-}$ mice is strongly upregulated at the protein level. $P2X7^{-/-}$ mice exhibited reduced lung inflammation with reduced fibrosis markers such as lung collagen [13]. Deletion of P2X7R is a protective factor in acute lung injury [14]. Through the upregulation of JAM-A and claudin-4 and -15 in a kinase-dependent manner, an improved barrier function of the oral epithelium could be demonstrated [21].

Our data suggest that increased constitutive JAM-A protein level may have a protective effect against BLM-induced lung injury in $P2X7^{-/-}$ mice. BLM-treated PCLS from $P2X7^{-/-}$ mice responded with a slighter increase in mRNA expression of JAM-A than BLM-treated PCLS from WT mice. The reduced level of JAM-A upregulation in the $P2X7^{-/-}$ mice in comparison to the WT mice indicates a lower sensitivity of this protein to the effects of BLM in the alveolar epithelium.

JAM-A is concentrated at epithelial and endothelial tight junctions and it has been shown that JAM-A localizes to claudin-based tight junction fibrils in epithelial cells [22]. It does not directly regulate the barrier between the cells, but rather interacts as a signaling molecule with divergent downstream target proteins [23]. Nevertheless, in various epithelial and endothelial cell lines including primary rat alveolar epithelial cells, it has been shown that siRNA mediated downregulation of JAM-A expression results in enhanced paracellular permeability, as determined by TER measurements [16].

Long-term treatment of PCLS (five days) with BLM showed a strong downregulation of JAM-A when compared to the untreated PCLS (own unpublished data).

To examine the consequences of decreased GSK-3β activity on JAM-A under BLM treatment, the GSK-3β inhibitor LiCl was used in this study. JAM-A is affected by the inhibition of GSK-3β. The initial upregulation of JAM-A under BLM treatment is prevented by the inactivation of GSK-3β. Inhibition of GSK-3β causes JAM-A expression to remain at levels comparable to that of the untreated cells.

This result indicates that inhibition of GSK-3β has a positive effect on the deregulatory changes in JAM-A expression under BLM treatment. Several studies have shown that the inhibition of GSK-3β reduces the development of acute lung injury and inflammation and has a protective effect on lung fibrosis induced by BLM [24,25]. The P2X7$^{-/-}$ mice, which showed no fibrotic changes under BLM treatment, had a high constitutive expression of GSK-3β(Ser9) [12], which is an indication of the protective effect of GSK-3β inhibition.

While the data on GSK-3β inhibition in acute lung injury are fairly clear, there are little data on its effect on TJ proteins. Severson et al. [20] have shown that endogenous GSK-3β activity is required for maintenance of the AJC, and therefore for epithelial barrier function by regulating the expression of transmembrane proteins claudin-1 and occludin. They also observed a differential decrease in the labeling of key AJC proteins following GSK-3β inhibition, a decrease in occludin, claudin-1, and E-cadherin protein levels, but they could not show any effect on JAM-A expression and localization. They reported that in both human intestinal (SK-CO15) and kidney (MDCK) epithelial cells, a decrease in GSK-3β activity interfered with epithelial cell–cell transitions, thereby increasing paracellular permeability.

It was previously shown by Bazzoni et al. [26] that the absence of JAM-A enhanced cell motility, increased membrane protrusions, affected microtubule stability, and reduced focal adhesions in endothelial cells. The consequences of JAM-A absence were reversed on treatment with GSK-3β inhibitors.

In this study, treatment with oxATP alone reduced the expression of P2X7R and increased JAM-A when compared to the untreated WT cells. After the addition of oxATP to BLM-treated cells, the P2X7R was downregulated, but a higher amount of JAM-A protein was still measured than in the untreated cells. In this case, JAM-A was also upregulated. Furthermore, inactivation of P2X7R by oxATP led to a substantial reduction in the constitutively present level of inactive GSK-3β in untreated and BLM-treated cells.

The inhibition of P2X7R under BLM treatment resulted in the opposite effect on GSK-3β(Ser9) when compared to the effect of the GSK-3β inhibitor LiCl. The inactivated form of GSK-3β, the GSK-3β(Ser9) was even further downregulated, which was expressed downstream in the upregulation of JAM-A. Figure 6 summarizes the data:

Interestingly, the inhibition of P2X7R under BLM did not lead to the upregulation of GSK-3β as found in P2X7$^{-/-}$ mice. The siRNA-mediated downregulation of P2X7R led in turn to the upregulation of GSK-3β in untreated alveolar epithelial cells [12]. The different effects on GSK-3β still have to be clarified. However, knockout or inhibition of P2X7R always leads to an increase in the JAM-A protein level, indicating a repressive effect of P2X7R on the expression of JAM-A.

Furthermore, we have shown that activation of P2X7R by BzATP resulted first in a very slight upregulation of JAM-A after 24 h, and then in a strong downregulation of the protein after 48 h in alveolar epithelial cells E10. Guo et al. [27] showed in E10 cells that activation of P2X7R by BzATP increased the phosphorylation of Y216 and decreased the phosphorylation at S9 in GSK-3β without affecting the total GSK-3β expression. This result indicates that BzATP stimulates GSK-3β activity.

It has been demonstrated that JAM-A has the ability to promote the assembly and remodeling of alveolar epithelial tight junctions in response to acute lung injury and plays a protective role in preventing lung damage and promoting fluid clearance [28]. Identifying pathways that increase the expression and function of JAM-A in acute lung injury may identify new approaches to promote barrier function in response to inflammation and injury.

We were able to show for the first time that P2X7R plays an important role in the regulation of JAM-A in the alveolar epithelium. Downregulation of P2X7R or the absence of the protein leads to upregulation of JAM-A, possibly resulting in an increase in barrier function. Conversely, stimulation of P2X7R leads to downregulation of the protein. A modulating effect on JAM-A has been demonstrated under BLM treatment for GSK-3β.

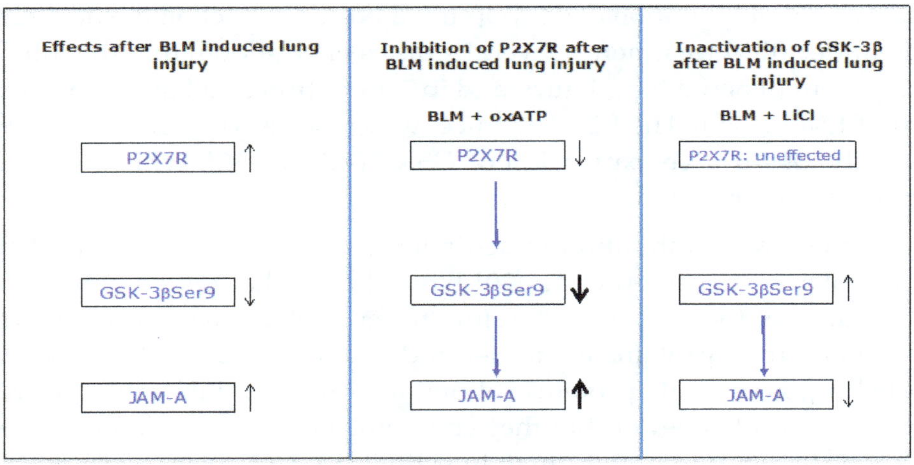

Figure 6. BLM treatment results in increased protein levels of P2X7R and JAM-A as well as in a reduced content of the inactive form of GSK-3β GSK-3β(Ser9). After inhibition of P2X7R by oxATP under BLM exposure, the effect on both proteins is further enhanced. Inactivating of the GSK-3β by LiCl under BLM exposure directly leads to a reduction of JAM-A. The influence of P2X7R on JAM-A is rather indirect.

4. Materials and Methods

4.1. Ethics Statement

All animal experiments were approved by the Ethics Committee of the Dresden University of Technology and the license for the removal of organs was provided by Landesdirektion Dresden (file no. 24-9168.24-1/2007-26; file no. 24-9168.24-1/2010-11).

4.2. Experimental Animals

WT mice were purchased from Charles River (C57BL/6; Charles River, Wilmington, USA) and the P2X7$^{-/-}$ mice were obtained from Pfizer (B6.129P2-P2rx7^{tm1Gab}/J; Pfizer, New York, NY, USA) [29]. Our animals were housed at the Animal Care Facility at the Medical Faculty "Carl Gustav Carus" of Dresden University of Technology and had steady free access to standard chow and water. All performed procedures were in accordance with the Technical University of Dresden Animal Care and Use Committee Guidelines. For our experiments, we examined the lung tissue of male and female mice with an age of 8 to 16 weeks.

4.3. Cell Line and Cell Culture

The mouse lung cell line E10 [30] was acquired by M. Williams (Pulmonary Center, Boston University School of Medicine, Boston, MA, USA). Cells were cultured in DMEM/Ham's F12 medium (1:1) purchased by Gibco (ThermoFisher Scientific, Waltham, MA, USA), supplemented with 5% (*v*/*v*) fetal bovine serum (Biochrom AG Seromed, Berlin, Germany) and 2.5 mM L-glutamine (Merck KGaA, Darmstadt, Germany). E10 cells were seeded at a density of 1.5×10^4 to 3×10^4 cells/mL and passaged three times a week up to 25 passages and were grown at 37 °C in a 5% CO_2 atmosphere up to a confluence of 60–80%.

For treatment of the cells, the medium was supplemented with 100 mU/mL BLM (Bleocell, STADA Arzneimittel AG, Bad Vilbel, Germany), 150 μM oxATP, 150 μM BzATP, and 10 mM LiCl (Sigma-Aldrich, Munich, Germany). OxATP and LiCl were added to the cells 1 h before BLM treatment.

4.4. Precision-Cut Lung Slices (PCLS) and Tissue Culture

To attain PCLS, we followed the procedure published by [31] with several modifications such as the process of obtaining, cutting, handling, and incubating the lung slices described in detail by [8]. After 24 h of incubation, the lung slices were homogenized for real-time reverse transcription PCR, Western blot analyses, or embedded in paraffin for immunohistochemistry.

4.5. RNA Isolation and Real-Time Reverse Transcription PCR (Real-Time RT PCR)

The isolation of total RNA was realized as previously described with some modification [8]. Primers applied for real-time RT PCR were: JAM-A (5′-TCCTGGGCTCTTTGGTACAAGG-3, 5′-TCCTGGGCTCTTTGGTACAAGG-3), mHmbs (5′-GCTTCGCTGCATTGCTGAAA-3′, 5′-CCAGTCAGGTACAGTTGCCC-3′), mRpl32 (5′-GCACCAGTCAGACCGATATGTG-3′, 5′-CTTCTCCGCACCCTGTTGTC-3′).

The identity of the PCR products was proven by melting point analysis. Using the ΔΔCT method at CFX Manager (Bio-Rad), the relative quantification of gene expression was performed with housekeeping genes *Hmbs* (hydroxymethylbilane synthase) and Rpl32 (ribosomal protein L32).

4.6. Western Blot Analysis

Total protein concentrations of the lysates of lung tissue and cells were determined by using the BCA Protein Assay Kit (ThermoFisher Scientific) according to the manufacture's guidelines. Murine tissue protein extraction was performed as described previously in [12] by using the Precellys 24 Homogenizer (PEQLAB, Erlangen, Germany) and lysis buffer including 0.02 M Tris, pH 8.5; 0.125 M NaCl; and 1% (*v*/*v*) Triton X-100 with protease inhibitor Complete Tablets, EDTA-free (Roche, Basel, Switzerland).

Cell protein extraction was performed by applying ice cold PBS buffer without Mg^{2+} and Ca^{2+} (Biochrom AG, Berlin, Germany) supplemented with protease inhibitor Complete Tablets, EDTA-free (Roche) into T75 flasks (Greiner Bio-one GmbH, Frickenhausen, Germany). The cells were scratched from the surface, collected, and pelleted at 500× *g* for 5 min. After adding lysis buffer including 0.02 M Tris, pH 7.5; 0.14 M NaCl; 1 mM EDTA, pH 8.0; and 1% (*v*/*v*) Triton X-100 with protease inhibitor Complete Tablets, EDTA-free (Roche), the lysate was incubated 45 min at 4 °C with slight motion and centrifuged at 10.000× *g* for 20 min at 4 °C to collect the supernatant containing the protein.

For SDS-PAGE, the samples were diluted to a homogeneous total protein concentration, transferred into 6× SDS sample buffer (300 mM Tris, pH 6.8; 100 mM Dithiothreitol; 0.1% (*w*/*v*); 30% (*w*/*v*) glycerol; 10% (*w*/*v*) SDS), boiled at 95 °C for 5 min and 10–50 μg of total protein per sample were loaded on a 12% SDS-polyacrylamide gel. Western blot analysis was performed as described [32] with minor modifications. The PVDF Immobilon-P Membrane (Merck Millipore, Billerica, USA) was blocked for 1 h in TBS-T buffer (17 mM Tris, pH 7.4; 2.7 mM KCl; 137 mM NaCl; 0.2% (*v*/*v*) Tween 20) including 5% (*w*/*v*) dried non-fat powdered milk (Carl Roth GmbH, Karlsruhe, Germany) and incubated at 4 °C overnight with the following primary antibodies: polyclonal rabbit anti-human JAM-A (A302-891A), dilution 1:1000 (Bethyl Laboratories Inc.); polyclonal rabbit anti mouse P2X7R (APR-004; Alomone Labs Inc.), dilution 1:500; monoclonal mouse anti-human GSK-3β (610202; BD Biosciences), dilution 1:1000; monoclonal rabbit anti-human Phospho-GSK-3β (Ser9) (#9323; Cell Signaling Technology Inc.), dilution 1:1000; and monoclonal mouse anti -tubulin (sc-8035; Santa Cruz Biotechnology Inc.), dilution 1:1000.

The following secondary antibodies were used at room temperature for 1 h: donkey anti-rabbit IgG, HRP-linked F(ab)2 fragment (GE Healthcare, Chalfont St Giles, Buckinghamshire, UK), and horse anti-mouse IgG, HRP-linked antibody (Cell Signaling, Danvers, MA, USA). The chemiluminescent signal was detected by using Immobilon Western Chemiluminescent HRP Substrate (Merck Millipore) by following the manufacturer's guidelines and Image Reader LAS-3000 (Fujifilm, Tokyo, Japan). Quantification was done with ImageJ 1.51 u free software (Wayne Rasband, National Institutes of Health, Bethesda, MD, USA) and each line was normalized to corresponding α-tubulin (α-Tub).

4.7. Immunohistochemistry

Fixation of 5 μm thin lung tissue in 4% (*v*/*v*) buffered formalin, embedding in paraffin, sectioning, and immunostaining were performed as described previously in [8,17]. The primary antibody against JAM-A was detected with a biotinylated secondary antibody, followed by incubation with the streptavidin/biotin-peroxidase complex (Vectastain Elite Kit, Serva, Heidelberg, Germany). As a negative control, the primary antibody was replaced with PBS or a non-immune serum.

4.8. Immunofluorescence

Immunofluorescence and double immunofluorescence staining on frozen cryostat sections of mouse lung tissue were performed, as previously described in Reference [33]. The following primary antibodies were used: polyclonal rabbit anti JAM-A and monoclonal mouse anti T1α clone E11, dilution 1:200, which was a kind gift from Dr. A. Wetterwald, Bern (Switzerland). As secondary antibodies, we used goat anti-rabbit IgG conjugated to fluorescein isothiocyanate (FITC, Dianova, Hamburg, Germany; dilution 1:100 (*v*/*v*)) and donkey anti-mouse IgG, Texas Red labelled (Dianova, Hamburg, Germany; dilution 1:100 (*v*/*v*)). Negative controls included the omission of the primary antibody. Acetone-methanol fixed monolayers of E10 cells were similarly incubated with the same dilution of the JAM-A antibody.

4.9. Statistical Analysis

One-way analysis of variance (ANOVA) was used to determine the results of Western blot analysis and real-time RT PCR with three or more groups, followed by the post hoc Bonferroni test in case significance was achieved. Statistical comparison of two groups was performed as a two tailed Student´s *t* test. Statistical analysis was done with GraphPad Prism 5.03 software (GraphPad Software, San Diego, CA, USA). We determined significance at * $p = 0{,}05$ and high significance at ** $p = 0.01$. A minimum of three independent experiments for each technique was performed.

Author Contributions: Conceptualization, K.B. and M.K.; Investigation, K-P.W. and A.S.; Data curation, K-P.W. and M.K.; Writing, K-P.W., M.K., and K.B.; Writing–review & editing, K.B.

Acknowledgments: The authors thank A. Neisser, S. Bramke, and D. Streichert for their expert technical assistance and Heinz Fehrenbach (Borstel, Germany) for his critical reading of the manuscript.

Abbreviations

BLM	Bleomycin
GSK-3β	Glycogen synthase kinase-3 beta
JAM-A	Junctional adhesion molecule-A
LiCl	Lithium chloride
PCLS	Precision-cut lung slices
PKC-β1	Protein kinase C-beta1
P2X7R	P2X7 receptor
WT	Wildtype

References

1. Johnson, M.D.; Widdicombe, J.H.; Allen, L.; Barbry, P.; Dobbs, L.G. Alveolar epithelial type i cells contain

transport proteins and transport sodium, supporting an active role for type i cells in regulation of lung liquid homeostasis. *Proc. Natl. Acad. Sci. USA* **2002**, *99*, 1966–1971. [CrossRef] [PubMed]

2. Kasper, M.; Barth, K. Potential contribution of alveolar epithelial type i cells to pulmonary fibrosis. *Biosci. Rep.* **2017**, *37*, 1–18. [CrossRef]
3. McElroy, M.C.; Kasper, M. The use of alveolar epithelial type i cell-selective markers to investigate lung injury and repair. *Eur. Respir. J.* **2004**, *24*, 664–673. [CrossRef]
4. Ramirez, M.I.; Millien, G.; Hinds, A.; Cao, Y.; Seldin, D.C.; Williams, M.C. T1alpha, a lung type i cell differentiation gene, is required for normal lung cell proliferation and alveolus formation at birth. *Dev. Biol.* **2003**, *256*, 61–72. [CrossRef]
5. Drab, M.; Verkade, P.; Elger, M.; Kasper, M.; Lohn, M.; Lauterbach, B.; Menne, J.; Lindschau, C.; Mende, F.; Luft, F.C.; et al. Loss of caveolae, vascular dysfunction, and pulmonary defects in caveolin-1 gene-disrupted mice. *Science* **2001**, *293*, 2449–2452. [CrossRef] [PubMed]
6. Englert, J.M.; Hanford, L.E.; Kaminski, N.; Tobolewski, J.M.; Tan, R.J.; Fattman, C.L.; Ramsgaard, L.; Richards, T.J.; Loutaev, I.; Nawroth, P.P.; et al. A role for the receptor for advanced glycation end products in idiopathic pulmonary fibrosis. *Am. J. Pathol.* **2008**, *172*, 583–591. [CrossRef]
7. Gabazza, E.C.; Kasper, M.; Ohta, K.; Keane, M.; D'Alessandro-Gabazza, C.; Fujimoto, H.; Nishii, Y.; Nakahara, H.; Takagi, T.; Menon, A.G.; et al. Decreased expression of aquaporin-5 in bleomycin-induced lung fibrosis in the mouse. *Pathol. Int.* **2004**, *54*, 774–780. [CrossRef] [PubMed]
8. Ebeling, G.; Blasche, R.; Hofmann, F.; Augstein, A.; Kasper, M.; Barth, K. Effect of p2x7 receptor knockout on aqp-5 expression of type i alveolar epithelial cells. *PLoS ONE* **2014**, *9*, e100282. [CrossRef] [PubMed]
9. Chen, Z.; Jin, N.; Narasaraju, T.; Chen, J.; McFarland, L.R.; Scott, M.; Liu, L. Identification of two novel markers for alveolar epithelial type i and ii cells. *Biochem. Biophys. Res. Commun.* **2004**, *319*, 774–780. [CrossRef] [PubMed]
10. Bowler, J.W.; Bailey, R.J.; North, R.A.; Surprenant, A. P2x4, p2y1 and p2y2 receptors on rat alveolar macrophages. *Br. J. Pharmacol.* **2003**, *140*, 567–575. [CrossRef]
11. Adinolfi, E.; Giuliani, A.L.; De Marchi, E.; Pegoraro, A.; Orioli, E.; Di Virgilio, F. The p2x7 receptor: A main player in inflammation. *Biochem. Pharmacol.* **2018**, *151*, 234–244. [CrossRef]
12. Barth, K.; Blasche, R.; Neisser, A.; Bramke, S.; Frank, J.A.; Kasper, M. P2x7r-dependent regulation of glycogen synthase kinase 3beta and claudin-18 in alveolar epithelial type i cells of mice lung. *Histochem. Cell Biol.* **2016**, *146*, 757–768. [CrossRef]
13. Riteau, N.; Gasse, P.; Fauconnier, L.; Gombault, A.; Couegnat, M.; Fick, L.; Kanellopoulos, J.; Quesniaux, V.F.; Marchand-Adam, S.; Crestani, B.; et al. Extracellular atp is a danger signal activating p2x7 receptor in lung inflammation and fibrosis. *Am. J. Respir. Crit. Care. Med.* **2010**, *182*, 774–783. [CrossRef]
14. Galam, L.; Rajan, A.; Failla, A.; Soundararajan, R.; Lockey, R.F.; Kolliputi, N. Deletion of p2x7 attenuates hyperoxia-induced acute lung injury via inflammasome suppression. *Am. J. Physiol. Lung Cell Mol. Physiol.* **2016**, *310*, L572–L581. [CrossRef]
15. Moncao-Ribeiro, L.C.; Cagido, V.R.; Lima-Murad, G.; Santana, P.T.; Riva, D.R.; Borojevic, R.; Zin, W.A.; Cavalcante, M.C.; Rica, I.; Brando-Lima, A.C.; et al. Lipopolysaccharide-induced lung injury: Role of p2x7 receptor. *Respir. Physiol. Neurobiol.* **2011**, *179*, 314–325. [CrossRef]
16. Monteiro, A.C.; Parkos, C.A. Intracellular mediators of jam-a-dependent epithelial barrier function. *Ann. N Y Acad. Sci.* **2012**, *1257*, 115–124. [CrossRef]
17. Bläsche, R.; Ebeling, G.; Perike, S.; Weinhold, K.; Kasper, M.; Barth, K. Activation of p2x7r and downstream effects in bleomycin treated lung epithelial cells. *Int. J. Biochem. Cell Biol.* **2012**, *44*, 514–524. [CrossRef]
18. Balda, M.S.; Gonzalez-Mariscal, L.; Matter, K.; Cereijido, M.; Anderson, J.M. Assembly of the tight junction: The role of diacylglycerol. *J. Cell Biol.* **1993**, *123*, 293–302. [CrossRef]
19. Tsujio, I.; Tanaka, T.; Kudo, T.; Nishikawa, T.; Shinozaki, K.; Grundke-Iqbal, I.; Iqbal, K.; Takeda, M. Inactivation of glycogen synthase kinase-3 by protein kinase c delta: Implications for regulation of tau phosphorylation. *FEBS Lett.* **2000**, *469*, 111–117. [CrossRef]
20. Severson, E.A.; Kwon, M.; Hilgarth, R.S.; Parkos, C.A.; Nusrat, A. Glycogen synthase kinase 3 (gsk-3) influences epithelial barrier function by regulating occludin, claudin-1 and e-cadherin expression. *Biochem. Biophys. Res. Commun.* **2010**, *397*, 592–597. [CrossRef]
21. Ye, P.; Yu, H.; Simonian, M.; Hunter, N. Ligation of cd24 expressed by oral epithelial cells induces kinase

dependent decrease in paracellular permeability mediated by tight junction proteins. *Biochem. Biophys. Res. Commun.* **2011**, *412*, 165–169. [CrossRef] [PubMed]

22. Liu, Y.; Nusrat, A.; Schnell, F.J.; Reaves, T.A.; Walsh, S.; Pochet, M.; Parkos, C.A. Human junction adhesion molecule regulates tight junction resealing in epithelia. *J. Cell Sci.* **2000**, *113 (Pt 13)*, 2363–2374.
23. Kostrewa, D.; Brockhaus, M.; D'Arcy, A.; Dale, G.E.; Nelboeck, P.; Schmid, G.; Mueller, F.; Bazzoni, G.; Dejana, E.; Bartfai, T.; et al. X-ray structure of junctional adhesion molecule: Structural basis for homophilic adhesion via a novel dimerization motif. *EMBO J.* **2001**, *20*, 4391–4398. [CrossRef]
24. Cuzzocrea, S.; Mazzon, E.; Esposito, E.; Muia, C.; Abdelrahman, M.; Di Paola, R.; Crisafulli, C.; Bramanti, P.; Thiemermann, C. Glycogen synthase kinase-3beta inhibition attenuates the development of ischaemia/reperfusion injury of the gut. *Intensive Care. Med.* **2007**, *33*, 880–893. [CrossRef] [PubMed]
25. Gurrieri, C.; Piazza, F.; Gnoato, M.; Montini, B.; Biasutto, L.; Gattazzo, C.; Brunetta, E.; Cabrelle, A.; Cinetto, F.; Niero, R.; et al. 3-(2,4-dichlorophenyl)-4-(1-methyl-1h-indol-3-yl)-1h-pyrrole-2,5-dione (sb216763), a glycogen synthase kinase-3 inhibitor, displays therapeutic properties in a mouse model of pulmonary inflammation and fibrosis. *J. Pharmacol. Exp. Ther.* **2010**, *332*, 785–794. [CrossRef]
26. Bazzoni, G.; Tonetti, P.; Manzi, L.; Cera, M.R.; Balconi, G.; Dejana, E. Expression of junctional adhesion molecule-a prevents spontaneous and random motility. *J. Cell Sci.* **2005**, *118*, 623–632. [CrossRef] [PubMed]
27. Guo, Y.; Xiao, L.; Sun, L.; Liu, F. Wnt/beta-catenin signaling: A promising new target for fibrosis diseases. *Physiol. Res.* **2012**, *61*, 337–346.
28. Mitchell, L.A.; Overgaard, C.E.; Ward, C.; Margulies, S.S.; Koval, M. Differential effects of claudin-3 and claudin-4 on alveolar epithelial barrier function. *Am. J. Physiol. Lung Cell Mol. Physiol.* **2011**, *301*, L40–L49. [CrossRef] [PubMed]
29. Solle, M.; Labasi, J.; Perregaux, D.G.; Stam, E.; Petrushova, N.; Koller, B.H.; Griffiths, R.J.; Gabel, C.A. Altered cytokine production in mice lacking p2x(7) receptors. *J. Biol. Chem.* **2001**, *276*, 125–132. [CrossRef]
30. Herzog, C.R.; Soloff, E.V.; McDoniels, A.L.; Tyson, F.L.; Malkinson, A.M.; Haugen-Strano, A.; Wiseman, R.W.; Anderson, M.W.; You, M. Homozygous codeletion and differential decreased expression of p15ink4b, p16ink4a-alpha and p16ink4a-beta in mouse lung tumor cells. *Oncogene* **1996**, *13*, 1885–1891. [PubMed]
31. Held, H.D.; Martin, C.; Uhlig, S. Characterization of airway and vascular responses in murine lungs. *Br. J. Pharmacol.* **1999**, *126*, 1191–1199. [CrossRef] [PubMed]
32. Linge, A.; Morishima, N.; Kasper, M.; Barth, K. Bleomycin induces caveolin-1 and -2 expression in epithelial lung cancer a549 cells. *Anticancer Res.* **2007**, *27*, 1343–1351. [PubMed]
33. Pfleger, C.; Ebeling, G.; Blasche, R.; Patton, M.; Patel, H.H.; Kasper, M.; Barth, K. Detection of caveolin-3/caveolin-1/p2x7r complexes in mice atrial cardiomyocytes in vivo and in vitro. *Histochem. Cell Biol.* **2012**, *138*, 231–241. [CrossRef] [PubMed]

10

On Top of the Alveolar Epithelium: Surfactant and the Glycocalyx

Matthias Ochs [1,2,*,†], Jan Hegermann [3,†], Elena Lopez-Rodriguez [1], Sara Timm [4], Geraldine Nouailles [5], Jasmin Matuszak [6], Szandor Simmons [6], Martin Witzenrath [2,5] and Wolfgang M. Kuebler [2,6]

1 Institute of Functional Anatomy, Charité-Universitätsmedizin Berlin, 10117 Berlin, Germany
2 German Center for Lung Research (DZL), 10117 Berlin, Germany
3 Research Core Unit Electron Microscopy and Institute of Functional and Applied Anatomy, Hannover Medical School, 30625 Hannover, Germany
4 Core Facility Electron Microscopy, Charité-Universitätsmedizin Berlin, 10117 Berlin, Germany
5 Department of Infectious Diseases and Respiratory Medicine, and Division of Pulmonary Inflammation, Charité-Universitätsmedizin Berlin, 10117 Berlin, Germany
6 Institute of Physiology, Charité-Universitätsmedizin Berlin, 10117 Berlin, Germany
* Correspondence: matthias.ochs@charite.de
† These authors contributed equally and share first authorship.

Abstract: Gas exchange in the lung takes place via the air-blood barrier in the septal walls of alveoli. The tissue elements that oxygen molecules have to cross are the alveolar epithelium, the interstitium and the capillary endothelium. The epithelium that lines the alveolar surface is covered by a thin and continuous liquid lining layer. Pulmonary surfactant acts at this air-liquid interface. By virtue of its biophysical and immunomodulatory functions, surfactant keeps alveoli open, dry and clean. What needs to be added to this picture is the glycocalyx of the alveolar epithelium. Here, we briefly review what is known about this glycocalyx and how it can be visualized using electron microscopy. The application of colloidal thorium dioxide as a staining agent reveals differences in the staining pattern between type I and type II alveolar epithelial cells and shows close associations of the glycocalyx with intraalveolar surfactant subtypes such as tubular myelin. These morphological findings indicate that specific spatial interactions between components of the surfactant system and those of the alveolar epithelial glycocalyx exist which may contribute to the maintenance of alveolar homeostasis, in particular to alveolar micromechanics, to the functional integrity of the air-blood barrier, to the regulation of the thickness and viscosity of the alveolar lining layer, and to the defence against inhaled pathogens. Exploring the alveolar epithelial glycocalyx in conjunction with the surfactant system opens novel physiological perspectives of potential clinical relevance for future research.

Keywords: lung; alveoli; air-blood barrier; epithelium; air-liquid interface; alveolar lining layer; glycocalyx; surfactant

---

1. The Alveolar Epithelium of the Lung and its Surfactant Lining

The architecture of the lung is optimized to serve its main function, gas exchange. A large surface area for air and blood (about 120 m^2) with minimal distance (about 2 μm) is distributed over hundreds of millions of alveoli. The wall separating neighbouring alveoli contains three tissue compartments that constitute the air-blood barrier: alveolar epithelium, capillary endothelium, and the interstitium in-between. The basic knowledge about the structure and function of the alveolar epithelium seems to be well established. It is a continuous layer constituted by a mosaic of two cell types with specific differentiation. While alveolar epithelial type I (AEI) cells are specialised lining cells, alveolar epithelial type II (AEII) cells are specialized secretory and progenitor cells. AEI cells, which are less frequent than AEII cells, cover the vast majority of the alveolar surface with their branched thin squamous cell extensions [1]. Interspersed are single cuboidal AEII cells, which are easily recognized by their characteristic secretory organelles, the surfactant-storing lamellar bodies. Epithelial renewal and repair of both cell types is provided by AEII cells (for review, see [2,3]).

Soon after the first demonstration of a continuous alveolar epithelium in the mammalian lung by electron microscopy (EM) [4,5], it became obvious that this epithelium is not naked. It is covered by a fluid alveolar lining layer consisting of two phases: a surface film and an aqueous hypophase [6,7]. Later cryo-EM studies have confirmed the existence of a thin and continuous alveolar lining layer [8]. Surfactant, the secretory product of AEII cells, is a central component of this layer, i.e., it exerts its functions at the air-liquid interface of lung alveoli (for review, see [2,9–13]).

Surfactant is complex, both biochemically and ultrastructurally. It consists of about 90% lipids (mainly saturated phospholipids) and about 10% proteins (including the surfactant proteins SP-A, SP-B, SP-C and SP-D). All surfactant components are synthesized, stored, secreted and to a large extent recycled by AEII cells. Intracellular surfactant (at least lipids and the hydrophobic SP-B and SP-C) is assembled in lamellar bodies prior to secretion. Intraalveolar surfactant includes the surface film and morphologically distinct subtypes in the hypophase. These subtypes largely correspond to different stages in surfactant metabolism and activity. According to current models, freshly secreted surface-active lamellar body material transforms into tubular myelin, which is a potential precursor of the surface film. Additional multilayered surface-associated surfactant reservoirs have also been suggested. Inactive surfactant is usually present as small unilamellar vesicles. These can either be taken up by AEII cells for recycling or degradation or taken up by alveolar macrophages for degradation. Thus, the hypophase of the alveolar lining layer provides both a substrate on which surfactant acts as well as a reservoir in which intermediates of surfactant metabolism (precursors and remnants) are located.

The functions of surfactant are biophysical as well as immunomodulatory, with its individual components contributing to these functions in different and specific ways. The hydrophobic SP-B and SP-C are assigned mainly biophysical relevance whereas the hydrophilic SP-A and SP-D, which belong to the protein family of collectins, are considered to serve mainly immunomodulatory functions. Regarding its biophysical functions, surfactant stabilizes alveolar dimensions and thus prevents alveolar collapse by a surface-area dependent reduction of alveolar surface tension. Moreover, the low surface tension at the alveolar air-liquid interface secured by surfactant also prevents intraalveolar edema formation. Surfactant is therefore essential for normal alveolar micromechanics and lung function by keeping alveoli homogeneously open, dry and clean (reviewed in [2,11,13]).

2. The Glycocalyx of the Alveolar Epithelium

The Greek term "glycocalyx" can be translated as "sweet husk" [14]. It is a sugar-rich external cell coat common in many cell types, in particular where facing a lumen. The glycocalyx is anchored to the apical cell membrane and consists of two main backbone molecule classes: proteoglycans with long unbranched glycosaminoglycan side chains and glycoproteins with short branched carbohydrate side chains. Proteoglycan core proteins can be attached to the cell membrane by a transmembrane domain (e.g., syndecans) or by a glycosylphosphatidylinositol anchor (e.g., glypicans). Glycosaminoglycans are long negatively charged polymers consisting of disaccharide subunits. Common glycosaminoglycans in the glycocalyx are heparan sulphate, chondroitin sulphate and the un-sulphated hyaluronan. Hyaluronan differs from the other glycosaminoglycans in that it is (at least in part) not directly bound to a core protein but either binds to its receptor CD44 or intercalates throughout the glycocalyx, thereby contributing to hydration and viscosity. Other molecules and ions are attached to this cell surface coat, thus forming a highly hydrated dynamic meshwork that can function as a regulator for barrier permeability by maintaining osmotic gradients, as a regulator for cell adhesion or as a mechanosensor (reviewed in [15–17]).

The pulmonary endothelial glycocalyx recently gained attention because of its role in various lung diseases such as acute respiratory distress syndrome and pulmonary arterial hypertension [17–20]. However, much less is known about the glycocalyx of the alveolar epithelium. Compared to the available literature on surfactant, it seems that it has almost been overlooked as a component of the epithelial lining in lung alveoli. Only few studies have focussed on or at least appreciated the existence of an alveolar epithelial glycocalyx. One finds some early EM studies which reported the visualization of an alveolar epithelial glycocalyx (see below). This line of research was not pursued further until recently. Based on previous reports on alveolar shedding of syndecans in models of lung injury [21,22], Haeger et al. reported the presence of heparan sulphate at the alveolar surface and its shedding into alveolar spaces, together with syndecans 1 and 4, in mice subjected to lipopolysaccharide-induced acute lung injury. This led to increased lung protein permeability and thus a loss of barrier function. The shedding of heparan sulphate was at least partly mediated by matrix metalloproteinases [23]. Possible implications of these findings, e.g., for mechanical ventilation or pathogen invasion during ventilator-associated pneumonia, have been highlighted [24].

Given these recent data and evidence from studies on the endothelial glycocalyx, it is obvious that the alveolar epithelial glycocalyx should have important functions in lung health and, when altered, in lung disease. These may include the regulation of alveolar fluid balance, the permeability of the air-blood barrier and the binding of inhaled pathogens. Based on the water binding capacity of glycocasaminoglycans like hyaluronan (where one molecule can bind up to 6000 molecules of water [25]), the alveolar epithelial glycocalyx must be involved in the regulation of the thickness and viscosity of the aqueous hypophase of the alveolar lining layer. This smooth lining layer has been estimated in rat lungs to have an area-weighted average thickness of 200 nm, with averages of 140 nm over flat parts of alveolar walls, 90 nm at alveolar junctions covering protrusions like capillaries and cell perikarya and 890 nm at alveolar junctions filling surface irregularities [8]. Using the area-weighted thickness of 200 nm and an alveolar surface area of 120 m^2 in the human lung, one can calculate the volume of the alveolar lining layer to be 24 mL or about 1/3 mL per kg body weight. These values are in very good agreement with other estimates (summarized in [26]). Since the thickness of this alveolar lining layer contributes to the effective thickness of the air-blood barrier, which has to be crossed by oxygen diffusion, it directly determines the efficiency of gas exchange. Moreover, it is this alveolar lining layer where surfactant functions as anti-atelectatic agent.

3. Interactions Between Surfactant and the Glycocalyx

Compared to other surfaces in the body, a unique feature of the alveolar epithelial surface are the potential interactions of the glycocalyx with components of the surfactant system. However, these interactions are so far basically unexplored although a direct topographical relationship is obvious (Figure 1). One main component of the glycocalyx, hyaluronan, known to be secreted by AEII cells in vitro [27,28], has been shown to improve the biophysical (surface tension reducing) activity of surfactant in vitro and in vivo [29–32]. Thus, hyaluronan may have therapeutic potential in lung diseases where surfactant inactivation is a major pathophysiological event. One example of particular interest is the sequence from acute lung injury to fibrosis where alterations of alveolar micromechanics (alveolar instability and collapse induration) due to surfactant dysfunction have been demonstrated [33–35](for review, see [36,37]). Moreover, hyaluronan can act as an important signal for AEII cell renewal and repair. Accordingly, in patients with severe pulmonary fibrosis, hyaluronan on the cell surface of AEII cells is reduced [38].

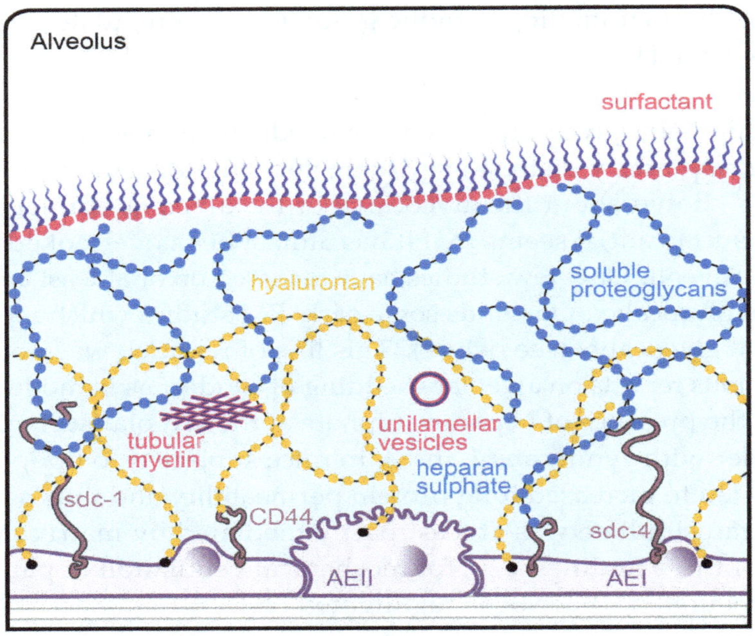

Figure 1. Schematic diagram of the alveolar lining layer with surfactant and glycocalyx components. Surfactant is present at the surface film and in the hypophase. Surfactant subtypes in the hypophase correspond to different stages in metabolism, shown here as active tubular myelin and inactive unilamellar vesicles. Proteoglycans of the glycocalyx can be attached to the apical membrane of type I (AEI) or type II (AEII) alveolar epithelial cells by syndecans like syndecan-1 (sdc-1) or syndecan-4 (sdc-4). Hyaluronan can bind either to its receptor CD44 or intercalates throughout the glyxcocalyx. The alveolar lining layer and its contents are not drawn to scale.

Based on these findings, one may speculate on the potential relevance of the alveolar epithelial glycocalyx for surfactant function in general, and vice versa. Glycocalyx components may not only influence the resistance of surfactant against inactivation in lung injury, but may also be involved in the regulation of surfactant homeostasis and in the maintenance of the micro-environment in which surfactant acts (e.g., by regulating the thickness and viscosity of the hypophase of the alveolar lining layer) under normal conditions.

The surfactant proteins, being "the smart molecules in the surfactant system" [39], deserve particular attention in this context. The hydrophilic environment created by the glycocalyx may facilitate interactions with the hydrophilic surfactant proteins. Thus, SP-A and SP-D are attractive candidates for interactions with the glycocalyx. Their known immunomodulatory functions include the binding and opsonization of pathogens, interactions with cells of the innate and adaptive immune system and direct antimicrobial activity. As lung collectins, their basic structural units are homo-trimers which are formed via the triple helix of their collagen domain. The monomers consist of four sub-units: an N-terminal domain, a collagen domain, an α-helical neck domain, and a C-terminal C-type lectin domain which is often referred to as the carbohydrate recognition domain (CRD). These homo-trimers usually multimerize to higher-order oligomers. SP-A forms octadecamers (6×3) arranged as a bouquet of flowers while SP-D forms dodecamers (4×3) where the trimers connect via their N-terminal domains to form a cruciform structure. This means that both SP-A and SP-D can bind sugars with their CRD, with higher affinity for clustered oligosaccharides than for single monosaccharides and with both common and distinct saccharide-binding activities (for review, see [40–44]). Thus, it seems plausible that SP-A and SP-D may interact with sugars of the glycocalyx, and that this interaction will influence their functional capacity.

The hydrophobic SP-B and SP-C (reviewed in [45,46]) may also have their role in this scenario. Because hyaluronan is known to interact with phospholipids and has hydrophobic regions which could bind to SP-B and SP-C, the hypothesis that hyaluronan interacts with surfactant components to form a viscous gel in the hypophase of the alveolar lining layer has been put forward [47]. By this, hyaluronan would contribute to smoothing alveolar epithelial surface irregularities (e.g., folds or cell projections) via locally varying the thickness of the hypophase, thereby resulting in a smoothly curved air-liquid interface—a phenomenon well described for the alveolar lining layer [8,48,49].

Another cell type of relevance in this context are alveolar macrophages. They reside as free cells in the aqueous hypophase of the alveolar lining layer where they exert their phagocytic activity. One of their major functions is the removal and degradation of spent intraalveolar surfactant material. Alveolar macrophages express the hyaluronan receptor CD44 and thus are coated with bound hyaluronan promoting their survival [50]. Moreover, alveolar macrophages lacking CD44 have impaired lipid homeostasis leading to an increase in intraalveolar surfactant lipids [51]. This indicates an important role for hyaluronan in surfactant catabolism.

Taken together, the coordinated interplay between surfactant and the glycocalyx is probably essential for alveolar micromechanics and lung function and thus deserves further attention.

4. Visualizing the Glycocalyx by Electron Microscopy

In order to gain a deeper understanding of the alveolar epithelial glycocalyx, one has to visualize it. The detailed architecture of the alveolar epithelium can only be resolved by EM (reviewed in [52]). Moreover, the high resolution offered by EM is also necessary to visualize the glycocalyx in its fine structural cell and tissue context. However, one has to bear in mind that no method of fixation for EM yields a "real in vivo" representation of lung structure. Although conventional chemical fixation for EM (based on glutaraldehyde and osmium tetroxide) results in good overall preservation of cell and tissue ultrastructure, the selective nature of the chemical interactions taking place during fixation, processing and dehydration (which are not very well understood) may induce artifacts. Therefore, morphological characteristics and differences observed in biological EM samples need to be interpreted with caution and knowledge of the preparation steps involved. This point is well appreciated in EM studies of lung surfactant (reviewed in [10,53]), but is at least as important for studies on the glycocalyx.

Theoretically, the method of choice for near in vivo preservation of the glycocalyx by EM is avoiding chemical fixatives and applying cryo-EM of vitreous sections (CEMOVIS) [54,55]. The cooling conditions necessary to avoid cryo-fixation artifacts in EM (in particular ice crystal formation) are achieved by freezing very small tissue samples (thickness only up to 200 μm, i.e., roughly the diameter of a single alveolus in the human lung) with very high pressure (around 2000 bar) [56]. CEMOVIS can be used in selected singular experiments, e.g., to visualize surfactant-containing lamellar bodies within AEII cells [57]. Cryo-methods have occasionally also been used to visualize the glycocalyx, e.g., the combination of slam freezing and freeze substitution of bovine aorta and rat fat pad endothelial cells in vitro [58]. However, high pressure freezing leads to forced collapse of alveoli and thus destruction of the delicate alveolar lining layer where both the alveolar epithelial glycocalyx and the intraalveolar surfactant film are located. Moreover, this approach is not suitable for quantitative microscopic analyses of whole lungs by stereology because it precludes adequate sampling for which the whole (fixed) organ should be available [59]. At current, this can only be achieved by chemical fixation of the whole lung under carefully controlled conditions, either by airway instillation or, preferably, by vascular perfusion, both of which also fulfil the criteria of consistent reproducibility in space (homogeneity) and time (repeatability) [60]. Thus, at least for the near future, chemical fixation approaches will remain the routine method(s) of choice to study the alveolar epithelial glycocalyx in large-scale experimental studies.

Classical early EM studies on the surface coat of cells (for organs other than the lung, see e.g., [61–63]) have since then been refined by various fixation agents and protocols. With respect to the EM visualization of the glycocalyx, routine chemical fixation protocols usually yield poor results. Thus, the addition of staining agents that bind to components of the glycocalyx is necessary. These agents, usually of high atomic number, provide an "electron-dense" dark contrast because they scatter beam electrons [64]. These cytochemical methods work fine as structural tools. However, a molecular interpretation is problematic because of a severely limited specificity of the staining agents. Moreover, based on studies on the endothelial glycocalyx (reviewed in [15,17]), it is highly likely that all of these methods underestimate the real height of the glycocalyx to some degree. Nevertheless, the actual height of the alveolar lining layer (see above) also has to be taken into account. Therefore, caution is necessary when transferring findings from the endothelial glycocalyx, which is facing a liquid lumen, to the completely different physiological situation in the alveolar space where there is only a very thin liquid alveolar lining layer.

Among the stains that have been used for the glycocalyx are ruthenium red, colloidal iron, phosphotungstic acid, lanthanum nitrate, alcian blue and lectins such as concanavalin A, wheat germ agglutinin, and peanut agglutinin [64]. Several of these methods have also been applied to the alveolar surface, e.g., colloidal iron [65,66], ruthenium red [67,68], phosphotungstic acid [69], and concanavalin A [68,70,71]. In some of them, a differential staining pattern between AEI and AEII cells was emphasized [66,69,70]. Lectin binding patterns for AEI and AEII cells have later been used as surface markers for these cell types (e.g., [72–74]), although results were not always consistent. These early studies have been nicely reviewed by Martins and Bairos [75].

One staining method of particular interest for the EM visualization of the glycocalyx is based on cationic hydrous thorium dioxide colloids ($cThO_2$), which has been shown to allow for better tissue penetration and more intense staining compared to other staining agents [76,77]. The size of the $cThO_2$ particles ranges from 1 to 1.7 nm. This approach has been applied successfully to study the glomerular endothelial glycocalyx in the kidney [78]. We have transferred this method to the lung in order to investigate the ultrastructure of the alveolar epithelial glycocalyx and potential associations with surfactant. Fixed samples of 1 to 2 mm edge length from mouse and human lungs were immersed in 100 mM sodium acetate buffer (NaAc) at pH 3.0 for 5 min, in 0.5% $cThO_2$ in NaAc for 5 min and again in NaAc for 5 min, followed by further post-fixation and embedding according to our routine lung EM protocol [79]. During immersion in NaAc and $cThO_2$, samples were gently massaged with a wooden skewer to allow the solutions to diffuse into the alveoli. The low pH increases the specificity for negatively charged glycocalyx components. Results based on this protocol are shown and described for mouse (Figures 2 and 3) and human (Figures 4–6) lung.

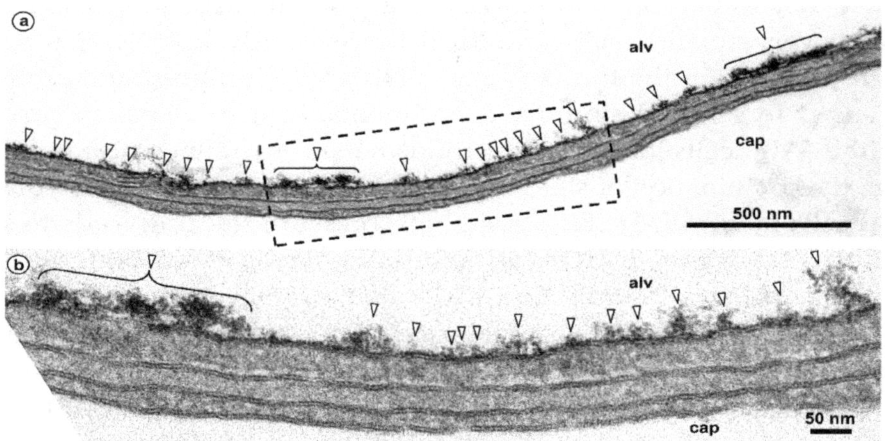

Figure 2. Mouse lung. Glycocalyx staining shown at lower (**a**) and higher (**b**) magnification. Alveolar lumen (alv) and capillary lumen (cap) are separated by the air-blood barrier consisting of a continuous alveolar epithelium, an interstitium and a continuous capillary endothelium. Here, a thin portion of the air-blood barrier is shown. The epithelium is made of thin extensions of alveolar epithelial type I cells. The interstitium is minimized to a common basal lamina shared by epithelium and endothelium. The endothelium is of the non-fenestrated type. The alveolar epithelial surface is clearly stained after treatment with colloidal thorium dioxide (arrowheads). The boxed area in (**a**) is shown in (**b**) at higher magnification.

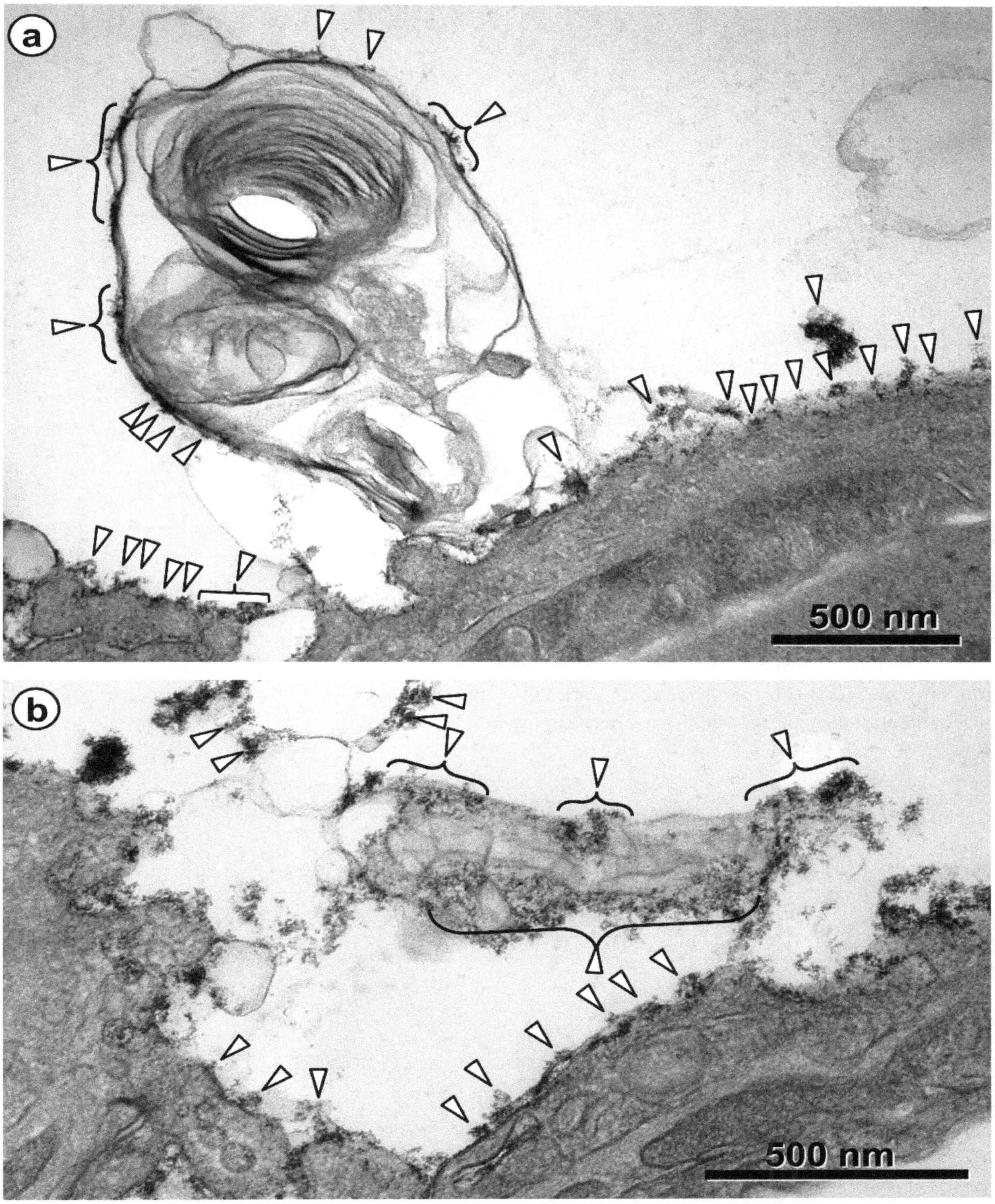

Figure 3. Mouse lung. Glycocalyx staining on intraalveolar surfactant. Intraalveolar surfactant material is visible on top of the alveolar epithelium as secreted lamellar body content (**a**) and as tubular myelin (**b**) with lattice-like structure. Both are stained, particularly at the outside, with thorium dioxide, like the surface of the alveolar epithelium (arrowheads).

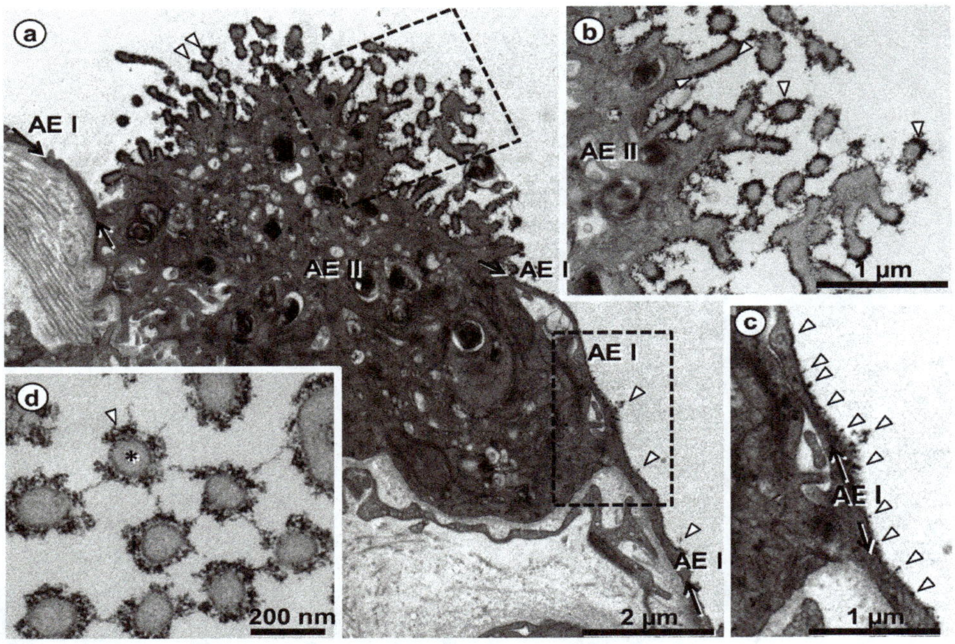

Figure 4. Human lung. Visualization of the glycocalyx on the surface of alveolar epithelial type I (AEI) and type II (AEII) cells. (**a**) Overview showing one AEII cell and neighboring thin AEI cell extensions, the lineage of the latter highlighted by arrows. The black lining and dots on the cell surfaces (arrowheads in (**a**)) depict the glycocalyx, marked by colloidal thorium dioxide. The boxed areas are shown in (**b**,**c**) at higher magnification. Note heavily stained microvilli (arrowheads in (**b**)) and staining at the apical cell membrane of AEI cell (arrowheads in (**c**)). (**d**) Profiles of cross-sectioned microvilli (one of them marked by asterisk) of an AEII cell. The glycocalyx (arrowhead in (**d**)) surrounds the microvilli and also appears as threads between them.

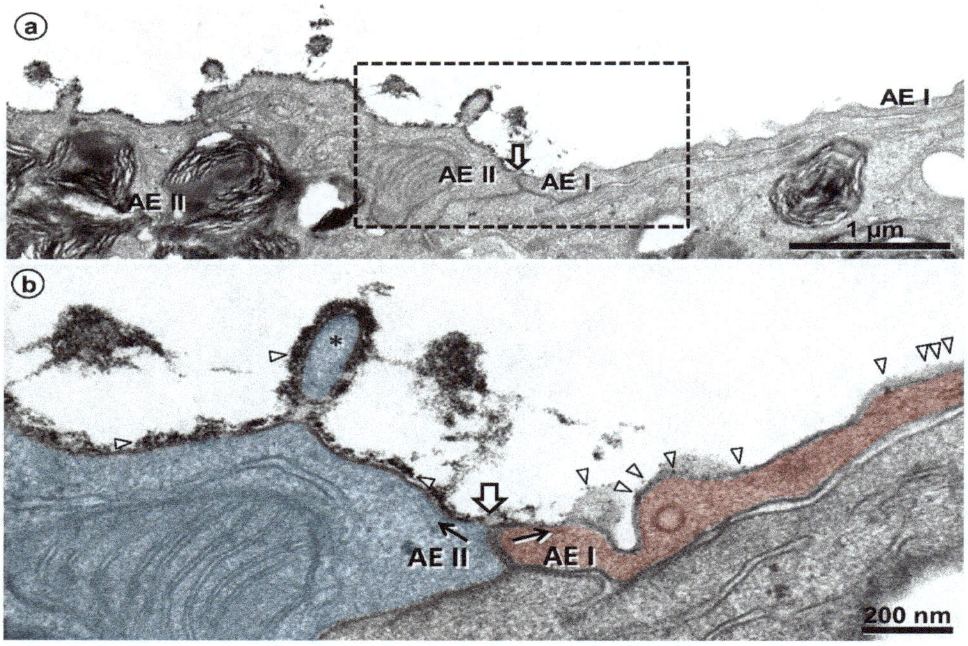

Figure 5. Human lung. Comparison of the glycocalyx of an alveolar epithelial type I (AEI) and type II (AEII) cell. (**a**) Alveolar surface depicted in sequence from an AEII cell (left) across the cell contact (block arrow) to an AEI cell (right). The boxed area is shown in (**b**) at higher magnification. (**b**) Different intensity of glycocalyx on the AEII (left, colored blue) and AEI (right, colored red) cell (along black arrows). The thorium dioxide deposition (marked by arrowheads) is intense on the AEII cell, forming a nearly continuous layer also visible on a microvillus (asterisk), while it appears rather punctual on the AEI cell.

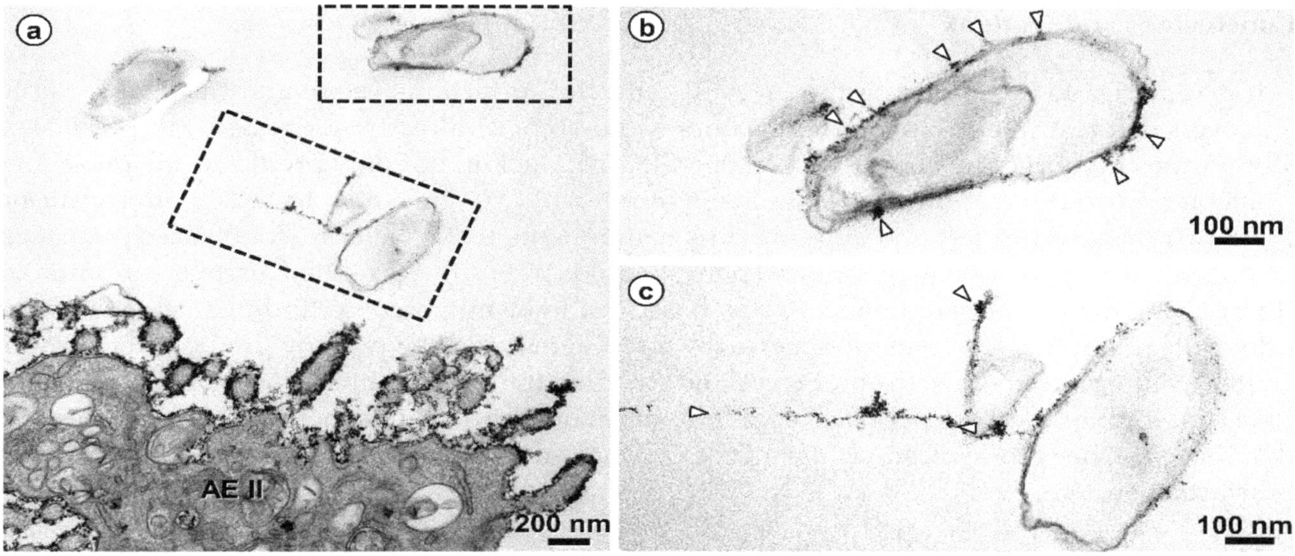

Figure 6. Human lung. Glycocalyx staining on intraalveolar surfactant. (**a**) Intraalveolar surfactant (boxed areas) in the airspace of an alveolus nearby an alveolar epithelial type II (AEII) cell is decorated by thorium dioxide. The boxed areas are shown in (**b**,**c**) at higher magnification. The stain on the intraalveolar surfactant (arrowheads) is less intense compared to the stain on the AEII cell, rather comparable with the punctual stain on an AEI cell (compare Figure 4).

Taken together, these findings indicate: (1) differences in the structure of the glycocalyx between the two cell types of the alveolar epithelium, with AEII cells showing a stronger staining, thus confirming earlier studies [66,69,70]; and (2) direct interactions of the alveolar epithelial glycocalyx with intraalveolar surfactant subtypes, including tubular myelin. These findings have several implications. In contrast to AEI cells, AEII cells possess numerous microvilli. Besides their function of providing an increased apical cell surface area, it is obvious that they are also effective as glycocalyx carriers. Interconnections between microvilli strongly contribute to the three-dimensional meshwork arrangement of the alveolar epithelial glycocalyx. Moreover, one has to take the topographical distribution of the two alveolar epithelial cell types into consideration. AEI cells, which cover about 95% of the alveolar surface, serve their lining function by providing thin cell extensions to the flat parts of the air-blood barrier that are optimized for efficient diffusion. On the other hand, the cuboidal AEII cells exert their secretory and renewal function mainly in the corners of alveoli where alveolar junctions are located. Thus, the well-known regional differences in the height of the alveolar lining layer between flat parts and junctions of alveoli (see above; [8]) are likely reflected in regional differences in the alveolar epithelial glycocalyx. Regarding the close association of the alveolar epithelial glycocalyx with intraalveolar surfactant, it is noteworthy that a similar staining pattern (i.e., at the outer lamellae of freshly secreted lamellar bodies and tubular myelin) has been shown by immunoelectron microscopy for SP-A in the human lung [80]. These morphological findings consolidate the notion of direct interactions of SP-A with components of the alveolar epithelial glycocalyx. This may be of particular relevance for tubular myelin, a still incompletely understood highly-ordered intraalveolar surfactant subtype. The characteristic lattice-like structure of tubular myelin requires the presence of SP-A which is located in the lattice with its CRD directed towards the corners [42,44,81], but an association of tubular myelin with carbohydrates has also been described [68,71]. Assumed to be an intermediate precursor of the surface film, tubular myelin may actually serve a dual function: not only as intraalveolar reservoir of surfactant lipids, but also as a "spider's web" for alveolar host defence that could be supported by the glycocalyx.

5. Conclusions and Outlook

It is remarkable that early studies on AEII cells, the surfactant system and the alveolar lining layer (even before these now common names were coined) already suggested the presence of carbohydrates in this context. In 1954, Charles Clifford Macklin not only predicted the presence of an "alveolar mucoid film", but also estimated ("arbitrarily") its thickness to be 200 nm (confirmed more than 40 years later [8]) and suggested its components to be "acid mucopolysaccharides and myelinogens", i.e., glycosaminoglycans and phospholipids [82]. After the actual discovery of surfactant by John Clements [83], Bolande and Klaus, based on light microscopic findings, suggested that, besides phospholipids, "a mucopolysaccharide fraction may also be present" in the alveolar lining layer [84]. Similarly, Groniowski and Biczyskowa studied the alveolar lining layer by EM and found evidence indicating "the existence of another component of the acidic mucopolysaccharide nature" [65]. In that sense, we have to reintroduce the glycocalyx into our concepts of the alveolar lining layer and the surfactant system.

The spatial interaction between surfactant and the glycocalyx at the alveolar epithelial surface may generate a "win-win" situation, where surfactant benefits from glycocalyx components such as hyaluronan, warranting its biophysical function. Conversely, surfactant may contribute to the integrity and function of the alveolar epithelial glycocalyx. It is unknown how the content of the alveolar hypophase is sensed, e.g., with respect to its volume, viscosity and surfactant pool size. This remains to be investigated both under normal and challenge conditions such as acute lung injury and pulmonary infection. Integrating the glycocalyx into our picture of the lung alveolus also offers attractive therapeutic perspectives, e.g., by adding glycocalyx components to exogenous surfactant preparations. Moreover, engineering of synthetic glycocalyx [85] provides a very promising approach for the preservation and/or reconstitution of the unique micro-environment on top of the alveolar surface. New developments in EM should be included in such studies, e.g., volume correlative light and electron microscopy techniques [86,87]. It seems timely to explore the structure and function of the alveolar epithelial glycocalyx, in particular its relations to the surfactant system. Given its potential importance, it should no longer remain an enigma.

Author Contributions: All authors contributed to the text and have read and agreed to the published version of the manuscript.

Acknowledgments: The authors thank Susanne Faßbender for excellent technical assistance. We acknowledge support from the German Research Federation (DFG) and the Open Access Publication Funds of Charité-Universitätsmedizin Berlin.

References

1. Schneider, J.P.; Wrede, C.; Hegermann, J.; Weibel, E.R.; Mühlfeld, C.; Ochs, M. On the topological complexity of human alveolar epithelial type 1 cells. *Am. J. Respir. Crit. Care Med.* **2019**, *199*, 1153–1156. [CrossRef]
2. Ochs, M.; Weibel, E.R. Functional design of the human lung for gas exchange. In *Fishman´s Pulmonary Diseases and Disorders*, 5th ed.; Grippi, M.A., Elias, J.A., Fishman, J.A., Kotloff, R.M., Pack, A.I., Senior, R.M., Eds.; McGraw-Hill: New York, NY, USA, 2015; pp. 20–62.
3. Hsia, C.C.W.; Hyde, D.M.; Weibel, E.R. Lung structure and the intrinsic challenges of gas exchange. *Compr. Physiol.* **2016**, *6*, 827–895. [PubMed]
4. Low, F.N. Electron microscopy of the rat lung. *Anat. Rec.* **1952**, *113*, 437–444. [CrossRef] [PubMed]
5. Low, F.N. The pulmonary alveolar epithelium of laboratory animals and man. *Anat. Rec.* **1953**, *117*, 241–264. [CrossRef] [PubMed]
6. Weibel, E.R.; Gil, J. Electron microscopic demonstration of an extracellular duplex lining layer of alveoli. *Respir. Physiol.* **1968**, *4*, 42–57. [CrossRef]
7. Gil, J.; Weibel, E.R. Improvements in demonstration of lining layer of lung alveoli by electron microscopy. *Respir. Physiol.* **1969**, *8*, 13–36. [CrossRef]

8. Bastacky, J.; Lee, C.Y.C.; Goerke, J.; Koushafar, H.; Yager, D.; Kenaga, L.; Speed, T.P.; Chen, Y.; Clements, J.A. Alveolar lining layer is thin and continuous: Low-temperature scanning electron microscopy of rat lung. *J. Appl. Physiol.* **1995**, *79*, 1615–1628. [CrossRef]
9. Perez-Gil, J. Structure of pulmonary surfactant membranes and films: The role of proteins and lipid-protein interactions. *Biochim. Biophys Acta* **2008**, *1778*, 1676–1695. [CrossRef]
10. Ochs, M. The closer we look the more we see? Quantitative microscopic analysis of the pulmonary surfactant system. *Cell. Physiol. Biochem* **2010**, *25*, 27–40. [CrossRef]
11. Orgeig, S.; Morrison, J.L.; Daniels, C.B. Evolution, development and function of the pulmonary surfactant system in normal and perturbed environments. *Compr. Physiol.* **2016**, *6*, 363–432.
12. Olmeda, B.; Martinez-Calle, M.; Perez-Gil, J. Pulmonary surfactant metabolism in the alveolar airspace: Biogenesis, extracellular conversions, recycling. *Ann. Anat.* **2017**, *209*, 78–92. [CrossRef] [PubMed]
13. Knudsen, L.; Ochs, M. The micromechanics of lung alveoli: Structure and function of surfactant and tissue components. *Histochem. Cell Biol.* **2018**, *150*, 661–676. [CrossRef] [PubMed]
14. Bennett, H.S. Morphological aspects of extracellular polysaccharides. *J. Histochem. Cytochem.* **1963**, *11*, 14–23. [CrossRef]
15. Reitsma, S.; Slaaf, D.W.; Vink, H.; van Zandvoort, M.A.M.J.; oude Egbrink, M.G.A. The endothelial glycocalyx: Composition, functions, and visualization. *Pfluegers Arch.* **2007**, *454*, 345–359. [CrossRef]
16. Tarbell, J.M.; Cancel, L.M. The glycocalyx and its significance in human medicine. *J. Intern. Med.* **2016**, *280*, 97–113. [CrossRef]
17. LaRiviere, W.B.; Schmidt, E.P. The pulmonary endothelial glycocalyx in ARDS: A critical role of heparan sulphate. *Curr. Top. Membr.* **2018**, *82*, 33–52.
18. Schmidt, E.P.; Yang, Y.; Janssen, W.J.; Gandjeva, A.; Perez, M.J.; Barthel, L.; Zemans, R.L.; Bowman, J.C.; Konayagi, D.E.; Yunt, Z.X.; et al. The pulmonary endothelial glycocalyx regulates neutrophil adhesion and lung injury during experimental sepsis. *Nat. Med.* **2012**, *18*, 1217–1223. [CrossRef]
19. Inagawa, R.; Okada, H.; Takemura, G.; Suzuki, K.; Takada, C.; Yano, H.; Ando, Y.; Usui, T.; Hotta, Y.; Miyazaki, N.; et al. Ultrastructural alteration of pulmonary capillary endothelial glycocalyx during endotoxemia. *Chest* **2018**, *154*, 317–325. [CrossRef]
20. Biasin, V.; Wygrecka, M.; Bärnthaler, T.; Jandl, K.; Jain, P.P.; Balint, Z.; Kovacs, G.; Leitinger, G.; Kolb-Lenz, D.; Kornmueller, K.; et al. Docking of meprin α to heparan sulphate protects the endothelium from inflammatory cell extravasation. *Thromb. Haemost.* **2018**, *118*, 1790–1802. [CrossRef]
21. Li, Q.; Park, P.W.; Wilson, C.L.; Parks, W.C. Matrilysin shedding of syndecan-1 regulates chemokine mobilization and transepithelial efflux of neutrophils in acute lung injury. *Cell* **2002**, *111*, 635–646. [CrossRef]
22. Pruessmeyer, J.; Martin, C.; Hess, F.M.; Schwarz, N.; Schmidt, S.; Kogel, T.; Hoettecke, N.; Schmidt, B.; Secht, A.; Uhlig, S.; et al. A disintegrin and metalloproteinase 17 (ADAM17) mediates inflammation-induced shedding of syndecan-1 and -4 by lung epithelial cells. *J. Biol. Chem.* **2010**, *285*, 555–564. [CrossRef] [PubMed]
23. Haeger, S.M.; Liu, X.; Han, X.; McNeil, J.B.; Oshima, K.; McMurty, S.A.; Yang, Y.; Ouyang, Y.; Zhang, F.; Nozik-Grayck, E.; et al. Epithelial heparan sulfate contributes to alveolar barrier function and is shed during lung injury. *Am. J. Respir. Cell Mol. Biol.* **2018**, *59*, 363–374. [CrossRef] [PubMed]
24. Weidenfeld, S.; Kuebler, W.M. Shedding first light on the alveolar epithelial glycocalyx. *Am. J. Respir. Cell Mol. Biol.* **2018**, *59*, 283–284. [CrossRef] [PubMed]
25. Allegra, L.; Patrona, S.D.; Petrigni, G. Hyaluronic acid: Perspectives in lung disease. *Handb. Exp. Pharmacol.* **2012**, *207*, 385–401.
26. Walters, D.V. Lung lining liquid—The hidden depths. *Biol. Neonate* **2002**, *81* (Suppl. 1), 2–5. [CrossRef]
27. Sahu, S.C.; Tanswell, A.K.; Lynn, W.S. Isolation and characterization of glycosaminoglycans secreted by human foetal lung type II pneumocytes in culture. *J. Cell Sci.* **1980**, *42*, 183–188.
28. Skinner, S.J.M.; Post, M.; Torday, J.S.; Stiles, A.D.; Smith, B.T. Characterization of proteoglycans synthesized by fetal rat lung type II pneumonocytes in vitro and the effects of cortisol. *Exp. Lung Res.* **1987**, *12*, 253–264. [CrossRef]
29. Lu, K.W.; Goerke, J.; Clements, J.A.; Taeusch, H.W. Hyaluronan decreases surfactant inactivation in vitro. *Pediatr. Res.* **2005**, *57*, 237–241. [CrossRef]
30. Taeusch, H.W.; de la Bernardino Serra, J.; Perez-Gil, J.; Alonso, C.; Zasadzinski, J.A. Inactivation of pulmonary

surfactant due to serum-inhibited adsorption and reversal by hydrophilic polymers: Experimental. *Biophys. J.* **2005**, *89*, 1769–1779. [CrossRef]

31. Wang, X.; Sun, Z.; Qian, L.; Guo, C.; Yu, W.; Wang, W.; Lu, K.W.; Taeusch, H.W.; Sun, B. Effects of hyaluronan-fortified surfactant in ventilated premature piglets with respiratory distress. *Biol. Neonate* **2006**, *89*, 15–24. [CrossRef]
32. Lopez-Rodriguez, E.; Cruz, A.; Richter, R.; Taeusch, H.W.; Perez-Gil, J. Transient exposure of pulmonary surfactant to hyaluronan promotes structural and compositional transformations into a highly active state. *J. Biol. Chem.* **2013**, *288*, 29872–29881. [CrossRef] [PubMed]
33. Lutz, D.; Gazdhar, A.; Lopez-Rodriguez, E.; Ruppert, C.; Mahavadi, P.; Günther, A.; Klepetko, W.; Bates, J.H.; Smith, B.; Geiser, T.; et al. Alveolar derecruitment and collapse induration as crucial mechanisms in lung injury and fibrosis. *Am. J. Respir. Cell Mol. Biol.* **2015**, *52*, 232–243. [CrossRef] [PubMed]
34. Steffen, L.; Ruppert, C.; Hoymann, H.G.; Funke, M.; Ebener, S.; Kloth, C.; Mühlfeld, C.; Ochs, M.; Knudsen, L.; Lopez-Rodriguez, E. Surfactant replacement therapy reduces acute lung injury and collapse induration related lung remodeling in the bleomycin model. *Am. J. Physiol. Lung Cell. Mol. Physiol.* **2017**, *313*, L313–L327. [CrossRef] [PubMed]
35. Zhou, T.; Yu, Z.; Jian, M.Y.; Ahmad, I.; Trempus, C.; Wagener, B.M.; Pittet, J.F.; Aggarwal, S.; Garantziotis, S.; Song, W.; et al. Instillation of hyaluronan reverses acid instillation injury to the mammalian blood gas barrier. *Am. J. Physiol. Lung Cell. Mol. Physiol.* **2018**, *314*, L808–L821. [CrossRef]
36. Todd, N.W.; Atamas, S.P.; Luzina, I.G.; Galvin, J.R. Permanent alveolar collapse is the predominant mechanism in idiopathic pulmonary fibrosis. *Expert Rev. Respir. Med.* **2015**, *9*, 411–418. [CrossRef]
37. Knudsen, L.; Ruppert, C.; Ochs, M. Tissue remodelling in pulmonary fibrosis. *Cell Tissue Res.* **2017**, *367*, 607–626. [CrossRef]
38. Liang, J.; Zhang, Y.; Xie, T.; Liu, N.; Chen, H.; Geng, Y.; Kurkciyan, A.; Stripp, B.R.; Jiang, D.; Noble, P.W.; et al. Hyaluronan and TLR4 promote surfactant-protein-C-positive alveolar progenitor cell renewal and prevent severe pulmonary fibrosis. *Nat. Med.* **2016**, *22*, 1285–1293. [CrossRef]
39. Hawgood, S.; Clements, J. Pulmonary surfactant and its apoproteins. *J. Clin. Investig.* **1990**, *86*, 1–6. [CrossRef]
40. Hawgood, S.; Poulain, F.R. The pulmonary collectins and surfactant metabolism. *Annu. Rev. Physiol.* **2001**, *63*, 495–519. [CrossRef]
41. Crouch, E.; Wright, J.R. Surfactant proteins A and D and pulmonary host defense. *Annu. Rev. Physiol.* **2001**, *63*, 521–554. [CrossRef]
42. McCormack, F.X.; Whitsett, J.A. The pulmonary collectins, SP-A and SP-D, orchestrate innate immunity in the lung. *J. Clin. Investig.* **2002**, *109*, 707–712. [CrossRef] [PubMed]
43. Wright, J.R. Immunoregulatory functions of surfactant proteins. *Nat. Rev. Immunol.* **2005**, *5*, 58–68. [CrossRef] [PubMed]
44. Kingma, P.S.; Whitsett, J.A. In defense of the lung: Surfactant protein A and surfactant protein B. *Curr. Opin. Pharmacol.* **2006**, *6*, 1–7. [CrossRef] [PubMed]
45. Weaver, T.E.; Conkright, J.J. Functions of surfactant proteins B and C. *Annu. Rev. Physiol.* **2001**, *63*, 555–578. [CrossRef]
46. Whitsett, J.A.; Weaver, T.E. Hydrophobic surfactant proteins in lung function and disease. *N. Engl. J. Med.* **2002**, *347*, 2141–2148. [CrossRef]
47. Bray, B.A. The role of hyaluronan in the pulmonary alveolus. *J. Theor. Biol.* **2001**, *210*, 121–130. [CrossRef]
48. Weibel, E.R.; Gil, J. Structure-Function Relationships at the Alveolar Level. In *Bioengineering Aspects of the Lung*; Lung Biology in Health and Disease; West, J.B., Ed.; Marcel Dekker: New York, NY, USA, 1977; Volume 3, pp. 1–81.
49. Rühl, N.; Lopez-Rodriguez, E.; Albert, K.; Smith, B.J.; Waever, T.E.; Ochs, M.; Knudsen, L. Surfactant protein B deficiency induced high surface tension: Relationship between alveolar micromechanics, alveolar fluid properties and alveolar epithelial cell injury. *Int. J. Mol. Sci.* **2019**, *20*, 4243. [CrossRef]
50. Dong, Y.; Poon, G.F.T.; Arif, A.A.; Lee-Sayer, S.S.M.; Dosanjh, M.; Johnson, P. The survival of fetal and bone-marrow monocyte-derived alveolar macrophages is promoted by CD44 and its interaction with hyaluronan. *Mucosal Immunol.* **2018**, *11*, 601–614. [CrossRef]
51. Dong, Y.; Arif, A.A.; Guo, J.; Ha, Z.; Lee-Sayer, S.S.M.; Poon, G.F.T.; Dosanjh, M.; Roskelley, C.D.; Huan, T.; Johnson, P. CD44 loss disrupts lung lipid surfactant homeostasis and exacerbates oxidized lipid-induced lung inflammation. *Front. Immunol.* **2020**, *11*, 29. [CrossRef] [PubMed]

52. Ochs, M.; Knudsen, L.; Hegermann, J.; Wrede, C.; Grothausmann, R.; Mühlfeld, C. Using electron microscopes to look into the lung. *Histochem. Cell Biol.* **2016**, *146*, 695–707. [CrossRef]
53. Gil, J. Histological preservation and ultrastructure of alveolar surfactant. *Annu. Rev. Physiol.* **1985**, *47*, 753–763. [CrossRef] [PubMed]
54. Al-Amoudi, A.; Chang, J.J.; Leforestier, A.; McDowall, A.; Salamin, L.M.; Norlen, L.P.O.; Richter, K.; Blanc, N.S.; Studer, D.; Dubochet, J. Cryo-electron microscopy of vitreous sections. *EMBO J.* **2004**, *23*, 3583–3588. [CrossRef] [PubMed]
55. Dubochet, J. Cryo-EM—The first 30 years. *J. Microsc.* **2011**, *245*, 221–224. [CrossRef] [PubMed]
56. Studer, D.; Humbel, B.; Chiquet, M. Electron microscopy of high pressure frozen samples: Bridging the gap between cellular ultrastructure and atomic resolution. *Histochem. Cell Biol.* **2008**, *130*, 877–889. [CrossRef] [PubMed]
57. Vanhecke, D.; Herrmann, G.; Graber, W.; Hillmann-Marti, T.; Mühlfeld, C.; Studer, D.; Ochs, M. Lamellar body ultrastructure revisited: High-pressure freezing and cryo-electron microscopy of vitreous sections. *Histochem. Cell Biol.* **2010**, *134*, 319–326. [CrossRef]
58. Ebong, E.E.; Macaluso, F.P.; Spray, D.C.; Tarbell, J.M. Imaging the endothelial glycocalyx in vitro by rapid freezing/freeze substitution transmission electron microscopy. *Arterioscler. Thromb. Vasc. Biol.* **2011**, *31*, 1908–1915. [CrossRef]
59. Hsia, C.C.W.; Hyde, D.M.; Ochs, M.; Weibel, E.R. An official research policy statement of the American Thoracic Society / European Respiratory Society: Standards for quantitative assessment of lung structure. *Am. J. Respir. Crit. Care Med.* **2010**, *181*, 394–418. [CrossRef]
60. Weibel, E.R. Morphometric and stereological methods in respiratory physiology, including fixation techniques. In *Techniques in the Life Sciences. Techniques in Respiratory Physiology*; Part 1; Otis, A.B., Ed.; Elsevier: Amsterdam, The Netherlands, 1984; pp. 1–35.
61. Ito, S. The enteric surface coat on cat intestinal microvilli. *J. Cell Biol.* **1956**, *27*, 475–491. [CrossRef]
62. Luft, J.H. Electron microscopy of cell extraneous coats as revealed by ruthenium red staining. *J. Cell Biol.* **1964**, *23*, 54A–55A.
63. Rambourg, A.; Leblond, C.P. Electron microscope observations on the carbohydrate-rich cell coat present at the surface of cells in the rat. *J. Cell Biol.* **1967**, *32*, 27–53. [CrossRef]
64. Hayat, M.A. *Stains and Cytochemical Methods*; Plenum Press: New York, NY, USA, 1993.
65. Groniowski, J.; Biczyskowa, W. Structure of the alveolar lining film of the lungs. *Nature* **1964**, *21*, 745–747. [CrossRef] [PubMed]
66. Kuhn, C., III. Cytochemistry of pulmonary alveolar epithelial cells. *Am. J. Pathol.* **1968**, *53*, 809–833. [PubMed]
67. Brooks, R.E. Ruthenium red stainable surface layer on lung alveolar cells; electron microscopic interpretation. *Stain Technol.* **1969**, *44*, 173–177. [CrossRef] [PubMed]
68. Bignon, J.; Faubert, F.; Jaurand, M.C. Plasma protein immunocytochemistry and polysaccharide cytochemistry at the surface of alveolar and endothelial cells in the rat lung. *J. Histochem. Cytochem.* **1976**, *24*, 1076–1084. [CrossRef] [PubMed]
69. Adamson, I.Y.R.; Bowden, D.H. The surface complexes of the lung. *Am. J. Pathol.* **1970**, *61*, 359–368. [PubMed]
70. Roth, J. Ultrahistochemical demonstration of saccharide components of complex carbohydrates at the alveolar cell surface and at the mesothelial cell surface of the pleura visceralis of mice by means of concanavalin A. *Exp. Pathol.* **1973**, *8*, 157–167.
71. Nir, I.; Pease, D.C. Polysaccharides in lung alveoli. *Am. J. Anat.* **1976**, *147*, 457–470. [CrossRef]
72. Meban, C. Ultrastructural visualisation of carbohydrate groups in the surface coating of hamster alveolar macrophages and pneumonocytes. *J. Anat.* **1986**, *146*, 131–139.
73. Taatjes, D.J.; Barcomb, L.; Leslie, K.O.; Low, R.B. Lectin binding patterns to terminal sugars of rat lung alveolar epithelial cells. *J. Histochem. Cytochem.* **1990**, *38*, 233–244. [CrossRef]
74. Iwatsuki, H.; Sasaki, K.; Suda, M.; Itano, C. Cell differentiation of alveolar epithelium in the developing rat lung: Ultrahistochemical studies of glycoconjugates on the epithelial cell surface. *Histochemistry* **1993**, *100*, 331–340. [CrossRef]
75. Martins, M.F.; Bairos, V.A. Glycocalyx of lung epithelial cells. *Int. Rev. Cytol.* **2002**, *216*, 131–173.
76. Groot, C.G. Positive colloidal thorium dioxide as an electron microscopical contrasting agent for glycosaminoglycans, compared with ruthenium red and positive colloidal iron. *Histochemistry* **1981**, *71*, 617–627. [CrossRef] [PubMed]

77. Lünsdorf, H.; Kristen, I.; Barth, E. Cationic hydrous thorium dioxide colloids—A useful tool for staining negatively charged surface matrices of bacteria for use in energy-filtered transmission electron microscopy. *BMC Microbiol.* **2006**, *6*, 59. [CrossRef] [PubMed]
78. Hegermann, J.; Lünsdorf, H.; Ochs, M.; Haller, H. Visualization of the glomerular endothelial glycocalyx by electron microscopy using cationic colloidal thorium dioxide. *Histochem. Cell Biol.* **2016**, *145*, 41–51. [CrossRef] [PubMed]
79. Mühlfeld, C.; Rothen-Rutishauser, B.; Vanhecke, D.; Blank, F.; Gehr, P.; Ochs, M. Visualization and quantitative analysis of nanoparticles in the respiratory tract by transmission electron microscopy. *Part. Fibre Toxicol.* **2007**, *4*, 11. [CrossRef]
80. Ochs, M.; Johnen, G.; Müller, K.M.; Wahlers, T.; Hawgood, S.; Richter, J.; Brasch, F. Intracellular and intraalveolar localization of surfactant protein A (SP-A) in the parenchymal region of the human lung. *Am. J. Respir. Cell Mol. Biol.* **2002**, *26*, 91–98. [CrossRef]
81. Voorhout, W.F.; Veenendaal, T.; Haagsman, H.P.; Verkleij, A.J.; Van Golde, L.M.G.; Geuze, H.J. Surfactant protein A is localized at the corners of the pulmonary tubular myelin lattice. *J. Histochem. Cytochem.* **1991**, *39*, 1331–1336. [CrossRef]
82. Macklin, C.C. The pulmonary alveolar mucoid film and the pneumonocytes. *Lancet* **1954**, *6822*, 1099–1104. [CrossRef]
83. Clements, J.A. Surface tension of lung extracts. *Proc. Soc. Exp. Biol. Med.* **1957**, *95*, 170–172. [CrossRef]
84. Bolande, R.P.; Klaus, M.H. The morphologic demonstration of an alveolar lining layer and its relationship to pulmonary surfactant. *Am. J. Pathol.* **1964**, *45*, 449–463.
85. Purcell, S.C.; Godula, K. Synthetic glycoscapes: Addressing the structural and functional complexity of the glycocalyx. *Interface Focus* **2019**, *9*, 20180080. [CrossRef] [PubMed]
86. Fang, T.; Lu, X.; Berger, D.; Gmeiner, C.; Cho, J.; Schalek, R.; Ploegh, H.; Lichtman, J. Nanobody immunostaining for correlated light and electron microscopy with preservation of ultrastructure. *Nat. Methods* **2018**, *15*, 1029–1032. [CrossRef] [PubMed]
87. Hegermann, J.; Wrede, C.; Fassbender, S.; Schliep, R.; Ochs, M.; Knudsen, L.; Mühlfeld, C. Volume-CLEM: A method for correlative light and electron microscopy in three dimensions. *Am. J. Physiol. Lung Cell. Mol. Physiol.* **2019**, *317*, L778–L784. [CrossRef] [PubMed]

11

miR-21-KO Alleviates Alveolar Structural Remodeling and Inflammatory Signaling in Acute Lung Injury

Johanna Christine Jansing [1,2], Jan Fiedler [3,4], Andreas Pich [5], Janika Viereck [3], Thomas Thum [3,4], Christian Mühlfeld [1,2] and Christina Brandenberger [1,2,*]

1 Institute of Functional and Applied Anatomy, Hannover Medical School, 30625 Hannover, Germany
2 Biomedical Research in Endstage and Obstructive Lung Disease Hannover (BREATH), Member of the German Center for Lung Research (DZL), 30625 Hannover, Germany; Johanna.C.Jansing@stud.mh-hannover.de (J.C.J.); muehlfeld.christian@mh-hannover.de (C.M.)
3 Institute of Molecular and Translational Therapeutic Strategies, Hannover Medical School, 30625 Hannover, Germany; fiedler.jan@mh-hannover.de (J.F.); viereck.janika@mh-hannover.de (J.V.); thum.thomas@mh-hannover.de (T.T.)
4 REBIRTH Center for Translational Regenerative Medicine, 30625 Hannover, Germany
5 Institute of Toxicology, Hannover Medical School, 30625 Hannover, Germany; pich.andreas@mh-hannover.de
* Correspondence: brandenberger.christina@mh-hannover.de

Abstract: Acute lung injury (ALI) is characterized by enhanced permeability of the air–blood barrier, pulmonary edema, and hypoxemia. MicroRNA-21 (miR-21) was shown to be involved in pulmonary remodeling and the pathology of ALI, and we hypothesized that miR-21 knock-out (KO) reduces injury and remodeling in ALI. ALI was induced in miR-21 KO and C57BL/6N (wildtype, WT) mice by an intranasal administration of 75 µg lipopolysaccharide (LPS) in saline ($n = 10$ per group). The control mice received saline alone ($n = 7$ per group). After 24 h, lung function was measured. The lungs were then excised for proteomics, cytokine, and stereological analysis to address inflammatory signaling and structural damage. LPS exposure induced ALI in both strains, however, only WT mice showed increased tissue resistance and septal thickening upon LPS treatment. Septal alterations due to LPS exposure in WT mice consisted of an increase in extracellular matrix (ECM), including collagen fibrils, elastic fibers, and amorphous ECM. Proteomics analysis revealed that the inflammatory response was dampened in miR-21 KO mice with reduced platelet and neutrophil activation compared with WT mice. The WT mice showed more functional and structural changes and inflammatory signaling in ALI than miR-21 KO mice, confirming the hypothesis that miR-21 KO reduces the development of pathological changes in ALI.

Keywords: acute lung injury; microRNA-21; alveolar micromechanics; structural remodeling; inflammatory signaling

---

1. Introduction

Acute lung injury (ALI) or acute respiratory distress syndrome (ARDS) results from severe alveolar injury with increased permeability of the alveolar–capillary barrier, which is most often caused by pneumonia or sepsis. The pathophysiology of the disease is characterized by a strong pulmonary inflammation with a diffuse alveolar damage and edema formation that leads to decreased pulmonary compliance, hypoxemia, and respiratory failure (reviewed in [1]). The mortality rate is still relatively high, and recovery is often associated with an increased risk of developing pulmonary fibrosis [2,3].

As of now, however, treatment options are limited to supportive care with mechanical ventilation, since pharmaceutical treatment options are still lacking [4].

MicroRNAs are small non-coding RNA sequences that regulate the gene expression of cellular processes, such as cell proliferation, differentiation, cell metabolism, or apoptosis, by forming complementary sequences to mRNAs and thereby inhibiting their translation (reviewed in [5,6]). MicroRNA-21 (miR-21) has been described to have pro-inflammatory, proliferative, and fibrotic activities in tumor development or fibrosis in a variety of different tissues and organs [7–9]. It was shown to be transcriptionally regulated via AP-1, STAT3, or NFκB signaling and interacting with a series of pathways such as PTEN/AKT, SMAD/TGFβ, PDCD4, and others (reviewed in [6,10]). In the lung, miR-21 was found to be upregulated and involved in the development of ALI and pulmonary fibrosis [11,12]. Patients with ARDS showed increased levels of miR-21 in the blood serum [13] and miR-21 was upregulated in different murine models of ALI [13–17]. This was also the case in patients with idiopathic pulmonary fibrosis (IPF) and in murine models of bleomycin-induced lung injury and fibrosis [12,18,19]. Previous studies have shown that the inhibition of miR-21 signaling improved lung function and oxygenation and reduced the formation of edema in ventilation-induced lung injury (VILI) or lipopolysaccharide- (LPS) induced ALI [13,17]. Other studies, however, also indicated that miR-21 could have beneficial effects on the development of ALI [20,21]. Together these studies provide evidence that miR-21 is involved in the development of ALI, however, its molecular role and the underlying mechanisms are still poorly understood.

While these previous studies have addressed the impact of miR-21 signaling in ALI by using synthetic overexpression (agomiR-21) or inhibition (antagomiR-21), in the current study miR-21 knock-out (KO) mice were used, with the advantage of a specific and permanent loss of miR-21 in the adult system. The impact of miR-21 was addressed in the acute phase of LPS-induced ALI, and we hypothesized that miR-21 KO ameliorates pulmonary inflammation and tissue damage.

2. Results

ALI was induced in male C57BL/6N wild-type (WT) mice and miR-21 knock-out (KO) mice by an intranasal application of 75 μg LPS per mouse ($n = 10$ per strain). Control mice received saline ($n = 7$ per strain). Twenty-four hours later, lung function was measured, mice were sacrificed, and lung injury, remodeling, and inflammation were analyzed. The MiR-21/snoRNA202 ratio was analyzed to measure relative miR-21 expression in the lung. In the KO mice, miR-21 expression was below assay sensitivity. In the WT controls, the ratio was 0.886/0.160 (mean/SD) and significantly ($p < 0.05$) increased with LPS exposure in WT mice (1.571/0.624).

2.1. Lung Function

The results of the lung function measurements are shown in Figure 1. The measurements revealed that static pulmonary compliance (Cst) and inspiratory capacity (IC) were significantly ($p < 0.05$) higher in WT compared with KO mice. This was equally apparent in the controls and LPS-treated mice. Significant differences with LPS exposure occurred only in WT mice, including increases in tissue resistance (G), hysteresivity (η), and hysteresis. No differences in tissue elastance (H) were measured between strains or with LPS treatment.

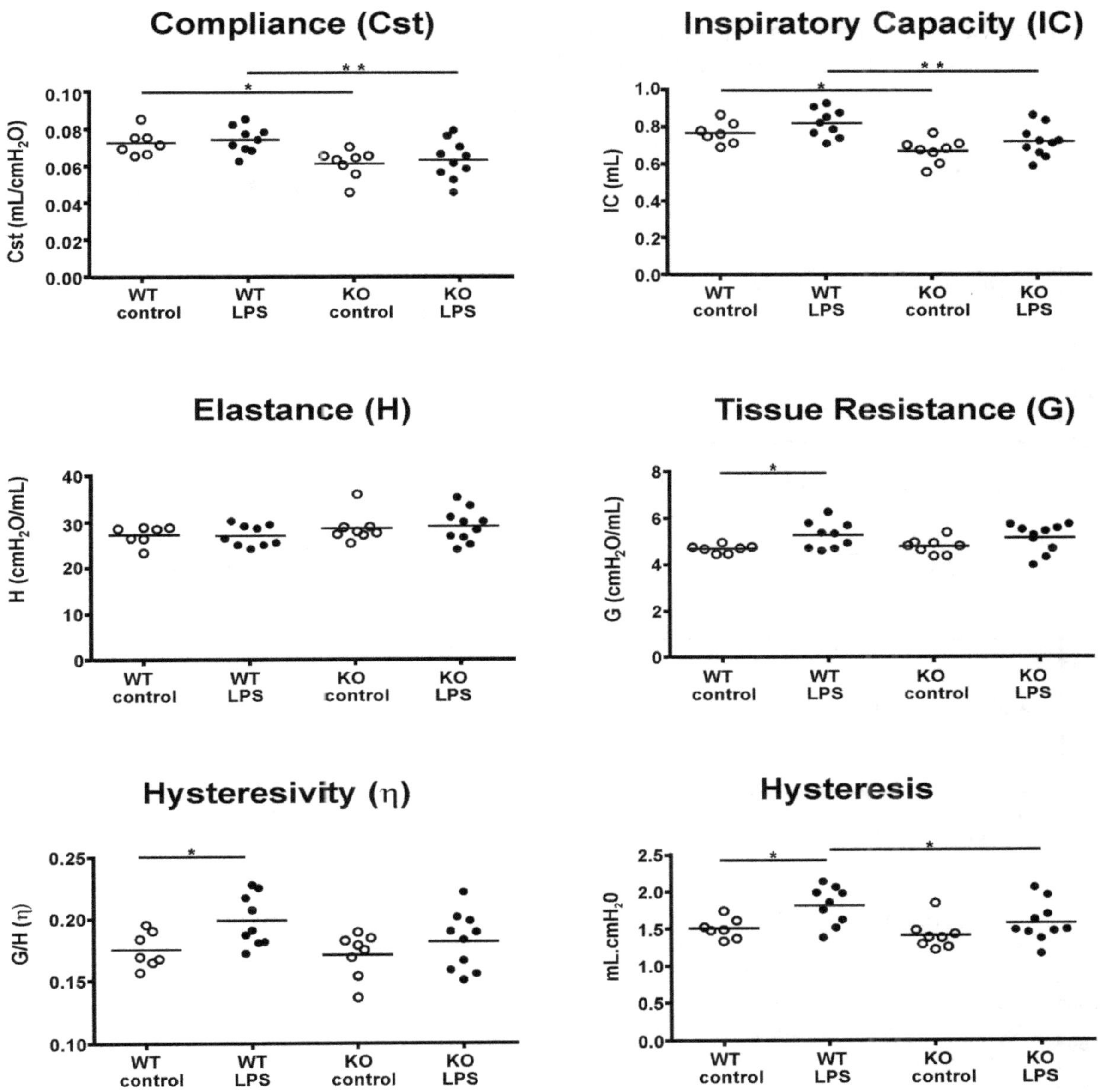

Figure 1. Lung function analysis. Pulmonary function and micromechanics were assessed at a positive end-expiratory pressure (PEEP) value of 3 cmH_2O with a mouse FlexiVent (SCIREQ) ventilator in wild-type (WT) and knock-out (KO) mice with and without acute lung injury (ALI). Each data point represents one animal; means are expressed by horizontal bars; lines indicate statistically significant differences between groups (* $p < 0.05$, ** $p < 0.01$).

2.2. Structural Changes

Structural changes in the lung parenchyma were assessed by stereology (Figure 2). LPS exposure caused an increase in lung volume in KO mice ($p = 0.002$) and in WT mice ($p = 0.054$) and a significant ($p < 0.05$) increase in the parenchymal volume of both WT and KO mice. Along with the parenchymal volume, significant increases were observed in alveolar volume and septal volume with LPS exposure in both strains. In the KO mice, the effect was also accompanied by a significant ($p = 0.04$) increase in the septal surface area, which was only manifested as a trend ($p = 0.07$) in WT mice. The main difference between the strains with ALI became apparent in septal thickness (τ(sept,par)). Here, a significant ($p = 0.004$) septal thickening upon LPS exposure was measured in WT mice, but not in

KO mice ($p = 0.32$). Histopathology (Figure 3) further revealed the recruitment of inflammatory cells, mostly neutrophils, into the lung tissue and alveolus.

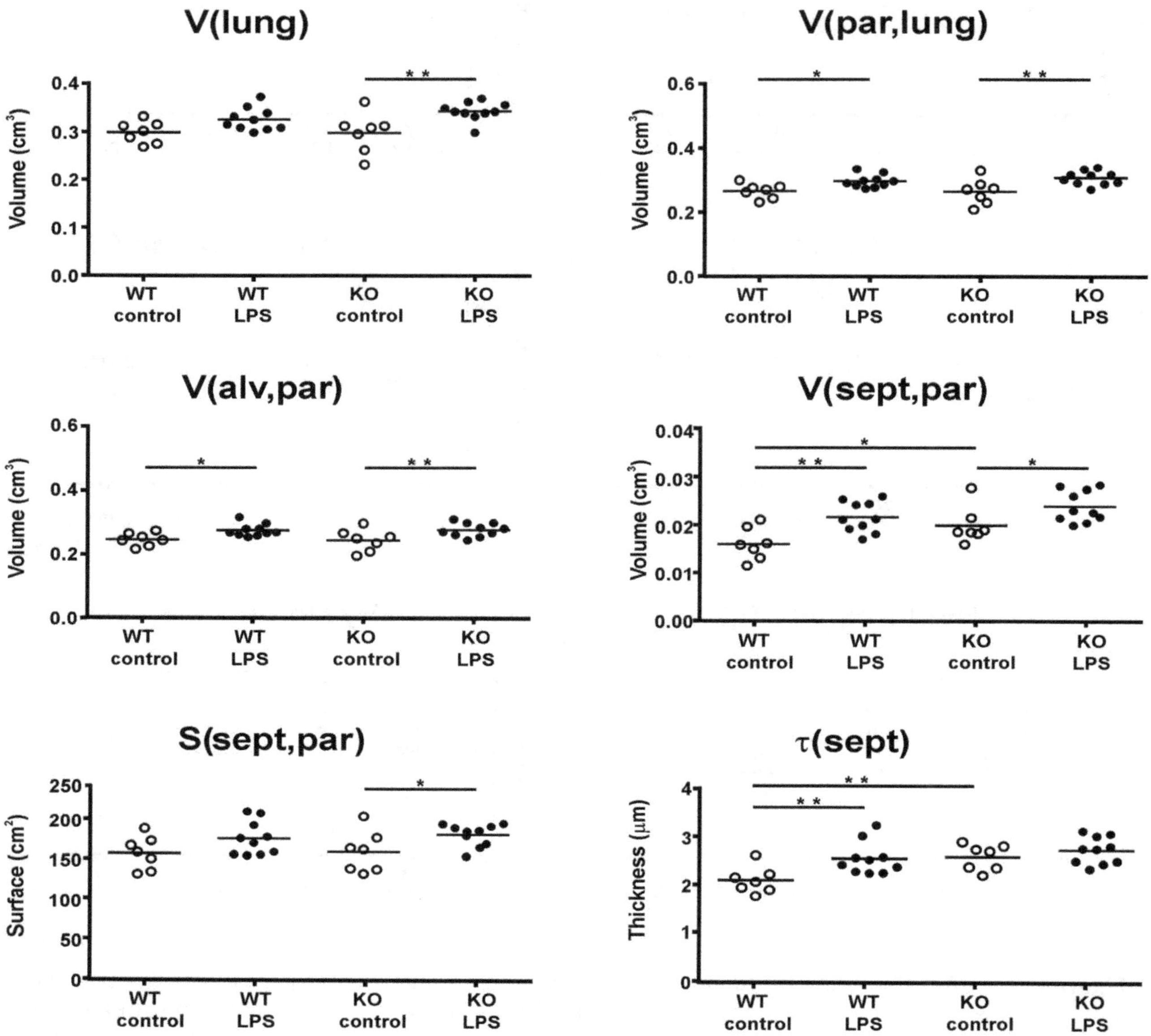

Figure 2. Structural alterations in lung tissue. Structural changes were assessed in the left lung lobe using stereology. The volume of the left lung lobe (V(lung)) was measured with volume displacement. The parenchymal content (V(par,lung)) and its alveolar volume (V(alv,par)) and septal volume (V(sept,par)) were estimated, as well as the septal surface area (S(sept,par)) and septal thickness (τ(sept)). Each data point represents one animal; means are expressed by horizontal bars; lines indicate statistically significant differences between groups (*$p < 0.05$, **$p < 0.01$).

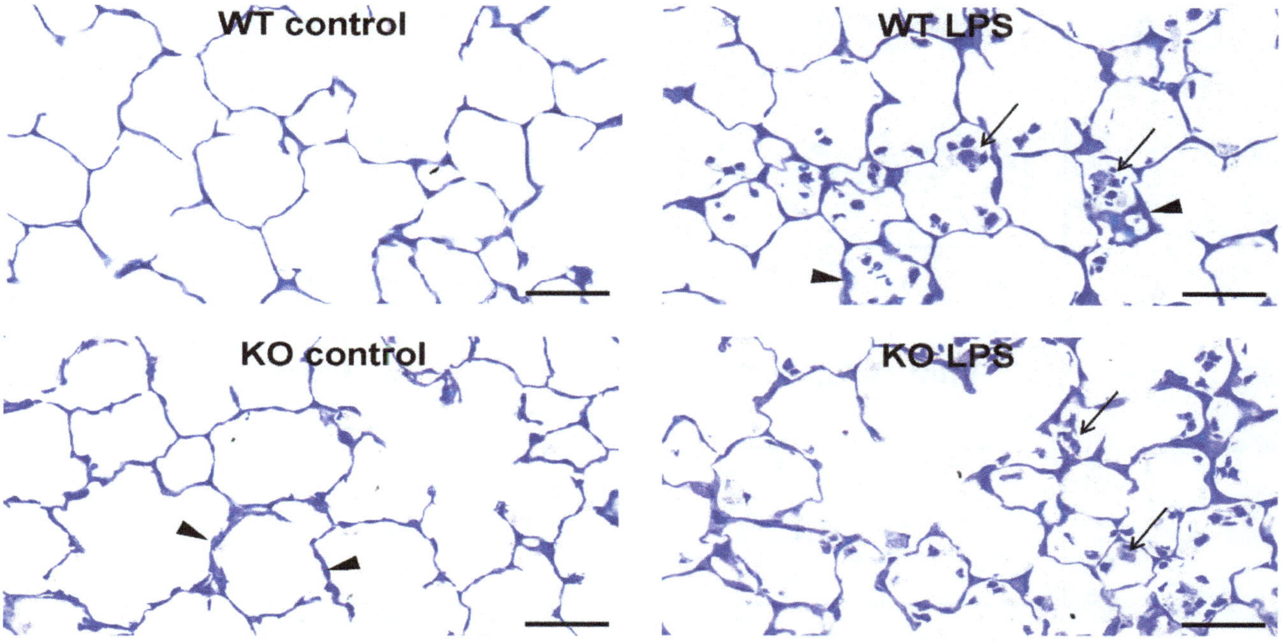

Figure 3. Representative light micrographs of toluidine blue stained lung parenchyma. The arrows indicate inflammatory cell infiltration, the arrow heads show septal thickening in the lung in the different experimental groups; scale bar = 50 μm.

2.3. *Ultrastructural Septal Remodeling*

Most changes between strains with ALI were apparent in the septa; therefore, the ultrastructural septal composition was further quantified with transmission electron microscopy (TEM) and stereology. As main septal compositions, the volume of alveolar epithelial cells (V(epi,sept)), endothelial cells (V(endo,sept)), interstitial cells, including fibroblasts and recruited inflammatory cells (V(int.cell,sept)), and extracellular matrix (ECM; V(ECM,sept)) were assessed (Figure 4A). Stereological quantification revealed that no differences between strains or with ALI were apparent in alveolar epithelial and endothelial cell volume, but the volume of interstitial cells increased significantly with ALI in both WT and KO mice. The increase in interstitial cells was mostly due to inflammatory cells recruited to the septa, as also shown in representative TEM images (Figure 4B). A significant strain-related difference in septal composition with LPS exposure was measured in the volume of septal ECM. The volume of ECM was generally lower in WT compared with KO mice, but only in WT mice was a significant ($p < 0.01$) increase found with LPS exposure. The changes in ECM composition were therefore sub-divided into collagen fibrils (V(collagen,sept)), elastic fibers (V(elastin,sept)) and other amorphous ECM (V(amorphous ECM,sept)), as shown in Table 1. The KO mice differed from the WT mice by an increased content of amorphous ECM in the septa. In WT mice, all three ECM compartments were significantly increased with LPS exposure, but no changes with LPS exposure were found in KO mice.

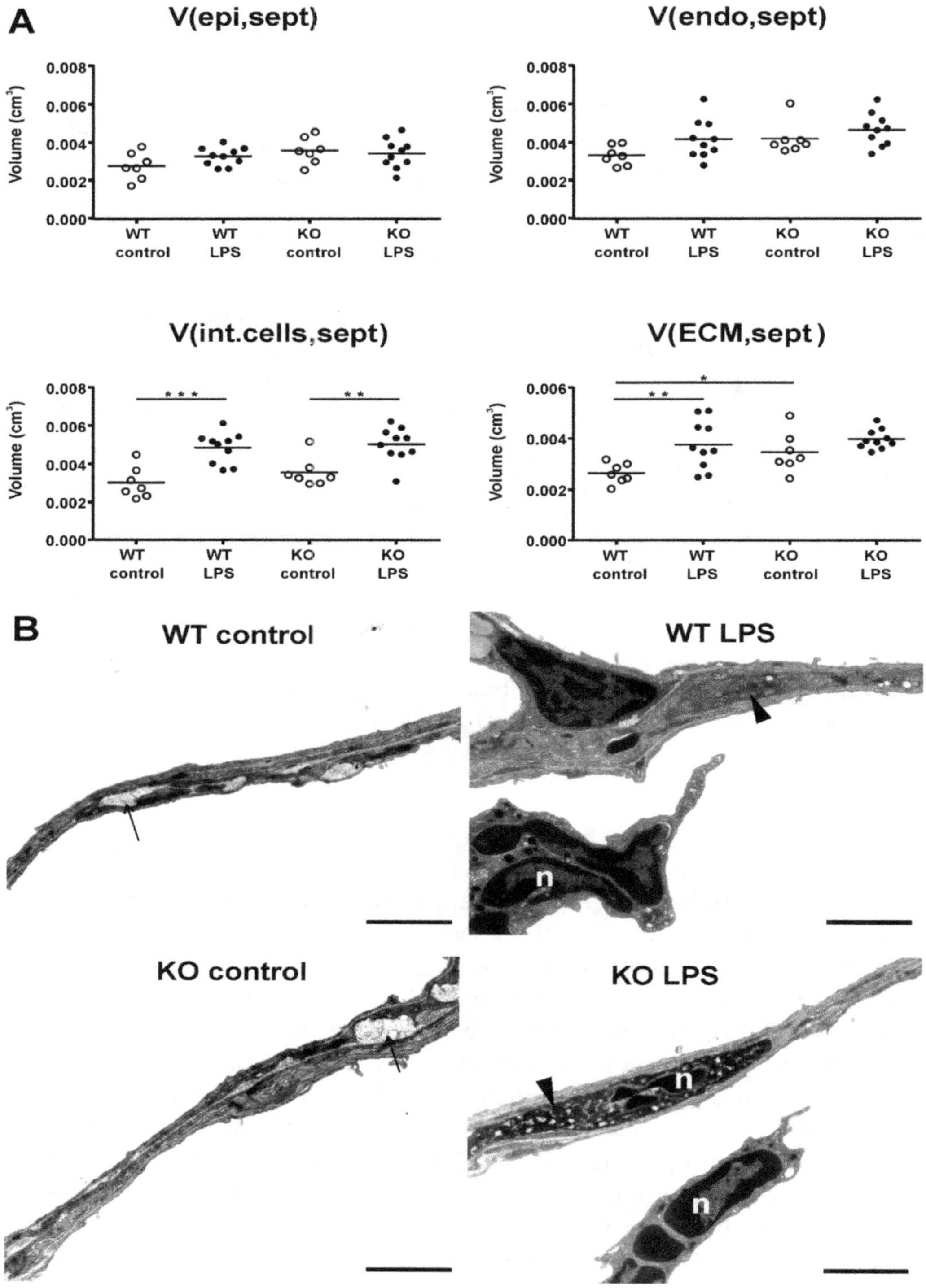

Figure 4. Ultrastructural changes in the pulmonary septa. The ultrastructural changes in the pulmonary septa of the left lung lobe were assessed using stereology (**A**). Analysis of the septal composition included the volume of alveolar epithelial cells (V(epi,sept)), endothelial cells (V(endo,sept)), interstitial cells (V(int.cells,sept), including fibroblasts and interstitial inflammatory cells, and ECM (V(ECM,sept) in the septa. Each data point represents one animal; means are expressed by horizontal bars; lines indicate statistically significant differences between groups (* $p < 0.05$, ** $p < 0.01$, *** $p < 0.001$). Representative transmission electron microscopy (TEM) images of the different experimental groups (**B**). The arrows show septal elastic fibers, the arrow heads point to interstitial cells, n = neutrophil, scale bar = 2 μm.

Table 1. Septal extracellular matrix (ECM) composition in the left lung lobe. Septal ECM compositions were ultrastructurally quantified as either collagen fibrils (V(collagen,sept)), elastic fibers (V(elastin,sept)), or other amorphous ECM (V(amorphous ECM,sept)). The results are displayed as mean / SD. **L** = significant lipopolysaccharide (LPS) effect in the respective strain group, **S** = significant strain effect in respective expcsure group; * $p < 0.05$, ** $p < 0.01$.

Group	V(collagen,sept) [mm^3]	V(elastin,sept) [mm^3]	V(amorphous ECM,sept) [mm^3]
WT control	0.3 / 0.10	0.9 / 0.15	1.5 / 0.28
WT LPS	0.4 / 0.13 **L****	1.3 / 0.40 **L****	2.0 / 0.51 **L***
KO control	0.4 / 0.16	1.0 / 0.29	2.0 / 0.46 **S***
KO LPS	0 5 / 0.14	1.3 / 0.19	2.2 / 0.26

2.4. Pulmonary Cytokine Expression

Inflammatory cytokine expression was measured in the lung tissue with a multiplex bead array. The levels of inflammatory cytokines (IFNγ, TNFα, IL-6, IL-1β, CXCL1, CCL2, and CCL5) were significantly increased with LPS exposure in both strains (Table 2). No differences were detected between strains in control mice and all cytokines, with the exception of CCL5, were equally induced in WT and KO mice after LPS exposure. CCL5, however, was 80% higher in WT compared with KO mice ($p < 0.001$).

Table 2. Inflammatory cytokine expression in lung tissue. Cytokine expression was normalized to total tissue protein concentration (pg/mg) and is displayed as mean / SD. **L** = significant LPS effect in the respective strain group, **S** = significant strain effect in respective exposure group; * $p < 0.05$, ** $p < 0.01$, *** $p < 0.001$.

Cytokines	WT Control	WT LPS	KO Control	KO LPS
IFNγ	0.08 / 0.01	11.94 / 16.67 **L***	0.08 / 0.04	10.07 / 9.81 **L***
TNFα	0.52 / 0.14	45.21 / 28.05 **L*****	0.50 / 0.21	41.51 / 28.25 **L*****
IL-6	1.43 / 0.37	43.60 / 31.16 **L****	1.19 / 0.49	32.05 / 14.97 **L****
IL-1β	21.37 / 3.84	88.85 / 40.58 **L*****	18.94 / 5.07	75.70 / 24.49 **L*****
CXCL1	10.19 / 4.18	1239.68 / 652.86 **L*****	12.15 / 10.72	1241.02 / 563.06 **L*****
CCL2	1.56 / 0.43	84.29 / 34.42 **L*****	1.85 / 0.67	67.63 / 23.20 **L*****
CCL5	68.49 / 16.19	269.64 / 60.60 **L*****	60.76 / 17.08	150.07 / 40.47 **L***/ S*****

2.5. Proteomics Analysis

A proteome analysis was conducted in WT and KO mice with LPS or control treatment (n = 3 per experimental group). The extracted proteins were digested with trypsin and analyzed with LC-MS, and proteins were identified and quantified. Overall, 4259 protein groups were identified and 3876 could be quantified in all replicates. Some missing values were imputated. Relative changes in WT mice with LPS are shown in Supplemental File 1 and changes in KO mice with LPS are shown in Supplemental File 2. With LPS exposure, 193 protein groups were significantly upregulated and 93 were significantly downregulated in samples of WT mice, while 118 protein groups were significantly upregulated and 74 were significantly downregulated in miR-21 KO mice. Principal component analysis and volcano plots of the data are shown in Figure 5. Of the significantly regulated protein groups, 70 were commonly regulated with LPS exposure in both WT and KO mice, while 212 were only regulated in WT and 121 in KO mice. A string database analysis (string-db.org) was performed for a potential pathway analysis, and the reactome pathways are shown in Table 3. The most significant reactome pathways in WT mice upon LPS exposure were "innate immune system", "neutrophil degranulation", and "platelet degranulation/activation". These were also present in the miR-21 KO mice but were much more attenuated. Some signaling molecules associated with neutrophil and platelet activation, ECM remodeling or coagulation cascade (e.g., EGFR, CD44, CD63, CD177, CTSG, MMP8, MMP9, ELA2, MPO, pro-thrombin, fibrinogen, or fibronectin) were only found to be significantly upregulated in WT, but not in miR-21 KO mice with ALI. Protein groups related to "platelet degranulation", "regulation of complement cascade", "immune system", and "neutrophil degranulation" were already attenuated in KO compared with WT mice without LPS exposure. Other protein groups related to "activation of DNA fragmentation", "formation of senescence-associated heterochromatin foci", or "apoptosis", however, were found to be more prominent in untreated KO mice. Relative changes in KO vs WT control mice are shown in Supplemental File 3.

Table 3. Transcriptomics pathway analysis. Data showing reactome pathway description extracted from string database analysis (false discovery rate $p < 0.01$).

WT GO-Term	Reactome Pathway Description	Count in Gene Set	False Discovery Rate
MMU-168249	Innate Immune System	70 of 879	1.67×10^{-32}
MMU-168256	Immune System	80 of 1523	3.30×10^{-26}
MMU-6798695	Neutrophil degranulation	47 of 476	6.37×10^{-25}
MMU-114608	Platelet degranulation	22 of 121	4.71×10^{-16}
MMU-76002	Platelet activation, signaling and aggregation	26 of 242	3.03×10^{-14}
MMU-109582	Hemostasis	34 of 489	1.26×10^{-13}
MMU-381426	Regulation of Insulin-like Growth Factor (IGF)transport and uptake	19 of 129	1.48×10^{-12}
MMU-977606	Regulation of Complement cascade	13 of 41	3.89×10^{-12}
MMU-8957275	Post-translational protein phosphorylation	17 of 114	2.16×10^{-11}
MMU-5686938	Regulation of TLR by endogenous ligand	8 of 13	3.26×10^{-9}
MMU-140877	Formation of Fibrin Clot (Clotting Cascade)	10 of 34	4.07×10^{-9}
MMU-1474244	Extracellular matrix organization	16 of 246	5.55×10^{-6}
MMU-216083	Integrin cell surface interactions	9 of 68	1.36×10^{-5}
MMU-6803157	Antimicrobial peptides	9 of 69	1.43×10^{-5}
MMU-140875	Common Pathway of Fibrin Clot Formation	6 of 20	1.72×10^{-5}
MMU-76009	Platelet Aggregation (Plug Formation)	6 of 29	0.0001
MMU-166665	Terminal pathway of complement	4 of 7	0.00018
MMU-140837	Intrinsic Pathway of Fibrin Clot Formation	5 of 20	0.00028
MMU-354192	Integrin alphaIIb beta3 signaling	5 of 22	0.0004
MMU-354194	GRB2: SOS provides linkage to MAPK signaling for integrins	4 of 11	0.00058
MMU-6799990	Metal sequestration by antimicrobial proteins	3 of 3	0.00073
MMU-372708	p130Cas linkage to MAPK signaling for integrins	4 of 12	0.00073
MMU-168898	Toll-like Receptor Cascades	9 of 131	0.0011
MMU-202733	Cell surface interactions at the vascular wall	8 of 103	0.0012
MMU-1566948	Elastic fiber formation	5 of 37	0.0027
MMU-1236973	Cross-presentation of particulate exogenous antigens (phagosomes)	3 of 7	0.0035
KO GO-term	**Reactome Pathway description**	**Count in Gene Set**	**False Discovery Rate**
MMU-6798695	Neutrophil degranulation	17 of 476	0.00024
MMU-168249	Innate Immune System	22 of 879	0.00088
MMU-76002	Platelet activation, signaling and aggregation	11 of 242	0.00094
MMU-2173782	Binding and Uptake of Ligands by Scavenger Receptors	5 of 31	0.00094
MMU-114608	Platelet degranulation	8 of 121	0.00094
MMU-2168880	Scavenging of heme from plasma	4 of 19	0.0016
MMU-168256	Immune System	27 of 1523	0.0073

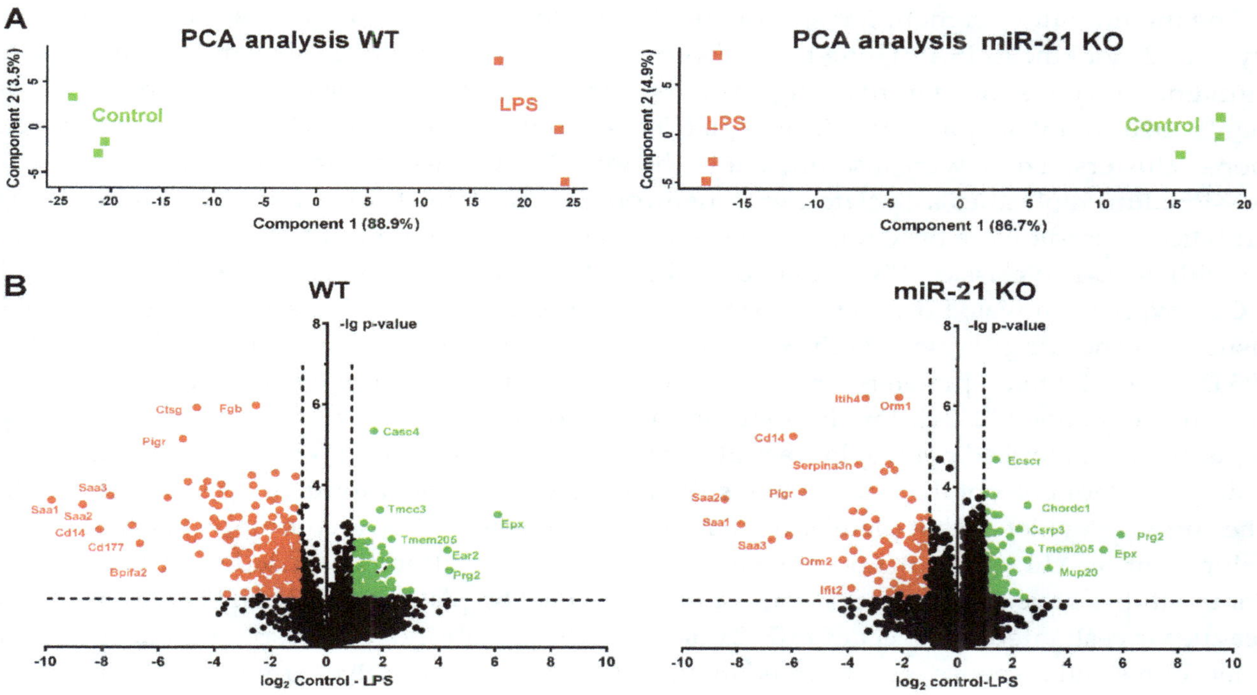

Figure 5. Proteome analyses of mice challenged with LPS. The total protein was isolated from the right lung lobes (n = 3 per experimental group) and proteome analyses were performed as described in the methods section. Principal component analyses of the regulated proteins showing separated groups of the replicate analyses (**A**). The volcano plots display the up- and down-regulated proteins (**B**). X-axes give the ratios of the mean protein intensities as $\log_2$-values. Y-axes show the –lg of the p-values. The proteins upregulated in the LPS-treated samples are shown in red, and proteins downregulated in the LPS samples are shown in green. Some selected proteins are indicated by the gene name.

3. Discussion

MiR-21 was shown to be involved in the acute inflammatory as well as in the chronic fibrotic phase of ALI [13,19]. Herein, we addressed the impact of miR-21 on early inflammatory response and early tissue damage in ALI by comparing the degree of ALI in miR-21 KO vs WT mice. As hypothesized, the genetic loss of miR-21 reduced structural remodeling, inflammatory signaling, and lung function decline in ALI.

Previous studies have addressed the impact of miR-21 signaling in ALI by using ago- or antagomiRs to regulate miR-21 signaling, however, with controversial results [13,17,20,21]. Vaporidi and colleagues showed that mice pretreated with anti-miR-21 before the induction of VILI had better oxygenation and lower BALF protein concentrations in comparison to mice that were not pretreated with anti-miR-21, suggesting that the downregulation of miR-21 ameliorated the development of VILI [17]. Qi and colleagues also showed that miR-21 supported the inhibition of ENaC-γ, an epithelial sodium channel that is essential for the removal of edematous fluid in ALI, through PTEN/AKT signaling, and downregulation of miR-21 reversed this effect [13]. However, other studies suggested a beneficial effect of miR-21, mediated either by its anti-apoptotic potential in ischemia/reperfusion induced lung injury or by inhibiting LPS-mediated NFκB signaling in rats with ALI [20,21]. The reasons for the different study outcomes could be related to the particular injury models as well as the time points and the read-out parameters, but also to the specificity of miR-21 targeting. In comparison to these previous studies, the advantage of the genetic knock-out of miR-21 is the full and homogeneous deletion of miR-21 and the lack of side effects due to the potential reaction of the anatogonists with unspecific targets. In line with the first two studies, our results provide evidence that inflammatory signaling, structural remodeling and impaired lung function in ALI was improved by the deletion of miR-21.

The inflammatory signaling response in ALI with miR-21 KO was addressed with proteomics analysis and cytokine ELISA in lung tissue. The results show that miR-21 KO significantly dampened the inflammatory response in the lung. The reactome pathway analysis showed "innate immune system", "neutrophil degranulation", and "platelet degranulation/activation" to be the most prominent response clusters. These were also present in the miR-21 KO mice, but much more attenuated, and some signaling molecules associated with neutrophil and platelet activation, ECM remodeling or coagulation cascade were only found to be significantly upregulated in WT but not in miR-21 KO mice with ALI. The classic LPS-mediated TLR4/MyD88/NFκB pathway that regulates TNFα, IL-6 or CCL2 expression was, however, not significantly affected by miR-21 KO. Among the cytokines measured in the lung tissue, CCL5 was the only one which was downregulated by miR-21 KO. CCL5 is one of the main platelet-derived chemokines involved in acute inflammatory response and neutrophil activation [22–24]. Previous studies have shown that platelet depletion or treatment with CCL5 antibodies reduced neutrophil recruitment and permeability in LPS-induced ALI [25] and that blocking platelet-neutrophil aggregation resulted in a reversal of acid-induced ALI [26]. Hence, these studies provide evidence that platelet-mediated neutrophil activation significantly contributes to the development of ALI, and our findings suggest that this activation is reduced in miR-21 KO mice. Previous studies have suggested that miR-21 has an impact on platelet activation [27,28]. Barwari and colleagues investigated the effect of miR-21 on platelets and fibrinogenic response and showed that platelet counts and response were lowered in miR-21 KO mice, while the pharmacological inhibition of miR-21 did not affect platelet numbers but significantly decreased the release of platelet granules [27]. We did not assess platelet counts in our study, but the previous findings still support our observations that miR-21 KO reduces the platelet activation cascade, contributing to the fibrinogenic response and neutrophil activation in ALI.

Structural changes with ALI included an increase in parenchymal lung volume in both strains (WT and KO), which was associated with an increase in alveolar volume and septal volume. An increase in septal thickness with LPS treatment was only found in WT mice. These changes fit with our observations in lung function measurements, where an increase in tissue resistance (G) and hysteresis was detected. G is an inverse measure of compliance in the parenchymal lung tissue and its increase in ALI, related to septal edema formation, has been shown previously [29]. Hysteresis might increase due to changes in tissue resistance and elastance or due to changes in surfactant composition [30,31]. We further analyzed the septal composition on the ultrastructural level to characterize changes in septal tissue composition, including cells and ECM. In both strains, we detected an increase in inflammatory cells—mostly neutrophils—that were recruited to the site of injury. However, the WT mice also showed an increase in ECM volume, consisting of increased volumes of collagen fibrils, elastic fibers, and amorphous ECM, which was not present in the KO mice. These findings suggest an increase in inter-septal fluid as well as early tissue remodeling in ALI in WT, but not in KO mice, with an impact on pulmonary micromechanics. Studies addressing miR-21 in lung tissue remodeling and fibrosis have also shown that treatment with anti-miR-21 or a pharmacological inhibitor of miR-21 reduced the development of fibrosis by attenuating TGF-β signaling [12,32]. TGF-β has been reported to be modulated by miR-21 and is related to tissue remodeling and the development of fibrosis [27,33,34]. In this study, we did not detect differences in TGF-β signaling between WT and KO mice with ALI. However, it has to be considered that 24 h is a very early time point to address tissue remodeling, and the development of fibrosis usually occurs several days after induction of injury. Hence, our study provides insight into early septal remodeling with impact on lung function in ALI that is improved by deletion of miR-21.

Besides attenuating the development of ALI, miR-21 KO also caused some general changes in lung structure and function. For example, lung compliance and inspiratory capacity was reduced in miR-21 KO compared with WT mice. The lung volume was, however, approximately the same in both strains. The major differences on the structural level between the two strains were a higher septal volume and thickness in the KO mice with an increased content of amorphous ECM. It seems likely that these structural changes affected lung compliance and inspiratory capacity in KO mice; however, other parameters, such as tissue resistance or tissue elastance, that are usually affected by changes in septal composition were the same in both strains. It is therefore likely that other mechanisms, which were not covered by our analysis, were responsible for the differences between the two strains in pulmonary micromechanics. Furthermore, it is not clear which regulatory processes led to structural changes in the miR-21 KO mice. Interestingly though, any differences in pulmonary micromechanics and lung structure between WT and KO mice disappeared with progressing age (18 month old mice, Supplementary Figures S1 and S2), so it seems that there exists a compensatory mechanism for miR-21 signaling in miR-21 KO mice. This might also be in line with other reports that showed decent effects of antagomiR-21 treatment but not of genetic miR-21 deletion in cardiac tissue remodeling [27], suggesting some adaptive response to miR-21 KO.

In summary, within this project, it was shown that miR-21 contributes to inflammatory signaling and septal remodeling in ALI. In particular, we could show that miR-21 KO reduced platelet and neutrophil degranulation and septal ECM remodeling in ALI. MiR-21 KO improved lung function and dampened the inflammation in ALI, and the recent data indicate that miR-21 could be a potential therapeutic non-coding RNA target in the treatment of ALI.

4. Material and Methods

4.1. Animal Model

Male C57BL/6N mice (WT) and miR-21 knock-out mice (KO; B6N-Mir21^{tm1Engl}) were bread and maintained at the local animal facility at Hannover Medical School. The KO mice were originally provided by Prof. Engelhardt, TU Munich, Germany, and the strain has been described previously in the literature by Chau et al. [35]. The mice were housed in standard cages in groups of 1–5 and had access to food and water ad libitum. At the age of 3 months, ALI was induced by intranasal administration of 75 μg LPS in 30 μL physiological saline solution ($n = 10$ per group). The control mice received equal volume of saline solution ($n = 7$ per group). The animals were sacrificed 24 h after the induction of ALI, as described previously [29]. All animal procedures were approved by the Lower Saxony State Office for Consumer Protection and Food Safety (LAVES; Authorization number: 33.9-42502-04-14/1623, Approval Date: 26/09/2014) in accordance with the German law for animal protection and with the European Directive, 2010/63/EU.

4.2. Lung Function Analysis

Lung function analysis was performed with a FlexiVent rodent ventilator FX1 for mice (SCIREQ) as described previously [29]. In brief, mice were tracheotomized under deep anesthesia and mechanically ventilated with a frequency of 100 breaths/min and a tidal volume of 10 mL/kg body weight. Pulmonary function was assessed by ventilation perturbations at a positive end-expiratory pressure (PEEP) value of 3 cmH_2O to estimate tissue elastance (H), tissue resistance (G), and hysteresivity (η) with the constant phase model to the impedance spectra. The inspiratory capacity (IC) was assessed by derecruitability maneuvers, static compliance (Cst), and hysteresis by recording quasi-static pressure-volume loops. The lung function measurement was only considered as valid if the heart was beating during measurements.

After lung function measurements, animals were killed by exsanguination and lungs were excised. The left lung lobe was chemically fixed via intra-tracheal instillation at a pressure of 20 cmH_2O with a fixative mixture of 1.5% paraformaldehyde and 1.5% glutaraldehyde in 0.15 M HEPES buffer for histopathology and stereological analysis. The right lung lobes were separated and immediately snap-frozen in liquid nitrogen for later processing for cytokine and proteomics analysis.

4.3. Histopathology and Stereology

The left lung lobes were stored for at least 24 h in the fixative solution, followed by lung volume measurement via volume displacement and systematic uniform random subsampling (SURS) as described previously [29,36]. In brief, lung tissue was sliced in 2 mm sections and every other section, with a random starting point, was processed and embedded in glycol methacrylate (Technovit 7100 resin, Kulzer GmbH) for light microscopic analysis. The remaining lung sections were further subsampled into tissue blocks of approximately 1 mm^3 size and embedded in epoxy resin (SERVA Electrophoresis GmbH) for electron microscopic and ultrastructural analysis. The embedding procedures were performed as described previously [29].

Stereological analyses were used to quantify the pulmonary structural characteristics and were performed in accordance with the ATS/ERS guidelines [37]. The following parameters were determined by stereology and bright-field light microscopy: volumes of parenchyma, septa, and alveoli, the surface of the alveoli, and the septal thickness as previously described in detail [29]. For the analysis, the samples embedded in glycol methacrylate were cut into 1.5 μm thick sections and stained with toluidine blue. The histological slides were then digitalized with a histological slide scanner (AxioScan.Z1, Zeiss) at a 20× magnification. The images for stereological analysis were obtained by SURS using the newCast acquisition software (Visiopharm). For parenchymal volume estimation, 50 images were sampled at a 5× magnification and analyzed with the SETPanizer software [38] with a test system of 36 points. For the other parameters, 60 images were sampled at a magnification of 20×. The images were analyzed with the STEPanizer software with a test system of 2 lines and a test system of 49 points to count alveolar airspace volume, septal volume, septal surface area, and septal thickness, as described in Kling et al. 2017 [29].

The ultrastructural analysis of the air–blood barrier was done by means of stereology and TEM assessing the following parameters: the volume of epithelial, endothelial, and interstitial cells, ECM, elastic fibers, and capillary lumen. Of the epon embedded tissue blocks, three per lung were randomly chosen, cut in ultrathin sections (60–80 nm thick), mounted on copper grids and stained with uranyl acetate and lead citrate. TEM images were acquired with a Morgagni 268 microscope (FEI) by SURS. Approximately 60 images of the air–blood barrier were recorded per tissue block at a magnification of 18,000x. The images were analyzed with the newCast software (Visiopharm, Hoersholm, Denmark) and a test system with 5 lines.

4.4. Gene Expression Analysis

Total RNA isolation was performed on the accessory lung lobe of the right lung with the NucleoSpin miRNA Kit (Macherey-Nagel) according to the manufacturer's protocol. To analyze miRNA expression, two-step RT-PCR primer sets from Applied Biosystems were used according to the manufacturer's protocol. SnoRNA-202 served as a housekeeping control. The quantification of miRNA was conducted using a VIIa7 Real-Time PCR cycler (Life Technologies, Waltham, MA, USA).

4.5. Cytokine Expression in Lung Tissue

For cytokine concentration analysis, tissue from the caudal lung lobe of the right lung was mixed with 10 ml/g cOmplete™ (Sigma–Aldrich, Taufkirchen, Germany) in PBS and was subsequently homogenized (Tissue Lyser, Qiagen, Germantown, MD, USA). Total protein concentration of the supernatant of the lung homogenate was examined with the Pierce™ BCA Protein Assay Kit (Thermo Fisher Scientific, Waltham, MA, USA). The cytokine concentration was then analyzed with the LEGENDplex bead array ELISA (# 740621, BioLegend, San Diego, CA, USA) according to the supplier's manual and as described previously [39]. Cytokine measurements (pg/mL) were then normalized to the total protein concentration (mg/mL) to pg/mg.

4.6. Sample Preparation for LC-MS Analysis

Protein isolation was done with the NucleoSpin RNA/Protein Kit (Macherey-Nagel) on the cranial and middle lobes of the right lung according to the manufacturer's protocol. The total protein concentration was measured with the Pierce BCA Protein Assay Kit (Thermo Fisher Scientific). Isolated protein suspension was then mixed with Laemmli buffer and incubated for 5 min at 95°C. Proteins were then alkylated by the addition of acrylamide up to a concentration of 2% and incubation at RT for 30 min. Afterwards, SDS-PAGE proteins were stained with Coomassie Brilliant Blue (CBB). Each lane was cut into four pieces, which were further minced into 1 mm^3 gel pieces. Further sample processing was done as described [40]. Briefly, gel pieces were destained two times with 200 µL 50% and 50 mM ammonium bicarbonate (ABC) at 37°C for 30 min and were then dehydrated with 100% ACN. The solvent was removed in a vacuum centrifuge and 100 µL 10 ng/ µL sequencing grade Trypsin (Promega) in 10% ACN, 40 mM ABC were added. Gels were rehydrated in trypsin solution for 1 hour on ice and then covered with 10% ACN, 40 mM ABC. Digestion was performed over night at 37°C and was stopped by adding 100 µL of 50% ACN, 0.1% TFA. After incubation at 37°C for 1 hour, the solution was transferred into a fresh sample vial. This step was repeated twice and extracts were combined and dried in a vacuum centrifuge. Dried peptide extracts were redissolved in 30 µL 2% ACN, 0.1% TFA, with shaking at 800 rpm for 20 min. After centrifugation at 20,000× *g*, aliquots of 12.5 µL each were stored at −20 °C.

4.7. LC-MS Analysis

LC-MS analyses were done as described elsewhere [40]. Briefly, peptide samples were separated with a nano-flow ultrahigh pressure liquid chromatography system (RSLC, Thermo Scientific) equipped with a trapping column (3 µm C18 particle, 2 cm length, 75 µm ID, Acclaim PepMap, Thermo Scientific) and a 50 cm separation column (2 µm C18 particle, 75 µm ID, Acclaim PepMap, Thermo Scientific). Peptide mixtures were injected, enriched, and desalted on the trapping column at a flow rate of 6 µL/min with 0.1% TFA for 5 min. The trapping column was switched online with the separating column and peptides were eluted from the separating column with a multi-step binary gradient of buffer A (0.1% formic acid) and buffer B (80% ACN, 0.1% formic acid). The flow rate was 250 nL/min and the column temperature was set to 45°C. The RSLC system was coupled online via a Nano Spray Flex Ion Soure II (Thermo Scientific) to an LTQ-Orbitrap Velos mass spectrometer that was operated in data-dependent acquisition mode. Overview scans were acquired at a resolution of 60k in the orbitrap analyzer. The top 10 most intensive ions were selected for CID fragmentation in the LTQ. Active exclusion was activated so that ions fragmented once were excluded from further fragmentation for 70 s within a mass window of 10 ppm of the specific m/z value.

The raw data were processed using Max Quant software [41] and the entries of mouse uniprot data base, including common contaminants. The proteins were identified by a false discovery rate of 0.01 on protein and peptide level and quantified by extracted ion chromatograms of all peptides. Data visualizations were done with Perseus [42] and GraphPad Prism software.

4.8. Statistical Analysis

Statistical analyses were conducted with the SigmaPlot software (SYSTAT Software Inc; San Jose, USA) by a two-way analysis of variance (ANOVA) followed by a pair-wise comparison with Bonferroni-test. The data that were not normally distributed were subject to a ln or square root transformation. If data normalization failed, ANOVA on Ranks followed by a Mann–Whitney U *t*-test with a Bonferroni correction was performed.

Author Contributions: J.C.J., J.F., T.T., C.M. and C.B. designed study, J.C.J., J.F., A.P., J.V. and C.B. performed experiments, J.C.J., J.F., A.P. and C.B. analyzed the results, J.C.J., T.T., C.M. and C.B. interpreted the results, J.C.J., A.P. and C.B. designed figures, C.B. drafted the manuscript, all authors edited and approved the manuscript. All authors have read and agreed to the published version of the manuscript

Acknowledgments: We thank Rita Lichatz, Susanne Kuhlmann, Annette Just and Melanie Bornemann for their excellent technical assistance.

References

1. Ware, L.; Matthay, M. The acute respiratory distress syndrome. *J. Clin. Invest.* **2012**, *122*, 2731–2740. [CrossRef]

2. Marshall, R.; Bellingan, G.; Laurent, G. The acute respiratory distress syndrome: Fibrosis in the fast lane: Editorial. *Thorax* **1998**, *53*, 815–817. [CrossRef]
3. Mineo, G.; Ciccarese, F.; Modolon, C.; Landini, M.P.; Valentino, M.; Zompatori, M. Post-ARDS pulmonary fibrosis in patients with H1N1 pneumonia: role of follow-up CT. *Radiol. Medica* **2012**, *117*, 185–200. [CrossRef]
4. Fan, E.; Brodie, D.; Slutsky, A.S. Acute respiratory distress syndrome advances in diagnosis and treatment. *JAMA J. Am. Med. Assoc.* **2018**, *319*, 698–710. [CrossRef] [PubMed]
5. Jonas, S.; Izaurralde, E. Towards a molecular understanding of microRNA-mediated gene silencing. *Nat. Rev. Genet.* **2015**, *16*, 421–433. [CrossRef] [PubMed]
6. Kumarswamy, R.; Volkmann, I.; Thum, T. Regulation and function of miRNA-21 in health and disease. *RNA Biol.* **2011**, *8*. [CrossRef] [PubMed]
7. Krichevsky, A.M.; Gabriely, G. miR-21: A small multi-faceted RNA. *J. Cell. Mol. Med.* **2009**, *13*, 39–53. [CrossRef]
8. Zhong, X.; Chung, A.C.K.; Chen, H.Y.; Dong, Y.; Meng, X.M.; Li, R.; Yang, W.; Hou, F.F.; Lan, H.Y. miR-21 is a key therapeutic target for renal injury in a mouse model of type 2 diabetes. *Diabetologia* **2013**, *56*, 663–674. [CrossRef]
9. Thum, T.; Gross, C.; Fiedler, J.; Fischer, T.; Kissler, S.; Bussen, M.; Galuppo, P.; Just, S.; Rottbauer, W.; Frantz, S.; et al. MicroRNA-21 contributes to myocardial disease by stimulating MAP kinase signalling in fibroblasts. *Nature* **2008**, *456*, 980–984. [CrossRef]
10. Sheedy, F.J. Turning 21: Induction of miR-21 as a key switch in the inflammatory response. *Front. Immunol.* **2015**, *6*, 1–9. [CrossRef]
11. Cao, Y.; Lyu, Y.; Tang, J.; Li, Y. MicroRNAs: Novel regulatory molecules in acute lung injury/acute respiratory distress syndrome (review). *Biomed. Reports* **2016**, *4*, 523–527. [CrossRef] [PubMed]
12. Liu, G.; Friggeri, A.; Yang, Y.; Milosevic, J.; Ding, Q.; Thannickal, V.J.; Kaminski, N.; Abraham, E. miR-21 mediates fibrogenic activation of pulmonary fibroblasts and lung fibrosis. *J. Exp. Med.* **2010**, *207*, 1589–1597. [CrossRef] [PubMed]
13. Qi, W.; Li, H.; Cai, X.H.; Gu, J.Q.; Meng, J.; Xie, H.Q.; Zhang, J.L.; Chen, J.; Jin, X.G.; Tang, Q.; et al. Lipoxin A4 activates alveolar epithelial sodium channel gamma via the microRNA-21/PTEN/AKT pathway in lipopolysaccharide-induced inflammatory lung injury. *Lab. Investig.* **2015**, *95*, 1258–1268. [CrossRef] [PubMed]
14. Mook Lee, S.; Choi, H.; Yang, G.; Park, K.C.; Jeong, S.; Hong, S. MicroRNAs mediate oleic acid-induced acute lung injury in rats using an alternative injury mechanism. *Mol. Med. Rep.* **2014**, *10*, 292–300.
15. Tan, K.S.; Choi, H.; Jiang, X.; Yin, L.; Seet, J.E.; Patzel, V.; Engelward, B.P.; Chow, V.T. Micro-RNAs in regenerating lungs: An integrative systems biology analysis of murine influenza pneumonia. *BMC Genomics* **2014**, *15*. [CrossRef] [PubMed]
16. Li, W.; Ma, K.; Zhang, S.; Zhang, H.; Liu, J.; Wang, X.; Li, S. Pulmonary microRNA expression profiling in an immature piglet model of cardiopulmonary bypass-induced acute lung injury. *Artif. Organs* **2015**, *39*, 327–335. [CrossRef]
17. Vaporidi, K.; Vergadi, E.; Kaniaris, E.; Hatziapostolou, M.; Lagoudaki, E.; Georgopoulos, D.; Zapol, W.M.; Bloch, K.D.; Iliopoulos, D. Pulmonary microRNA profiling in a mouse model of ventilator-induced lung injury. *AJP Lung Cell. Mol. Physiol.* **2012**, *303*, L199–L207. [CrossRef]
18. Li, P.; Zhao, G.Q.; Chen, T.F.; Chang, J.X.; Wang, H.Q.; Chen, S.S.; Zhang, G.J. Serum miR-21 and miR-155 expression in idiopathic pulmonary fibrosis. *J. Asthma* **2013**, *50*, 960–964. [CrossRef]
19. Makiguchi, T.; Yamada, M.; Yoshioka, Y.; Sugiura, H.; Koarai, A.; Chiba, S.; Fujino, N.; Tojo, Y.; Ota, C.; Kubo, H.; et al. Serum extracellular vesicular miR-21-5p is a predictor of the prognosis in idiopathic pulmonary fibrosis. *Respir. Res.* **2016**, *17*. [CrossRef]
20. Zhu, W.D.; Xu, J.; Zhang, M.; Zhu, T.M.; Zhang, Y.H.; Sun, K.E. Microrna-21 inhibits lipopolysaccharide-induceacute lung injury by targeting nuclear factor-κb. *Exp. Ther. Med.* **2018**, *16*, 4616–4622.
21. Li, J.; Wei, L.; Han, Z.; Chen, Z. Mesenchymal stromal cells-derived exosomes alleviate ischemia/reperfusion injury in mouse lung by transporting anti-apoptotic miR-21-5p. *Eur. J. Pharmacol.* **2019**, *852*, 68–76. [CrossRef] [PubMed]
22. Yu, C.; Zhang, S.; Wang, Y.; Zhang, S.; Luo, L.; Thorlacius, H. Platelet-derived CCL5 regulates CXC chemokine

formation and neutrophil recruitment in acute experimental colitis. *J. Cell. Physiol.* **2016**, *231*, 370–376. [CrossRef] [PubMed]

23. De Stoppelaar, S.F.; van 't Veer, C.; van der Poll, T. The role of platelets in sepsis. *Thromb. Haemost.* **2014**, *112*, 666–677. [PubMed]
24. Page, C.; Pitchford, S. Neutrophil and platelet complexes and their relevance to neutrophil recruitment and activation. *Int. Immunopharmacol.* **2013**, *17*, 1176–1184. [CrossRef] [PubMed]
25. Grommes, J.; Drechsler, M.; Soehnlein, O. CCR5 and FPR1 mediate neutrophil recruitment in endotoxin-induced lung injury. *J. Innate Immun.* **2014**, *6*, 111–116. [CrossRef] [PubMed]
26. Zarbock, A.; Singbartl, K.; Ley, K. Complete reversal of acid-induced acute lung injury by blocking of platelet-neutrophil aggregation. *J. Clin. Invest.* **2006**, *116*, 3211–3219. [CrossRef] [PubMed]
27. Barwari, T.; Eminaga, S.; Mayr, U.; Lu, R.; Armstrong, P.C.; Chan, M.V.; Sahraei, M.; Fernández-Fuertes, M.; Moreau, T.; Barallobre-Barreiro, J.; et al. Inhibition of profibrotic microRNA-21 affects platelets and their releasate. *JCI Insight* **2018**, *3*. [CrossRef]
28. Li, Y.; Yan, L.; Zhang, W.; Hu, N.; Chen, W.; Wang, H.; Kang, M.; Ou, H. MicroRNA-21 inhibits platelet-derived growth factor-induced human aortic vascular smooth muscle cell proliferation and migration through targeting activator protein-1. *Am. J. Transl. Res.* **2014**, *6*, 507–516.
29. Kling, K.M.; Lopez-Rodriguez, E.; Pfarrer, C.; Mühlfeld, C.; Brandenberger, C. Aging exacerbates acute lung injury induced changes of the air-blood barrier, lung function and inflammation in the mouse. *Am. J. Physiol. Lung Cell. Mol. Physiol.* **2017**, *312*, L1–L12. [CrossRef]
30. Suki, B.; Bartolák-Suki, E. Biomechanics of the Aging Lung Parenchyma. In *Mechanical Properties of Aging Soft Tissues*; Derby, B., Akhtar, R., Eds.; Springer International Publishing: New York, NY, USA, 2014; pp. 95–133.
31. Schulte, H.; Mühlfeld, M.; Brandenberger, C. Age-related structural and functional changes in the mouse lung. *Front. Physiol.* **2019**, *10*, 1466. [CrossRef]
32. Gao, Y.; Lu, J.; Zhang, Y.; Chen, Y.; Gu, Z.; Jiang, X. Baicalein attenuates bleomycin-induced pulmonary fibrosis in rats through inhibition of miR-21. *Pulm. Pharmacol. Ther.* **2013**, *26*, 649–654. [CrossRef] [PubMed]
33. Wang, J.; He, F.; Chen, L.; Li, Q.; Jin, S.; Zheng, H.; Lin, J.; Zhang, H.; Ma, S.; Mei, J.; et al. Resveratrol inhibits pulmonary fibrosis by regulating miR-21 through MAPK/AP-1 pathways. *Biomed. Pharmacother.* **2018**, *105*, 37–44. [CrossRef] [PubMed]
34. Kumarswamy, R.; Volkmann, I.; Jazbutyte, V.; Dangwal, S.; Park, D.H.; Thum, T. Transforming growth factor-β-induced endothelial-to-mesenchymal transition is partly mediated by MicroRNA-21. *Arterioscler. Thromb. Vasc. Biol.* **2012**, *32*, 361–369. [CrossRef] [PubMed]
35. Chau, B.N.; Xin, C.; Hartner, J.; Ren, S.; Castano, A.P.; Linn, G.; Li, J.; Tran, P.T.; Kaimal, V.; Huang, X.; et al. MicroRNA-21 promotes fibrosis of the kidney by silencing metabolic pathways. *Sci. Transl. Med.* **2012**, *4*, 121ra18. [CrossRef] [PubMed]
36. Brandenberger, C.; Ochs, M.; Mühlfeld, C. Assessing particle and fiber toxicology in the respiratory system: the stereology toolbox. *Part. Fibre Toxicol.* **2015**, *12*, 1–15. [CrossRef] [PubMed]
37. Hsia, C.C.W.; Hyde, D.M.; Ochs, M.; Weibel, E.R. An official research policy statement of the American Thoracic Society/European Respiratory Society: standards for quantitative assessment of lung structure. *Am. J. Respir. Crit. Care Med.* **2010**, *181*, 394–418. [CrossRef] [PubMed]
38. Tschanz, S.A.; Burri, P.H.; Weibel, E.R. A simple tool for stereological assessment of digital images: the STEPanizer. *J Microsc* **2011**, *243*, 47–59. [CrossRef]
39. Brandenberger, C.; Kling, K.M.; Vital, M.; Mühlfeld, C. The role of pulmonary and systemic immunosenescence in acute lung injury. *Aging Dis.* **2018**, *9*, 553–565. [CrossRef]
40. Jochim, N.; Gerhard, R.; Just, I.; Pich, A. Impact of clostridial glucosylating toxins on the proteome of colonic cells determined by isotope-coded protein labeling and LC-MALDI. *Proteome Sci.* **2011**, *9*, 1–12. [CrossRef]
41. Cox, J.; Mann, M. MaxQuant enables high peptide identification rates, individualized p.p.b.-range mass accuracies and proteome-wide protein quantification. *Nat. Biotechnol.* **2008**, *26*, 1367–1372. [CrossRef]
42. Tyanova, S.; Temu, T.; Sinitcyn, P.; Carlson, A.; Hein, M.Y.; Geiger, T.; Mann, M.; Cox, J. The Perseus computational platform for comprehensive analysis of (prote)omics data. *Nat. Methods* **2016**, *13*, 731–740. [CrossRef] [PubMed]

12

The Hen or the Egg: Impaired Alveolar Oxygen Diffusion and Acute High-altitude Illness?

Heimo Mairbäurl [1,*], Christoph Dehnert [2], Franziska Macholz [3], Daniel Dankl [3], Mahdi Sareban [4] and Marc M. Berger [3]

1 Translational Lung Research Center (TLRC), part of the German Center for Lung Research (DZL), University of Heidelberg, 69120 Heidelberg, Germany
2 Medbase Checkup Center, 8400 Zürich, Switzerland
3 Department of Anesthesiology, Perioperative and General Critical Care Medicine, University Hospital Salzburg, 5020 Salzburg, Austria
4 University Institute of Sports Medicine, Prevention and Rehabilitation, and Research Institute of Molecular Sports Medicine and Rehabilitation, Paracelsus Medical University, 5020 Salzburg, Austria
* Correspondence: heimo.mairbaeurl@med.uni-heidelberg.de

Abstract: Individuals ascending rapidly to altitudes >2500 m may develop symptoms of acute mountain sickness (AMS) within a few hours of arrival and/or high-altitude pulmonary edema (HAPE), which occurs typically during the first three days after reaching altitudes above 3000–3500 m. Both diseases have distinct pathologies, but both present with a pronounced decrease in oxygen saturation of hemoglobin in arterial blood (SO_2). This raises the question of mechanisms impairing the diffusion of oxygen (O_2) across the alveolar wall and whether the higher degree of hypoxemia is in causal relationship with developing the respective symptoms. In an attempt to answer these questions this article will review factors affecting alveolar gas diffusion, such as alveolar ventilation, the alveolar-to-arterial O_2-gradient, and balance between filtration of fluid into the alveolar space and its clearance, and relate them to the respective disease. The resultant analysis reveals that in both AMS and HAPE the main pathophysiologic mechanisms are activated before aggravated decrease in SO_2 occurs, indicating that impaired alveolar epithelial function and the resultant diffusion limitation for oxygen may rather be a consequence, not the primary cause, of these altitude-related illnesses.

Keywords: high-altitude pulmonary edema; acute mountain sickness; oxygen diffusion limitation

1. Introduction

Acute mountain sickness (AMS) and high-altitude pulmonary edema (HAPE) can develop within hours to days after arrival at high-altitude. Although AMS and HAPE are diseases with different pathologies, data from studies performed at the Capanna Regina Margherita at an altitude of 4559 m in the Monte Rosa mountain range, where speed and time-course of ascent were always standardized to minimize the impact of confounding factors, show that one to two days after ascent subjects suffering from AMS and/or HAPE shared a significantly higher degree of hypoxemia than individuals tolerating this altitude well. In fact, in both altitude illnesses the arterial oxygen saturation (SO_2) was approximately 10% lower than in the healthy individuals at an altitude of 4559 m at the Capanna Margherita (AMS: e.g., [1]; HAPE: e.g., [2]), where the similarity in the magnitude of decrease is likely pure coincidence. The aggravated decrease in SO_2 can be caused by a variety of mechanisms, including impaired ventilation, which might result in decreased alveolar PO_2, hindrance of oxygen diffusion from the alveolar space into blood due to alveolar and interstitial edema, ventilation/perfusion mismatch, and altered oxygen affinity of hemoglobin. However, it is unclear whether the decreased

SO_2 is a prerequisite for causing high-altitude illness, or whether it is a consequence that rather aggravates severity.

Studies on the pathophysiology of AMS and HAPE have been performed on mountaineers after (rapid) ascent to altitudes >3000 m by driving, using a cable car, going on foot, and their combinations, most of which quite closely resemble mountaineering and high-altitude tourism. Studies have also been performed in chambers where in most instances exposure to normobaric hypoxia begun instantly by just stepping into a pre-adjusted hypoxic atmosphere. Both approaches have their advantages and disadvantages. Chamber studies allow for exactly-timed laboratory and clinical assessments under tightly controlled laboratory conditions. They also allow use of equipment that is not available in many high-altitude settings. By contrast, results from field studies are of course most relevant for mountaineering but are often affected by confounding factors like the physical effort of climbing a mountain, the slowly raising degree of hypoxia during the ascent, and (adverse) weather conditions. Thus it is possible that pathophysiologic mechanisms causing AMS and HAPE are different in field and laboratory conditions. Despite this possible limitation, data from these two situations will be combined in this review in order to obtain a timeline of the development of AMS and HAPE and to compare the early phase (hours, chamber studies) with the later phase (days) in field/mountain conditions. This approach might help dissect different pathophysiologic mechanisms and clarify the possible involvement of the alveolar epithelium and lung fluid balance in the pathogenesis of these diseases.

2. High-altitude Pulmonary Edema

HAPE typically occurs 24 to 72 h after rapid ascent to altitudes higher than 3000 m (for a comprehensive review see [3]). The incidence is approximately 5% in non-selected, not-acclimatized individuals after ascent to 4559 m [4,5]. Slow ascent rates and pre-acclimatization decrease the risk of occurrence, while the prevalence is highly increased (>60%) in individuals with HAPE during previous exposures to high-altitude indicating individual susceptibility [6].

Clinical symptoms of HAPE are dyspnea during exercise and later also at rest, cyanosis and hypoxemia, gurgling, and white, and as the illness progresses, pink, frothy sputum. X-ray images of the thorax show visible infiltrates [7]. Doppler-echocardiographic [8] and right-heart catheter [9,10] evaluations indicate exaggerated hypoxic pulmonary vasoconstriction (HPV) and increased capillary pressure [10] caused by venoconstriction or uneven distribution of blood flow [10,11]. Broncho-alveolar lavage fluid contains significant numbers of blood cells and plasma proteins but lacks typical inflammation markers [12], indicating that the alveolar leak is induced by high pressure rather than by inflammation [4]. This notion is supported by the fact that HAPE can be prevented by decreasing pulmonary arterial systolic pressure (sPAP) with, for example, nifedipine [13] and tadalafil [2]. The reasons for the exaggerated pressure response in HAPE-susceptible individuals have not been fully explored. They might include mechanisms decreasing the PO_2 at the pulmonary micro-vasculature, such as impaired ventilation and oxygen diffusion, where the diffusion limitation might be caused by an imbalance between filtration and alveolar fluid reabsorption, but might also be based on altered sensitivity to hypoxic vasoconstriction and vasodilatory mechanisms.

2.1. HAPE and Ventilation

Changes in ventilation upon exposure to hypoxia follow a distinct pattern [14], showing fast stimulation followed by ventilatory decline within minutes, after which ventilation increases in the course of the next few hours and days (ventilatory acclimatization). Oxygen saturation during exposure changes accordingly. The degree of stimulation of ventilation is often used to test the sensitivity of the ventilatory drive in hypoxia. However, this test often covers only the early phase of stimulation of ventilation by hypoxia because the test procedure often lasts less than 10 min. Hohenhaus et al. [15] have shown that in the early phase of ventilatory adjustments to hypoxia, HAPE-susceptibles have a decreased isocapnic hypoxic ventilatory response (HVR) at rest, which persists during exercise. Ventilation was found to be increased by 1.5 L/min per percent decrease in SO_2 in healthy controls but only by 0.8 L/min in HAPE-susceptible individuals. Both at rest and during exercise there was also a tendency towards lower poikilocapnic HVR in HAPE-susceptibles [15]. Thus it is possible that a blunted hypoxic ventilatory drive results in a decreased alveolar PO_2 relative to healthy individuals. This would result in an even further decreased PO_2 at pulmonary arterial smooth muscle cells and subsequently exaggerated hypoxic vasoconstriction, which is a hallmark of HAPE-susceptibility [13].

It is interesting to note that despite decreased HVR arterial partial pressure of carbon dioxide (PCO_2) was not increased in HAPE-susceptibles at high-altitude (4559 m) but tended to be slightly decreased [2]. Similarly, during 2 h of exposure to normobaric hypoxia equivalent to 4559 m of altitude HAPE-susceptibles showed decreased end-tidal PCO_2 (Figure 1). Together these results on PCO_2 obtained in poikilocapnic conditions after 10 min to 2 h of exposure to a constant level of hypoxia indicate stimulated rather than blunted ventilation upon exposure to hypoxia for hours to days, which is in contrast to the decreased isocapnic HVR mentioned above during the HVR-test [15]. It might be that the difference in time course of reaching certain levels of hypoxia and the duration of exposure to hypoxia explains this discrepancy. A hyperventilation induced decrease in PCO_2 might to some extent protect from exaggerated hypoxic pulmonary hypertension because low PCO_2 acts as a vasodilator on pulmonary arteries [16], but effects of CO_2 on HAPE-susceptibility have not been studied. Together these results show that alveolar ventilation is not abnormally low in HAPE-susceptibles during prolonged exposure to hypoxia and that a low alveolar PO_2 is not the reason for more pronounced hypoxemia and exaggerated HPV.

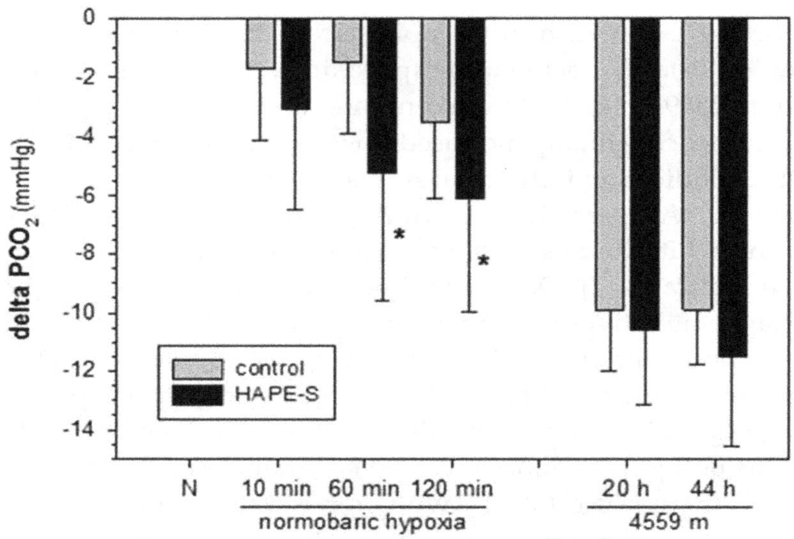

Figure 1. Time-course of decrease in partial pressure of carbon dioxide (PCO_2) in controls and high-altitude pulmonary edema –susceptibles (HAPE-S) in hypoxia. The decrease in PCO_2 was calculated as the difference between normoxia and the time-points in hypoxia for the respective studies. Data for normobaric hypoxia (equivalent to 4550 m) are so far unpublished end-tidal PCO_2 values from 15 controls and 17 HAPE-S from a study on the time course of change in systolic pulmonary arterial pressure reported in acute hypoxia reported in [17]). Data on high-altitude at the Capanna Margherita (4559 m) represent the arterial PCO_2 on day 2 of the sojourn from 10 controls and 9 HAPE-S from a study reported in [2]. Mean values ± standard deviation. N normoxia; * indicate significant difference between controls and HAPE-susceptibles.

2.2. *HAPE, Alveolar Fluid Clearance, and Pulmonary Arterial Hypertension*

Small amounts of fluid can easily be removed from the alveolar surface. This reabsorption is driven by an osmotic gradient generated by the reabsorption of Na^+ across the alveolar epithelium, where Na^+ passively enters alveolar epithelial cells via epithelial Na-channels (ENaC) inserted into the apical plasma membrane. Na^+ is then removed actively across the basolateral membrane by the Na/K-ATPase in exchange with K^+ [18]. Hypoxia of cultured primary alveolar epithelial cells inhibits active Na-reabsorption [19] by decreasing mRNA [20,21] and surface expression of both ENaC [22,23] and of the Na/K-ATPase [24]. Also the removal of fluid instilled into the lung was blunted when rats had been exposed to hypoxia [21,25,26], resulting in pulmonary edema indicated by increased lung water content of hypoxic rats. Measurements of alveolar reabsorption on ex-vivo human lungs have also been performed showing ENaC and Na/K-ATPase mediated active reabsorption [27], similar to rat lungs, but the effects of hypoxia have not been studied. In vivo measurements of reabsorption on the human lung are difficult. Indirect evidence can be derived from changes in the protein content of broncho-alveolar lavage fluid, which indicated a significant role of fluid clearance on clinical outcome of patients with acute respiratory distress syndrome (ARDS) [28]. However, rates of water flux cannot be quantified with this method. This approach is not applicable to HAPE because of increased filtration of protein-rich fluid, whereas epithelia appear tight to protein in healthy individuals [12].

Based on these findings on the relation between active Na-reabsorption and pulmonary edema in rats it appears possible that alveolar Na^+ reabsorption also plays a role in HAPE. Thus, a high basal activity of reabsorption would compensate excessive fluid accumulation caused by enhanced filtration, whereas insufficient reabsorption activity might promote alveolar edema [29].

Indirect evidence suggests that HAPE-susceptibles might have decreased Na-reabsorption in the lung. However, measurements were not possible at the alveolar epithelium, but at the nasal mucosa. This technique has been used to diagnose defective Cl-transport in cystic fibrosis [30,31], where the activity of Cl-secretion is decreased due to genetic variations of a Cl-channel called cystic fibrosis transmembrane regulator (CFTR) [32]. Use of this method on HAPE-susceptible subjects showed that the potential difference across the nasal mucosa (NPD) was lower in HAPE-susceptibles than in non-susceptibles in normoxia at low altitude [33]. Later, we confirmed this result [34] and also showed that the portion of the NPD caused by active Na-transport was lower, and that nasal epithelial Na-transport decreased even further at high-altitude (4559 m). If in fact these results indicate decreased Na-reabsorption in the alveoli, then exposure to hypoxia might start a vicious cycle in HAPE-susceptibles: hypoxic vasoconstriction increases fluid filtration into the alveolar space and intrinsically low Na-reabsorption in combination with hypoxic inhibition of transepithelial ion transport causes alveolar fluid accumulation. This further impairs oxygen diffusion and aggravates hypoxic pulmonary vasoconstriction. In sum, these events will eventually end in full-blown HAPE.

Indirect evidence for a protective role of an increased activity of Na-transport comes from treatment studies, where the inhaled β-adrenergic agonist salmeterol [33] and oral dexamethasone [2], both strong stimulators of alveolar epithelial reabsorption [21,35,36], significantly reduced the incidence of HAPE in HAPE-susceptible individuals. However, neither of these studies presented evidence for treatment-induced improvement of Na- and water-reabsorption. Furthermore, arguments for beneficial effects of improved alveolar reabsorption on pulmonary vascular tone in hypoxia are contradictory. Sartori et al. [33] found a pronounced improvement of arterial SO_2 and PO_2 in HAPE-susceptibles who received inhaled salmeterol during ascent and at high-altitude (4559 m) in comparison with a placebo group. Importantly, the treatment significantly reduced the incidence of HAPE in susceptible individuals. Yet, exaggerated sPAP did not decrease. For this reason the authors claimed that impaired alveolar Na-transport may cause HAPE-susceptibility, whereas improved Na-transport protects from HAPE [33]. However, this hypothesis has to be put into question. Less-severe hypoxic pulmonary arterial vasoconstriction and thus lower sPAP would be expected when stimulated reabsorption improves oxygenation. In fact, the authors of this study themselves published decreased sPAP in HAPE-susceptibles at high-altitude with salmeterol-inhalation in an abstract [37]. The discrepancy between results in the abstract [37] and their paper [33] has never been resolved. By contrast, oral dexamethasone [2] improved oxygenation and significantly decreased sPAP in HAPE-susceptibles. However, the action of this drug is not specific enough to conclude that stimulated alveolar reabsorption was the sole reason for improvement.

Along these lines, an interesting experiment has been performed on rats [38], where an aerosol containing the ENaC-inhibitor amiloride was administered to normoxic anesthetized rats at a dose that decreased alveolar fluid reabsorption by approximately 50%. This resulted in a significant increase in lung water within the first hour, decreased femoral arterial PO_2, and increased right ventricular pressure. This finding is in accordance with the above mentioned hypothesis. However, although showing increased lung water and elevated right ventricular pressure also in hypoxic rats, this study did not demonstrate additivity of amiloride and hypoxia, a situation supposed to mimic the situation of HAPE-susceptibles, that is, intrinsically low Na-transport and hypoxic inhibition of reabsorption. Lack of additivity weakens the argument of a role of impaired Na-reabsorption as a cause of exaggerated hypoxic pulmonary vasoconstriction.

2.3. Oxygen Saturation and Pulmonary Vasoconstriction

If lung water and subsequent impairment of oxygen diffusion for whatever reason were the only mechanism accounting for exaggerated pulmonary arterial vasoconstriction then the increase in sPAP in HAPE might be estimated from the relation between SO_2 and sPAP in healthy individuals determined by Luks et al. [39]. In this study arterial SO_2 was varied by having subjects breathe hyperoxic and hypoxic gas mixtures both at sea level and at different locations at high-altitude. Their results indicate that the mean tricuspid-valve pressure gradient (TVPG) was higher at a given SO_2 at the Everest Base Camp than at sea level, which may indicate some vascular remodeling during the slow ascent to high-altitude. However, the slope of the relationship between SO_2 and TVPG was the same at either location indicating that the responsiveness to oxygen had not changed. Their results showed an increase in sPAP of approximately 6 mmHg per decrease in SO_2 of 10% (Figure 2 in [39]). Applying this relation to studies performed in the Capanna Margherita (4559 m), a decrease in SO_2 by 15%, which is quite normal at this altitude, would cause an increase in sPAP by approximately 9 mmHg, which is slightly less than measured values. The additional decrease in SO_2 of approximately 10% found in HAPE would therefore account for an additional increase in sPAP of approximately 6 mmHg. However, sPAP values measured in HAPE are much higher, reaching values up to 100 mmHg. Furthermore, there appears to be no clear relation between sPAP and SO_2 in HAPE (Figure 2).

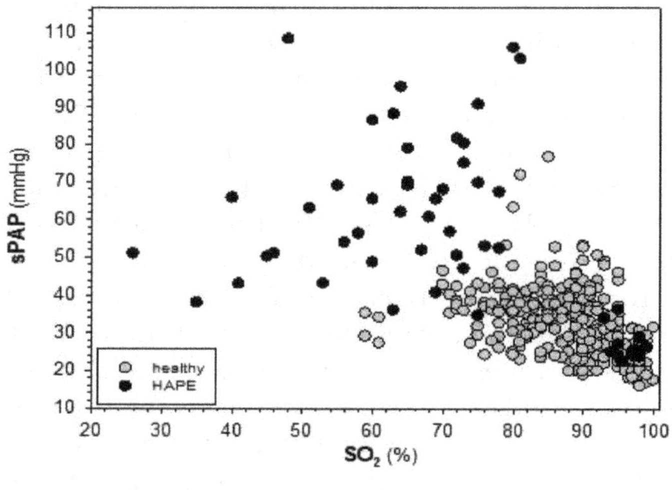

Figure 2. Lack of correlation between systolic pulmonary arterial pressure (sPAP) and SO_2 in HAPE. Individual values from published studies [2,12,40,41], which had all been performed at the Capanna Margherita (4559 m), where subjects ascended by cable car to an altitude of 3200 m and climbed then to the Capanna Gnifetti (3600 m) in the afternoon and spent the night at this altitude. On the next morning they climbed to the Capanna Margherita (4559 m), where they spent two nights.

Also results from short-term exposure to normobaric hypoxia point to altered vaso-reactivity in HAPE-susceptibles independent of differences in SO_2. Dehnert et al. [17] have shown that sPAP was significantly higher in HAPE-susceptibles than in controls as early as 10 min after exposure to hypoxia, and that this gap widens with prolonged hypoxic exposure. At this early time-point there was no difference in SO_2 (Figure 3) between these two groups indicating no diffusion limitation for oxygen and thus no accumulation of significant amounts of edema-fluid in the alveoli. Together these results point to some mechanism intrinsic to vascular smooth muscle cells exaggerating the pressure response in HAPE-susceptibles and that the diffusion limitation for oxygen is the consequence but not the initial trigger for HAPE. Mechanisms are not fully understood. It is unclear, to which extent an inhomogeneity of pulmonary vasoconstriction contributes to this setting [11,42]. Prevention of HAPE with tadalafil [2] and nifedipine [13,43] indicate altered NO-, cGMP-, and Ca-signaling. Interestingly, HAPE-susceptibles show impaired reactivity of peripheral arteries to the vasodilator acetylcholine in hypoxia, but not in normoxia, which might point to endothelial dysfunction and supports this notion [44], which might point to altered function of voltage-sensitive potassium channels. Lung vascular reactivity has not been studied using a similar approach.

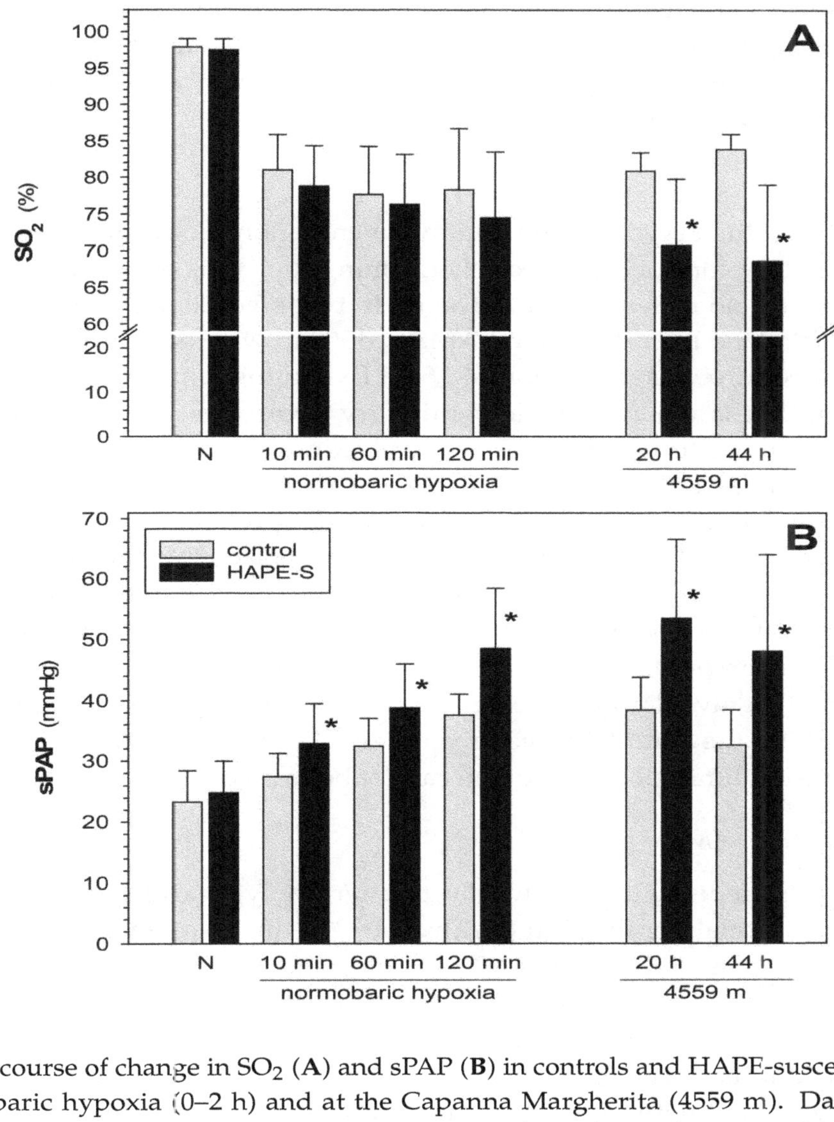

Figure 3. Time course of change in SO_2 (**A**) and sPAP (**B**) in controls and HAPE-susceptibles (HAPE-S) during normobaric hypoxia (0–2 h) and at the Capanna Margherita (4559 m). Data on short-term normobaric hypoxia are from 15 controls and 17 HAPE-S from the study reported in [17], those from exposure to high-altitude (4559 m) are from 10 controls and 9 HAPE-S from reference [2]. In both studies, systolic pulmonary arterial pressure (sPAP) has been measured by Doppler echo-cardiography. Oxygen saturation (SO_2) was measured by pulse-oximetry. Mean values ± standard deviation; N: normoxia; * indicates difference between controls and HAPE.

3. Acute Mountain Sickness (AMS)

AMS may occur within the first 5 to 12 h after ascent to altitudes >2500 m with a prevalence of up to 25% below 3000 m. Prevalence is much higher at higher altitudes (e.g., ~50–85% at altitudes between 4500 and 5500 m) [6]. As with HAPE, slow ascent and pre-acclimatization decrease the risks, whereas individual susceptibility, that is, AMS in previous sojourns at high-altitude, increases the risk of developing AMS [45].

Symptoms are subjective. They are best evaluated with scoring systems like the Lake Louise score and the Environmental Symptoms Questionnaire (ESQ; AMS-C) [46,47]. The leading symptom of AMS is headache [48]. Accompanying symptoms are light-headedness, dizziness, loss of appetite, nausea, vomiting, fatigue, lassitude, trouble sleeping, and peripheral edema [49]. Successful prevention with acetazolamide and dexamethasone [6] allows no clear conclusion on the pathophysiology.

Many studies report decreased SO_2 in hypoxia in individuals suffering from AMS in comparison with healthy controls, some of which suggest that decreased SO_2 might be predictive of AMS (e.g., [1,50–54]). However, even in healthy individuals there is great variability in SO_2 at high-altitude, which challenges this argument. Nevertheless, this finding raises the questions whether diffusion limitation for oxygen and the resulting aggravated hypoxemia are causal for the disease, and which mechanisms explain impaired oxygen diffusion.

3.1. AMS and Ventilation

As mentioned above, the degree of stimulation of ventilation is often measured as an indicator of the sensitivity of ventilatory control in hypoxia. Performing such tests on AMS-susceptible individuals provided varying results: no difference in the acute hypoxic ventilatory response (HVR) between controls and individuals who later developed AMS at 4559 m was found when exposure to hypoxia during the testing procedure was very short [15,55]. Extending exposure to the different levels of oxygen to 20–30 min, that is when hypoxic ventilatory depression can be expected to occur [14], a significantly lower SO_2 was found in AMS-susceptible individuals in comparison to controls [50], which might indicate enhanced ventilatory depression in AMS. Also on days one to three at the Capanna Margherita (4559 m), Bärtsch et al. [55] found that poikilocapnic HVR did not increase in individuals who developed AMS, which one would have expected from the time course of ventilatory acclimatization and what had actually been found in healthy controls in this study [55]. Interestingly, end-tidal PCO_2 was no different between controls and AMS despite the decreased HVR. Importantly, alveolar PO_2 calculated from published data (Table 3 in [55]) using the alveolar gas equation was also no different, indicating that alveolar PO_2 was within the normal range for this specific altitude. These results indicate normal (for the altitude) alveolar ventilation in AMS despite differences in HVR, which indicates that the diffusion limitation for oxygen cannot be caused by decreased alveolar PO_2.

3.2. Lung Water Content and AMS

Bärtsch et al. [55] also report a higher alveolar-to-arterial oxygen difference ($AaDO_2$) in those with severe AMS. Because of normal (for the altitude) alveolar PO_2 this result indicates a diffusion limitation for oxygen resulting in decreased SO_2 in AMS, which might be due to interstitial and/or alveolar edema. Extravascular lung water estimated from radiological and clinical tests and by measuring the closing volume was found to be higher in individuals with increased AMS-scores but without signs of HAPE at the Capanna Margherita (4559 m) [56]. However, in this study no difference in SO_2 was found between individuals with and without indications of subclinical edema [56]. In a study performed at 3810 m, a small but significant association between AMS and lung water assessed with the B-line score from ultrasound measurements was reported [57]. However, also in this study there was no significant correlation between the B-line score and the change in SO_2. This is surprising because a small increase in lung water is already thought to be sufficient to impair oxygen diffusion. This is in contradiction with the direct relation between the Lake Louise score and the $AaDO_2$ mentioned above [55].

The reason for increased lung water in AMS is not clear. Increased filtration of fluid due to elevated capillary pressure and increased permeability, impaired lymphatic drainage, and impaired alveolar clearance might all contribute. Results on most of those mechanisms are scarce. Indirect evidence for increased filtration can be derived from a significant correlation between decreased SO_2 in acute hypoxia and at high-altitude and increased sPAP in healthy individuals [39]. Based on an approximately 10% lower SO_2 in AMS on day 2 at the Capanna Margherita (4559 m) [55], one might expect an elevation in sPAP in AMS too. Plotting (Figure 4) the results from the placebo group from a study performed at the Capanna Margherita (4559 m) showing that inhaled budesonide did not prevent AMS [41] indicates that the dependency of sPAP on SO_2 was the same in healthy controls and in subjects with AMS and that this relation was very similar to the one reported by Luks et al. for healthy individuals [39]. In this study, SO_2 was approximately 8% lower in AMS ($p < 0.001$), while sPAP was only 3 mmHg higher in AMS than in healthy individuals ($p = 0.117$). In a study performed at 3450 m in the Jungfraujoch Research Station on a possible protective effect of remote ischemic preconditioning [58], there was no significant difference in SO_2 (0.386) and in sPAP ($p = 0.934$) between healthy subjects and those with AMS from the placebo group on the first morning after ascent. While on day three at high-altitude the difference in SO_2 between controls and AMS was increased slightly (+3%; $p = 0.041$), there was no difference in sPAP between both groups. This indicates that despite clear symptoms of AMS (Lake Louise score >4 and AMS-C >0.7) there was only a mild impairment of oxygen diffusion at this altitude. The degree of hypoxia at 3450 m might have been too small to allow the detection of a difference in sPAP between controls and AMS with typical clinical approaches. Another reason might be the mode of ascent: while subjects ascended to the Capanna Margherita (4559 m) on foot, ascent to the Jungfraujoch Research Station (3450 m) occurred by train and lasted only 2 h, which raises the question of a possible impact of physical exercise on the degree of AMS and other physiological and clinical parameters.

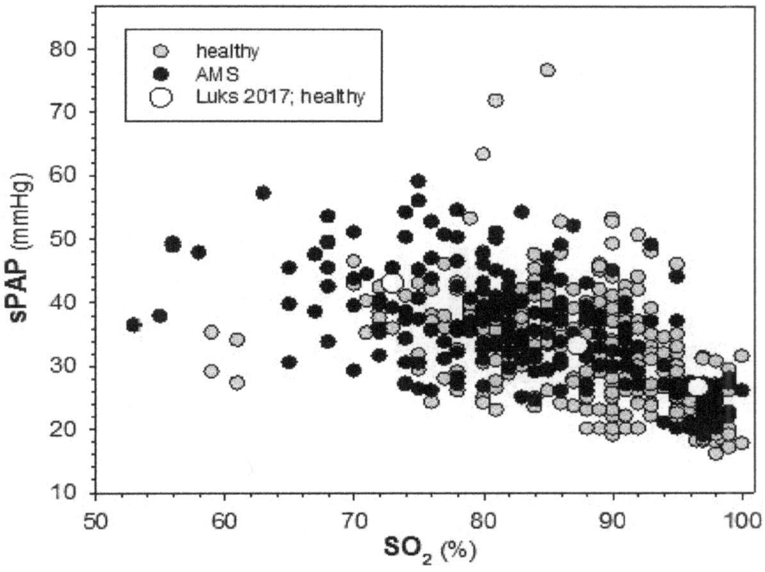

Figure 4. Relation between sPAP and SO_2 in acute mountain sickness (AMS) and in healthy controls. Individual values from the placebo-group of a study on effects of ischemic preconditioning performed at 3450 m at the Jungfraujoch Research Station [58] and from the placebo group of a study on effects of inhaled budesonide at the Capanna Margherita (4559 m) [41]. Data split by AMS have not been reported in these publications. Ascent to 3450 m was by train, to 4559 m by cable car and climbing (see legend to Figure 1). Open circles are the mean values reported in [39], for comparison.

It is unclear whether increased lung water indicated by decreased SO_2 in some studies is a requirement for the occurrence of AMS. Looking at earlier time points is necessary to answer this question, which is only possible by comparison of results from high-altitude with chamber studies performed at equivalent degrees of hypoxia. Figure 5 summarizes the results from the placebo group of a study on short-term effects of ischemic preconditioning in normobaric hypoxia [59] and shows the time course of changes in the Lake Louise score for AMS and the respective change in SO_2, and compares them with results from the placebo group from a study on the action of inhaled budesonide performed at an altitude of 4559 m [41]. It shows that symptoms of AMS become apparent already after 5 h in normobaric hypoxia and become stronger with prolonged stay. Also, at high-altitude symptoms were evident throughout the sojourn. However, in these early time-points in normobaric hypoxia there is no difference in SO_2 between AMS and controls. Lower SO_2 in subjects with AMS compared to controls seems to develop slowly after 18 h in normobaric hypoxia but is then present throughout the stay at high-altitude. Therefore, if SO_2 in fact indicates a diffusion limitation for oxygen, likely by formation of subclinical edema, then these results indicate that AMS-symptoms appear before this diffusion limitation develops. Thus, aggravated decrease in SO_2 appears not to be the primary trigger for AMS but rather a consequence.

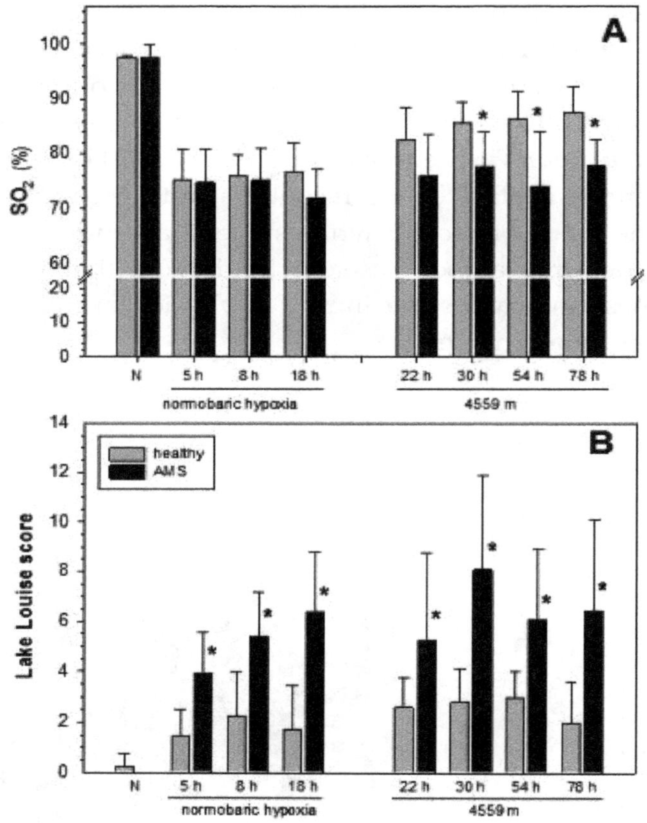

Figure 5. Time course of change in SO_2 (**A**) and in the Lake Louise score (**B**) in controls and individuals developing AMS during normobaric hypoxia and at the Capanna Margherita (4559 m). Data on normobaric hypoxia are from a study on effects of remote ischemic pre-conditioning from 6 controls and 8 subjects with AMS reported in [17,59,60], those from exposure to high-altitude (4559 m) are from 6 controls and 8 subjects with AMS as reported in [41]. Oxygen saturation (SO_2) was measured by pulse-oximetry. Mean values ± SD; N: normoxia; * indicates difference between controls and AMS.

4. Conclusions

Studying high-altitude-related illness in mountaineering settings includes gradually increasing severity of hypoxia and exertion during ascent. Often, complex measurements are not possible during ascent. In contrast, studies in normobaric hypoxia allow instant exposure to a constant level of decreased inspiratory oxygen, but in most cases physical exertion is lacking. Thus, results on physiological measures and on the development of high-altitude and hypoxia-related illness may be different between these two settings. Yet, combining them is the only way to assess the early phase of development of the illness and compare with the situation at high-altitude. This represents a major limitation of the analysis presented here.

Combination of these two settings indicates that SO_2, which is a surrogate measure of oxygen diffusion across the alveolar wall when alveolar PO_2 is normal (for the respective altitude), decreases slower than the illness develops; symptoms of AMS may appear hours before SO_2 drops to levels that are normal for the altitude. Also, the exaggerated increase in sPAP, likely the main trigger causing HAPE, well precedes the decrease in SO_2. Likely in both cases decreased SO_2 indicative of (sub)-clinical edema develops after the initial trigger. This indicates that enhanced filtration from the pulmonary capillaries, impaired removal of lung water by impaired lymphatic drainage and by inhibited alveolar Na- and water reabsorption are likely not the cause of edema development. However, a pre-existing defect in one of those systems might act as an amplifier by increasing the degree of hypoxemia. Whereas it is quite obvious that increased lung water in HAPE is caused by enhanced filtration due to individual susceptibility to exaggerated hypoxic pulmonary arterial vasoconstriction, the reason for subclinical edema in AMS is less clear, and multiple pathophysiologic mechanisms have to be assumed. For both diseases, AMS and HAPE, those amplifying mechanisms require clarification because the resultant aggravation of hypoxemia might advance the illness.

References

1. Berger, M.M.; Macholz, F.; Schmidt, P.; Fried, S.; Perz, T.; Dankl, D.; Niebauer, J.; Bärtsch, P.; Mairbäurl, H.; Sareban, M. Inhaled Budesonide Does Not Affect Hypoxic Pulmonary Vasoconstriction at 4559 Meter of Altitude. *High Alt. Med. Biol.* **2018**, *19*, 52–59. [CrossRef]
2. Maggiorini, M.; Brunner-La Rocca, H.P.; Peth, S.; Fischler, M.; Böhm, T.; Bernheim, A.; Kiencke, S.; Bloch, K.E.; Dehnert, C.; Naeije, R.; et al. Both tadalafil and dexamethasone may reduce the incidence of high-altitude pulmonary edema. *Ann. Intern. Med.* **2006**, *145*, 497–506. [CrossRef] [PubMed]
3. Swenson, E.R.; Bärtsch, P. High-altitude pulmonary edema. *Compr. Physiol.* **2012**, *2*, 2753–2773.
4. Dehnert, C.; Berger, M.M.; Mairbäurl, H.; Bärtsch, P. High-altitude pulmonary edema: A pressure-induced leak. *Respir. Physiol. Neurobiol.* **2007**, *158*, 266–273. [CrossRef] [PubMed]
5. Bärtsch, P.; Mairbäurl, H.; Maggiorini, M.; Swenson, E.R. Physiological aspects of high-altitude pulmonary edema. *J. Appl. Physiol.* **2005**, *98*, 1101–1110. [CrossRef]
6. Bärtsch, P.; Swenson, E.R. Clinical practice: Acute high-altitude illnesses. *New Engl. J. Med.* **2013**, *368*, 2294–2302. [CrossRef]
7. Bärtsch, P. High-altitude pulmonary edema. *Med. Sci. Sports Exerc.* **1999**, *31*, S23–S27. [CrossRef]
8. Vock, P.; Fretz, C.; Franciolli, M.; Bärtsch, P. High-altitude pulmonary edema: Findings at high-altitude chest radiography and physical examination. *Radiology* **1989**, *170*, 661–666. [CrossRef]
9. Hultgren, H.N.; Lopez, C.E.; Lundberg, E.; Miller, J. Physiologic studies of pulmonary edema at high-altitude. *Circulation* **1964**, *29*, 393–408. [CrossRef] [PubMed]
10. Maggiorini, M.; Melot, C.; Pierre, S.; Pfeiffer, F.; Greve, I.; Sartori, C.; Lepori, M.; Hauser, M.; Scherrer, U.; Naeije, R. High-altitude pulmonary edema is initially caused by an increase in capillary pressure. *Circulation* **2001**, *103*, 2078–2083. [CrossRef] [PubMed]
11. Dehnert, C.; Risse, F.; Ley, S.; Kuder, T.A.; Buhmann, R.; Puderbach, M.; Menold, E.; Mereles, D.; Kauczor, H.U.; Bärtsch, P.; et al. Magnetic resonance imaging of uneven pulmonary perfusion in hypoxia in humans. *Am. J. Respir. Crit. Care Med.* **2006**, *174*, 1132–1138. [CrossRef]
12. Swenson, E.R.; Maggiorini, M ; Mongovin, S.; Gibbs, J.S.R.; Greve, I.; Mairbäurl, H.; Bärtsch, P. Pathogenesis of high-altitude pulmonary edema: Inflammation is not an etiologic factor. *J. Am. Med. A* **2002**, *287*, 2228–2235. [CrossRef]
13. Bärtsch, P.; Maggiorini, M.; Ritter, M.; Noti, C.; Vock, P.; Oelz, O. Prevention of high-altitude pulmonary edema by nifedipine. *New Engl. J. Med.* **1991**, *325*, 1284–1289. [CrossRef]
14. Powell, F.L.; Milsom, W.K.; Mitchell, G.S. Time domains of the hypoxic ventilatory response. *Respir. Physiol.* **1998**, *112*, 123–134. [CrossRef]
15. Hohenhaus, E.; Paul, A.; McCullough, R.E.; Kücherer, H.; Bärtsch, P. Ventilatory and pulmonary vascular response to hypoxia and susceptibility to high-altitude pulmonary oedema. *Eur. Respir. J.* **1995**, *8*, 1825–1833. [CrossRef]

16. Barer, G.R.; Howard, P.; Shaw, J.W. Stimulus-response curves for the pulmonary vascular bed to hypoxia and hypercapnia. *J. Physiol.* **1970**, *211*, 139–155. [CrossRef]
17. Dehnert, C.; Grunig, E.; Mereles, D.; Von Lennep, N.; Bärtsch, P. Identification of individuals susceptible to high-altitude pulmonary oedema at low altitude. *Eur. Respir. J.* **2005**, *25*, 545–551. [CrossRef] [PubMed]
18. Mutlu, G.M.; Sznajder, J.I. Mechanisms of pulmonary edema clearance. *Am. J. Physiol.* **2005**, *289*, L685–L695. [CrossRef]
19. Mairbäurl, H.; Mayer, K.; Kim, K.J.; Borok, Z.; Bärtsch, P.; Crandall, E.D. Hypoxia decreases active Na transport across primary rat alveolar epithelial cell monolayers. *Am. J. Physiol.* **2002**, *282*, L659–L665. [CrossRef]
20. Wodopia, R.; Ko, H.S.; Billian, J.; Wiesner, R.; Bärtsch, P.; Mairbäurl, H. Hypoxia decreases proteins involved in transepithelial electrolyte transport of A549 cells and rat lung. *Am. J. Physiol.* **2000**, *279*, L1110–L1119.
21. Guney, S.; Schuler, A.; Ott, A.; Höschele, S.; Baloglu, E.; Bärtsch, P.; Mairbäurl, H. Dexamethasone prevents transport inhibition by hypoxia in rat lung and alveolar epithelial cells by stimulating activity and expression of Na/K-ATPase and ENaC. *Am. J. Physiol.* **2007**, *293*, L1332–L1338.
22. Planes, C.; Escoubet, B.; BlotChabaud, M.; Friedlander, G.; Farman, N.; Clerici, C. Hypoxia downregulates expression and activity of epithelial sodium channels in rat alveolar epithelial cells. *Am. J. Respir. Cell Mol. Biol.* **1997**, *17*, 508–518. [CrossRef] [PubMed]
23. Planes, C.; BlotChabaud, M.; Matthay, M.A.; Couette, S.; Uchida, T.; Clerici, C. Hypoxia and beta(2)-agonists regulate cell surface expression of the epithelial sodium channel in native alveolar epithelial cells. *J. Biol. Chem.* **2002**, *277*, 47318–47324. [CrossRef]
24. Dada, L.A.; Chandel, N.S.; Ridge, K.M.; Pedemonte, C.; Bertorello, A.M.; Sznajder, J.I. Hypoxia-induced endocytosis of Na,K-ATPase in alveolar epithelial cells is mediated by mitochondrial reactive oxygen species and PKC-zeta. *J. Clin. Investig.* **2003**, *111*, 1057–1064. [CrossRef]
25. Sakuma, T.; Hida, M.; Nambu, Y.; Osanai, K.; Toga, H.; Takahashi, K.; Ohya, N.; Inoue, M.; Watanabe, Y. Effects of hypoxia on alveolar fluid transport capacity in rat lungs. *J. Appl. Physiol.* **2001**, *91*, 1766–1774. [CrossRef] [PubMed]
26. Vivona, M.L.; Matthay, M.A.; Chabaud, M.B.; Friedlander, G.; Clerici, C. Hypoxia reduces alveolar epithelial sodium and fluid transport in rats: Reversal by beta-adrenergic agonist treatment. *Am. J. Respir. Cell Molec. Biol.* **2001**, *25*, 554–561. [CrossRef]
27. Sakuma, T.; Pittet, J.F.; Jayr, C.; Matthay, M.A. Alveolar liquid and protein clearance in the absence of blood flow or ventilation in sheep. *J. Appl. Physiol.* **1993**, *74*, 176–185. [CrossRef] [PubMed]
28. Ware, L.B.; Matthay, M.A. Alveolar fluid clearance is impaired in the majority of patients with acute lung injury and the acute respiratory distress syndrome. *Am. J. Respir. Crit. Care Med.* **2001**, *163*, 1376–1383. [CrossRef] [PubMed]
29. Höschele, S.; Mairbäurl, H. Alveolar flooding at high-altitude: Failure of reabsorption? *News Physiol. Sci.* **2003**, *18*, 55–59. [CrossRef] [PubMed]
30. Knowles, M.R.; Paradiso, A.M.; Boucher, R.C. In vivo nasal potential difference: Techniques and protocols for assessing efficacy of gene transfer in cystic fibrosis. *Hum. Gene Ther.* **1995**, *6*, 445–455. [CrossRef]
31. Middleton, P.G.; Geddes, D.M.; Alton, E.W.F.W. Protocols for in vivo measurements of the ion transport defects in cystic fibrosis nasal epithelium. *Eur. Respir. J.* **1994**, *7*, 2050–2056. [PubMed]
32. Davies, J.C.; Alton, E.W.; Bush, A. Cystic fibrosis. *BMJ* **2007**, *335*, 1255–1259. [CrossRef] [PubMed]
33. Sartori, C.; Allemann, Y.; Duplain, H.; Lepori, M.; Egli, M.; Lipp, E.; Hutter, D.; Turini, P.; Hugli, O.; Cook, S.; et al. Salmeterol for the prevention of high-altitude pulmonary edema. *New Engl. J. Med.* **2002**, *346*, 1631–1636. [CrossRef] [PubMed]
34. Mairbäurl, H.; Weymann, J.; Möhrlein, A.; Swenson, E.R.; Maggiorini, M.; Gibbs, J.S.R.; Bärtsch, P. Nasal epithelium potential difference at high-altitude (4559 m): Evidence for secretion. *Am. J. Respir. Crit. Care Med.* **2003**, *167*, 862–867. [CrossRef] [PubMed]
35. Matthay, M.A.; Clerici, C.; Saumon, G. Active fluid clearance from distal airspaces. *J. Appl. Physiol.* **2002**, *93*, 1533–1541. [CrossRef] [PubMed]
36. Baloglu, E.; Reingruber, T.; Bärtsch, P.; Mairbäurl, H. beta2-Adrenergics in hypoxia desensitize receptors but blunt inhibition of reabsorption in rat lungs. *Am. J. Respir. Cell Mol. Biol.* **2011**, *45*, 1059–1068. [CrossRef]
37. Sartori, C.; Lipp, E.; Duplain, H.; Egli, M.; Hutter, D.; Allemann, Y.; Nicod, P.; Scherrer, U. Prevention

of high-altitude pulmonary edema by beta-adrenergic stimulation of the alveolar transepithelial sodium transport. *Am. J. Respir. Crit. Care Med.* **2000**, *161*, A415.
38. Davieds, B.; Gross, J.; Berger, M.M.; Baloglu, E.; Bärtsch, P.; Mairbäurl, H. Inhibition of alveolar Na transport and LPS causes hypoxemia and pulmonary arterial vasoconstriction in ventilated rats. *Physiol. Rep.* **2016**, *4*, e12985. [CrossRef]
39. Luks, A.M.; Levett, D.; Martin, D.S.; Goss, C.H.; Mitchell, K.; Fernandez, B.O.; Feelisch, M.; Grocott, M.P.; Swenson, E.R.; Caudwell Xtreme Everest, I. Changes in acute pulmonary vascular responsiveness to hypoxia during a progressive ascent to high-altitude (5300 m). *Exp. Physiol.* **2017**, *102*, 711–724. [CrossRef]
40. Dehnert, C.; Luks, A.M.; Schendler, G.; Menold, E.; Berger, M.M.; Mairbäurl, H.; Faoro, V.; Bailey, D.M.; Castell, C.; Hahn, G.; et al. No evidence for interstitial lung oedema by extensive pulmonary function testing at 4559 m. *Eur. Respir. J.* **2010**, *35*, 812–820. [CrossRef]
41. Berger, M.M.; Macholz, F.; Sareban, M.; Schmidt, P.; Fried, S.; Dankl, D.; Niebauer, J.; Bärtsch, P.; Mairbäurl, H. Inhaled budesonide does not prevent acute mountain sickness after rapid ascent to 4559 m. *Eur. Respir. J.* **2017**, *50*, 1700982. [CrossRef] [PubMed]
42. Hopkins, S.R.; Garg, J.; Bolar, D.S.; Balouch, J.; Levin, D.L. Pulmonary blood flow heterogeneity during hypoxia and high-altitude pulmonary edema. *Am. J. Respir. Crit. Care Med.* **2005**, *171*, 83–87. [CrossRef] [PubMed]
43. Oelz, O.; Maggiorini, M.; Ritter, M.; Waber, U.; Jenni, R.; Vock, P.; Bärtsch, P. Nifedipine for high-altitude pulmonary oedema. *Lancet* **1989**, *334*, 1241–1244. [CrossRef]
44. Berger, M.M.; Hesse, C.; Dehnert, C.; Siedler, H.; Kleinbongard, P.; Bardenheuer, H.J.; Kelm, M.; Bärtsch, P.; Haefeli, W.E. Hypoxia Impairs Systemic Endothelial Function in Individuals Prone to High-Altitude Pulmonary Edema. *Am. J. Respir. Crit. Care Med.* **2005**, *172*, 763–767. [CrossRef] [PubMed]
45. Schneider, M.; Bernasch, D.; Weymann, J.; Holle, R.; Bärtsch, P. Acute mountain sickness: Influence of susceptibility, preexposure, and ascent rate. *Med. Sci. Sports Exerc.* **2002**, *34*, 1886–1891. [CrossRef] [PubMed]
46. Sampson, J.B.; Cymerman, A.; Burse, R.J.; Maher, J.T.; Rock, P.B. Procedures for the measurement of acute mountain sickness. *Aviat. Space Environ. Med.* **1983**, *54*, 1063–1073. [PubMed]
47. Dellasanta, P.; Gaillard, S.; Loutan, L.; Kayser, B. Comparing questionnaires for the assessment of acute mountain sickness. *High. Alt. Med. Biol.* **2007**, *8*, 184–191. [CrossRef]
48. Schneider, M.; Bärtsch, P. Characteristics of Headache and Relationship to Acute Mountain Sickness at 4559 Meters. *High. Alt. Med. Biol.* **2018**, *19*, 321–328. [CrossRef] [PubMed]
49. Bärtsch, P.; Bailey, D.M. Acute Mountain Sickness and High-altitude Cerebral Edema. In *High-altitude. Human Adaptation to Hypoxia*; Swenson, E.R., Bärtsch, P., Eds.; Springer: New York, NY, USA, 2014; pp. 379–404.
50. Burtscher, M.; Flatz, M.; Faulhaber, M. Prediction of susceptibility to acute mountain sickness by SaO_2 values during short-term exposure to hypoxia. *High. Alt. Med. Biol.* **2004**, *5*, 335–340. [CrossRef] [PubMed]
51. Richalet, J.P.; Larmignat, P.; Poitrine, E.; Letournel, M.; Canoui-Poitrine, F. Physiological risk factors for severe high-altitude illness: A prospective cohort study. *Am. J. Respir. Crit. Care Med.* **2012**, *185*, 192–198. [CrossRef]
52. Roach, R.C.; Greene, E.R.; Schoene, R.B.; Hackett, P.H. Arterial oxygen saturation for prediction of acute mountain sickness. *Aviat. Space Environ. Med.* **1998**, *69*, 1182–1185.
53. Burtscher, M.; Philadelphy, M.; Gatterer, H.; Burtscher, J.; Faulhaber, M.; Nachbauer, W.; Likar, R. Physiological Responses in Humans Acutely Exposed to High-altitude (3480 m): Minute Ventilation and Oxygenation Are Predictive for the Development of Acute Mountain Sickness. *High. Alt. Med. Biol.* **2019**, *20*, 192–197. [CrossRef] [PubMed]
54. Bailey, D.M.; Kleger, G.R.; Holzgraefe, M.; Ballmer, P.E.; Bärtsch, P. Pathophysiological significance of peroxidative stress, neuronal damage, and membrane permeability in acute mountain sickness. *J. Appl. Physiol.* **2004**, *96*, 1459–1463. [CrossRef] [PubMed]
55. Bärtsch, P.; Swenson, E.R.; Paul, A.; Julg, B.; Hohenhaus, E. Hypoxic ventilatory response, ventilation, gas exchange, and fluid balance in acute mountain sickness. *High. Alt. Med. Biol.* **2002**, *3*, 361–376. [CrossRef] [PubMed]
56. Cremona, G.; Asnaghi, P.; Baderna, P.; Brunetto, A.; Brutsaert, T.; Cavallaro, C.; Clark, T.M.; Cogo, A.; Donis, R.; Lanfranchi, P.; et al. Pulmonary extravascular fluid accumulation in recreational climbers: A prospective study. *Lancet* **2002**, *359*, 303–309. [CrossRef]

57. Alsup, C.; Lipman, G.S.; Pomeranz, D.; Huang, R.W.; Burns, P.; Juul, N.; Phillips, C.; Jurkiewicz, C.; Cheffers, M.; Evans, K.; et al. Interstitial Pulmonary Edema Assessed by Lung Ultrasound on Ascent to High-altitude and Slight Association with Acute Mountain Sickness: A Prospective Observational Study. *High. Alt. Med. Biol.* **2019**, *20*, 150–156. [CrossRef] [PubMed]
58. Berger, M.M.; Macholz, F.; Lehmann, L.; Dankl, D.; Hochreiter, M.; Bacher, B.; Bärtsch, P.; Mairbaurl, H. Remote ischemic preconditioning does not prevent acute mountain sickness after rapid ascent to 3450 m. *J. Appl. Physiol.* **2017**, *123*, 1228–1234. [CrossRef] [PubMed]
59. Berger, M.M.; Kohne, H.; Hotz, L.; Hammer, M.; Schommer, K.; Bartsch, P.; Mairbaurl, H. Remote ischemic preconditioning delays the onset of acute mountain sickness in normobaric hypoxia. *Physiol. Rep.* **2015**, *3*, e12325. [CrossRef] [PubMed]
60. Schommer, K.; Hammer, M.; Hotz, L.; Menold, E.; Bärtsch, P.; Berger, M.M. Exercise intensity typical of mountain climbing does not exacerbate acute mountain sickness in normobaric hypoxia. *J. Appl. Physiol.* **2012**, *113*, 1068–1074. [CrossRef] [PubMed]

13

Regeneration of Pulmonary Tissue in a Calf Model of Fibrinonecrotic Bronchopneumonia Induced by Experimental Infection with *Chlamydia psittaci*

Elisabeth M. Liebler-Tenorio [1,*], Jacqueline Lambertz [1,2], Carola Ostermann [1], Konrad Sachse [1,3] and Petra Reinhold [1]

1 Institute for Molecular Pathogenesis, Friedrich-Loeffler-Institut, Federal Research Institute for Animal Health, Naumburgerstr. 96a, 07743 Jena, Germany; Jacqueline.Lambertz@cvua-rrw.de (J.L.); Carola.Heike.Ostermann@googlemail.com (C.O.); konrad.sachse@gmx.net (K.S.); Petra.Reinhold@fli.de (P.R.)

2 Chemisches und Veterinäruntersuchungsamt Rhein-Ruhr-Wupper (CVUA-RRW), Deutscher Ring 100, 47798 Krefeld, Germany

3 Institute of Bioinformatics, Friedrich-Schiller-Universität Jena, Leutragraben 1, 07743 Jena, Germany

* Correspondence: Elisabeth.Liebler-Tenorio@fli.de

Abstract: Pneumonia is a cause of high morbidity and mortality in humans. Animal models are indispensable to investigate the complex cellular interactions during lung injury and repair in vivo. The time sequence of lesion development and regeneration is described after endobronchial inoculation of calves with *Chlamydia psittaci*. Calves were necropsied 2–37 days after inoculation (dpi). Lesions and presence of *Chlamydia psittaci* were investigated using histology and immunohistochemistry. Calves developed bronchopneumonia at the sites of inoculation. Initially, *Chlamydia psittaci* replicated in type 1 alveolar epithelial cells followed by an influx of neutrophils, vascular leakage, fibrinous exudation, thrombosis and lobular pulmonary necrosis. Lesions were most extensive at 4 dpi. Beginning at 7 dpi, the number of chlamydial inclusions declined and proliferation of cuboidal alveolar epithelial cells and sprouting of capillaries were seen at the periphery of necrotic tissue. At 14 dpi, most of the necrosis had been replaced with alveoli lined with cuboidal epithelial cells resembling type 2 alveolar epithelial cells and mild fibrosis, and hyperplasia of organized lymphoid tissue were observed. At 37 dpi, regeneration of pulmonary tissue was nearly complete and only small foci of remodeling remained. The well-defined time course of development and regeneration of necrotizing pneumonia allows correlation of morphological findings with clinical data or treatment regimen.

Keywords: lung; pneumonia; necrotizing; regeneration; model; bovine; chlamydia

---

1. Introduction

Pneumonia affects large proportions of the human population worldwide [1]. Community acquired pneumonia (CAP), which is defined as infection not acquired during hospitalization or ventilation, is the most common type of pneumonia and the most frequent cause of morbidity and mortality by infection in developed countries [2]. The annual incidence in adults is 1.5–1.7 per 1000 in Europe [3]. CAP can be caused by viral and bacterial pathogens. Infections with *Streptococcus pneumoniae* and *Haemophilus influenzae* are especially frequent [2,4], but a variety of other bacteria including the intracellular pathogens, *Mycoplasma pneumoniae, Chlamydia (C.) pneumoniae, C. psittaci, Coxiella burnetii* and *Legionella pneumophila* can also be involved [3]. Studies focusing on *Chlamydia* and *Mycoplasma* in patients with CAP indicate that these infections are more frequent than commonly reported, especially in children [5–7]. Infections with *C. psittaci* are about twice as frequent as with *C. pneumoniae* [6].

Infection models involving these pathogens are relevant to elucidate host reactions to the pathogen, development and resolution of tissue lesions and to evaluate treatment options. Only animal models can truly reflect the complex cellular interactions during lung injury and repair [8,9]. The search for appropriate animal models of respiratory disease in humans has a long history and is still ongoing [10]. Criteria to optimize experimental research were redefined recently [11]. While mouse models are most frequently used for being cost and time efficient and offering many options for genetic tracing and immunological monitoring, models in domestic animal species, as presented here, possess their own specific advantages, i.e., lung physiology and structure resembling more closely that of humans and spontaneous disease and lesions being comparable to those occurring in humans [8,11,12].

Symptoms of pneumonia are the result of pulmonary alveoli filling with exudate and thus preventing gas exchange. One of the complications of bacterial CAP is necrotizing pneumonia [13,14]. In humans, necrotizing pneumonia is most commonly seen in *Staphylococcus aureus*, *Streptococcus pneumoniae* or *Klebsiella pneumoniae* infections and may occur in both children and adults [13,15]. Conservative versus surgical treatment is subject to controversial debate [13,16,17]. While long-term effects with higher rates of mortality have been reported in elderly patients [18], full resolution within a few months occurred in most children [16].

In cattle and pigs, necrotizing lesions are observed in a number of bacterial pneumonias. The progression to necrotizing lesions may be due to virulence factors of microorganisms or to host reactions, which are more exudative especially in cattle [13]. Experimental infection of calves with *C. psittaci* was reported to progress to necrotizing lesions, with clinical course, pulmonary dysfunction and systemic host reactions having been well characterized [19–22]. In contrast to the general consensus that the outcome of pulmonary necrosis consists of fibrotic scars, sequestra or abscesses, complete healing was observed. In the following, the time sequence from tissue injury to regeneration is described based on qualitative histological data with the aim of providing a fundamental characterization of a necrotizing pneumonia model.

2. Results

2.1. Clinical Signs, Acute Phase Response and Pulmonary Dysfunctions

Details of clinical signs and pulmonary dysfunctions induced by the pathogen were reported elsewhere [19–22]. In brief, intrabronchial inoculation of 10^8 inclusion forming units (ifu) of *C. psittaci* per calf resulted in acute respiratory illness characterized by fever, dyspnea, dry cough, hyperemic conjunctivae and enlarged mandibular lymph nodes. Respiratory signs were accompanied by signs of a systemic inflammatory response, i.e., elevated heart rates (mild tachycardia), reduced appetite and dullness.

During the period of acute illness (i.e., 2–4 days post inoculation, dpi), blood gas analysis revealed hypoxemia. Pulmonary function testing indicated both obstructive and restrictive pulmonary disorders. The resulting pattern of spontaneous breathing was characterized by a reduction of tidal volume by about 25%, a doubling of respiratory rate, and consequently by a significant increase of minute ventilation to about 150%. Although acute clinical signs decreased and general health improved rapidly from 5 dpi onwards, alterations in respiratory mechanics, acute phase reaction (decreased blood concentrations of albumin and elevated blood concentration of lipopolysaccharide binding protein) and disorders in acid-base equilibrium lasted until 10–11 dpi. By the end of this study (37 dpi), the remaining three calves appeared clinically inconspicuous.

Data of rectal temperature, respiratory rate and tidal volume are given in Table S1 in absolute numbers, while relative changes of these parameters are included in Table 1.

Table 1. Clinical data, respiratory function, volume and characteristics of pulmonary lesions.

Day of Necropsy in dpi	Absolute Change in Rectal Temperature [1] in °C, Median {min; max}	Relative Change in Respiratory Rate [2]	Relative Change in Tidal Volume per kg b.wW. [3]	Volume of Pulmonary Lesions	Histologic Characteristics of Pulmonary Lesions
		in %, Median {min; max}			
2 (n = 3)	+2.5 {+1.8; +2.6}	+150 {+133; +285}	n.a. [4]	17 {17; 30}	purulent bronchopneumonia
3 (n = 3)	+ 2.4 {+1.9;+2.8}	+200 {+83; +173}	−19 {−38; −3}	25 {11; 31}	fibrinopurulent bronchopneumonia
4 (n = 3)	+1.0 {+0.5; +1.5}	+104 {+82; +127}	−27 {−31; −23}	25 {20; 27}	fibrinopurulent to necroticzing bronchopneumonia
7 (n = 3)	−0.6 {−0.7; +0.5}	+20 {0; +23}	−2 {−11; −1}	20 {14; 22}	first signs of organization, macrophage infiltration
10 (n = 3)	−0.1 {−0.7; +2.0}	0 {−4; 0}	+13 {−3; +19}	8 {8; 11}	cuboidal alveolar epithelial cells, new capillaries
14 (n = 3)	+0.1 {−0.1; +0.2}	+23 {+13; +67}	+19 {−1; +40}	0.5 {0.3; 3.3}	progressed organization, lymphocyte infiltration
35/37 (n = 3)	-0.1 {−0.4; +0.9}	−22 {−33; −11}	+2 {−2; +6}	0.3 {0.2; 1.5}	regeneration, remodeling (in lesions)

[1] Absolut change of rectal temperature between the average rectal temperature measured at two different days in the week before challenge (baseline) and the rectal temperature measured at the day of necropsy. [2] Respiratory rate was counted in resting animals (in stable). The relative change of respiratory rate was calculated between baseline values (= mean of individual measurements at two different days in the week before challenge) and the respiratory rate counted at the day of necropsy. [3] body weight; [4] not available (calves necropsied at 2 dpi were too sick to undergo pulmonary function testing).

2.2. *Pulmonary Lesions*

2.2.1. At 2 dpi

In two calves 17% of pulmonary tissue and in one calf 30% of pulmonary tissue were dark red, firm with a wet cut surface and pus draining from airways indicating purulent bronchopneumonia (Figures 1 and 2A). Lesions were located around bronchioles at the inoculation sites and often had cylindrical shape (Figure 2B). They were associated with mild fibrinous pleuritis in two calves.

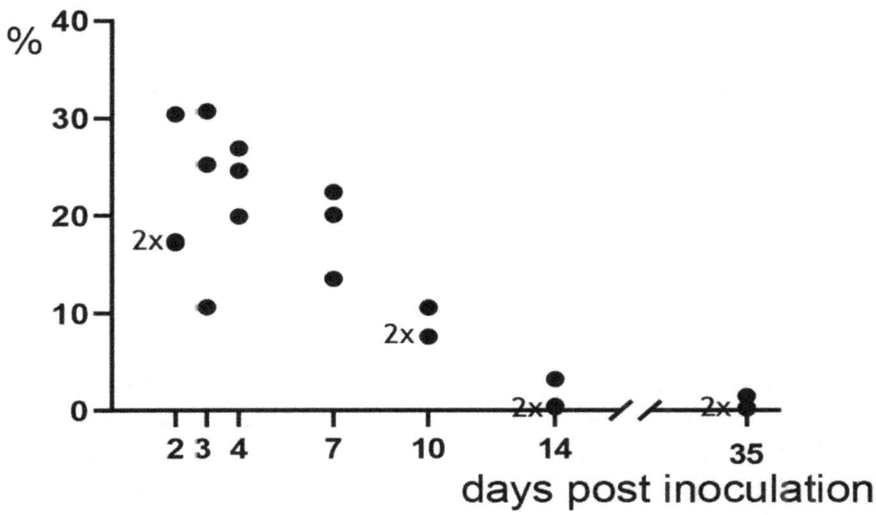

Figure 1. Percentage of pulmonary tissue with lesions at 2, 3, 4, 7, 10, 14 and 35/37 dpi. Each point in the diagram represents one or two (2×) individual calves.

By histology, lesions had a lobular distribution with numerous neutrophils and protein-rich exudate in alveoli, bronchioli and bronchi (Figure 2C,D). The walls and perivascular spaces of small arterioles at the periphery of lesions were thickened by protein-rich edema, fibrin precipitates and neutrophils (Figure 2C,E). Fibrin thrombi obstructed blood vessels. There were areas of necrosis in the vascular walls. Lymphatics in subpleural and interlobular connective tissue contained fibrin thrombi and a few neutrophils. Low numbers of chlamydial inclusions were found in type 1 alveolar epithelial cells (AEC1) and occasionally in neutrophils and macrophages in the exudate (Figure 2F).

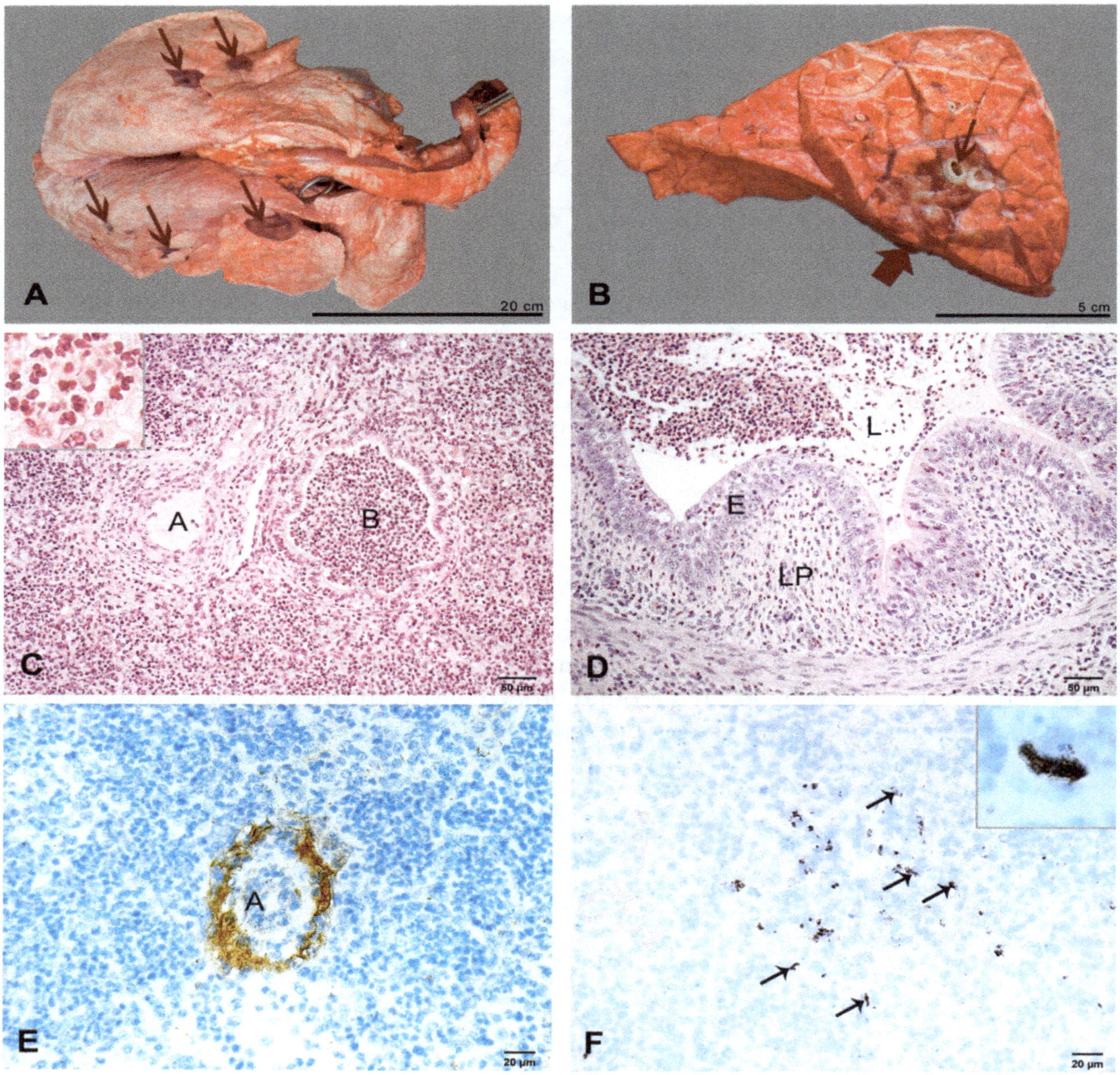

Figure 2. Pulmonary lesions at 2 dpi. (**A**) Macroscopic appearance and distribution of pulmonary lesions (dark red, arrows). (**B**) Section through the left basal lobe. A circumscribed, dark red and sunken lesion (thick arrow) is centered around a bronchus (thin arrow). (**C**) A bronchiolus (B) and the surrounding alveoli are distended by neutrophils. The wall of the arteriole (A) is infiltrated with neutrophils. Inset: higher magnification of neutrophils in an alveolus. HE-stain. (**D**) Numerous neutrophils in the lamina propria (LP), epithelium (E) and lumen (L) of a bronchus. HE-stain. (**E**). Fibrin precipitates (brown) surrounding a small arteriole (A). IHC, factor VIII. (**F**) Few chlamydial inclusions in type 1 alveolar epithelial cells (arrows, examples). Inset: higher magnification of a chlamydial inclusion. IHC, chlamydia.

2.2.2. At 3 dpi

The extent of pulmonary lesions varied from 11% to 31% (Figure 1). Lesions were firm, grey-red marbled, had a dry cut-surface and were associated with fibrinous pleuritis.

By histology, the fibrinopurulent pneumonia and severe vasculopathy had a lobar distribution and were more extensive than at 2 dpi (Figure 3A,B). Foci of necrosis were more frequent in bronchiolar epithelium and vascular walls (Figure 3B,C). There were small areas of complete necrosis of pulmonary tissue. In these areas, diffuse labeling of fibrin using immunohistochemistry for factor VIII was seen (Figure 3C), but no epithelial cells were labeled for cytokeratin.

Lesions in interlobular septa and pleura had increased in severity. Chlamydial inclusions were numerous in neutrophils and macrophages (Figure 3E), but rare in alveolar epithelial cells.

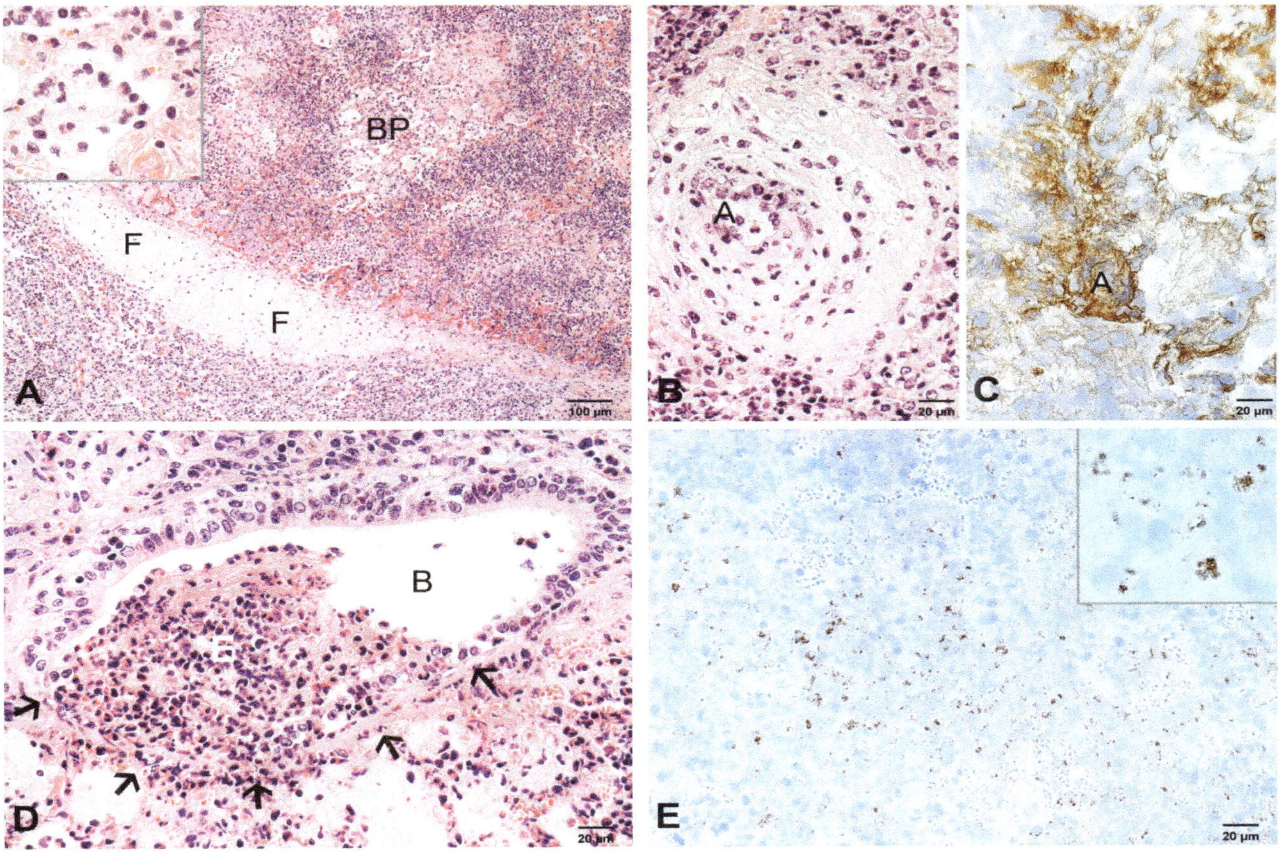

Figure 3. Pulmonary lesions at 3 dpi. (**A**) Lobular fibrinopurulent bronchopneumonia (BP) and fibrin thrombi (F) in interlobular lymphatics. Inset: higher magnification of an alveolus filled with fibrin and neutrophils. HE-stain. (**B**) Severe exudation throughout the wall and in the perivascular space of an arteriole (A). HE-stain. (**C**) Diffuse precipitates of fibrin (brown) in the wall and perivascular space of an arteriole (A) extending into the alveoli. IHC, factor VIII. (**D**) Necrosis (arrows) in the wall of a bronchiolus (B). The lumen is filled with exudate (E). HE-stain. (**E**) Numerous small chlamydial inclusions (brown) in neutrophils and macrophages. Inset: higher magnification of multiple chlamydial inclusions. IHC, chlamydia.

2.2.3. At 4 dpi

Pulmonary lesions varied between 20% and 27% (Figure 1). They were firm, grey-red marbled, bulging and associated with fibrinous pleuritis (Figure 4A).

By histology, lesions in airways, blood vessels and pleura were as described at 3 dpi. Areas of necrosis had expanded (Figure 4B). The inflammatory exudate consisted of neutrophils, fibrin and cellular detritus (Figure 4B). There was a more extensive loss of alveolar epithelial cells than at 3 dpi

(Figure 4C,D). Labeling of factor VIII revealed massive accumulations of fibrin in the walls and around arterioles and in the capillaries of interalveolar septa (Figure 4E,F). Several bronchioles and blood vessels were completely obstructed by fibrin. Chlamydial inclusions were numerous in neutrophils, macrophages and detritus in areas of necrosis.

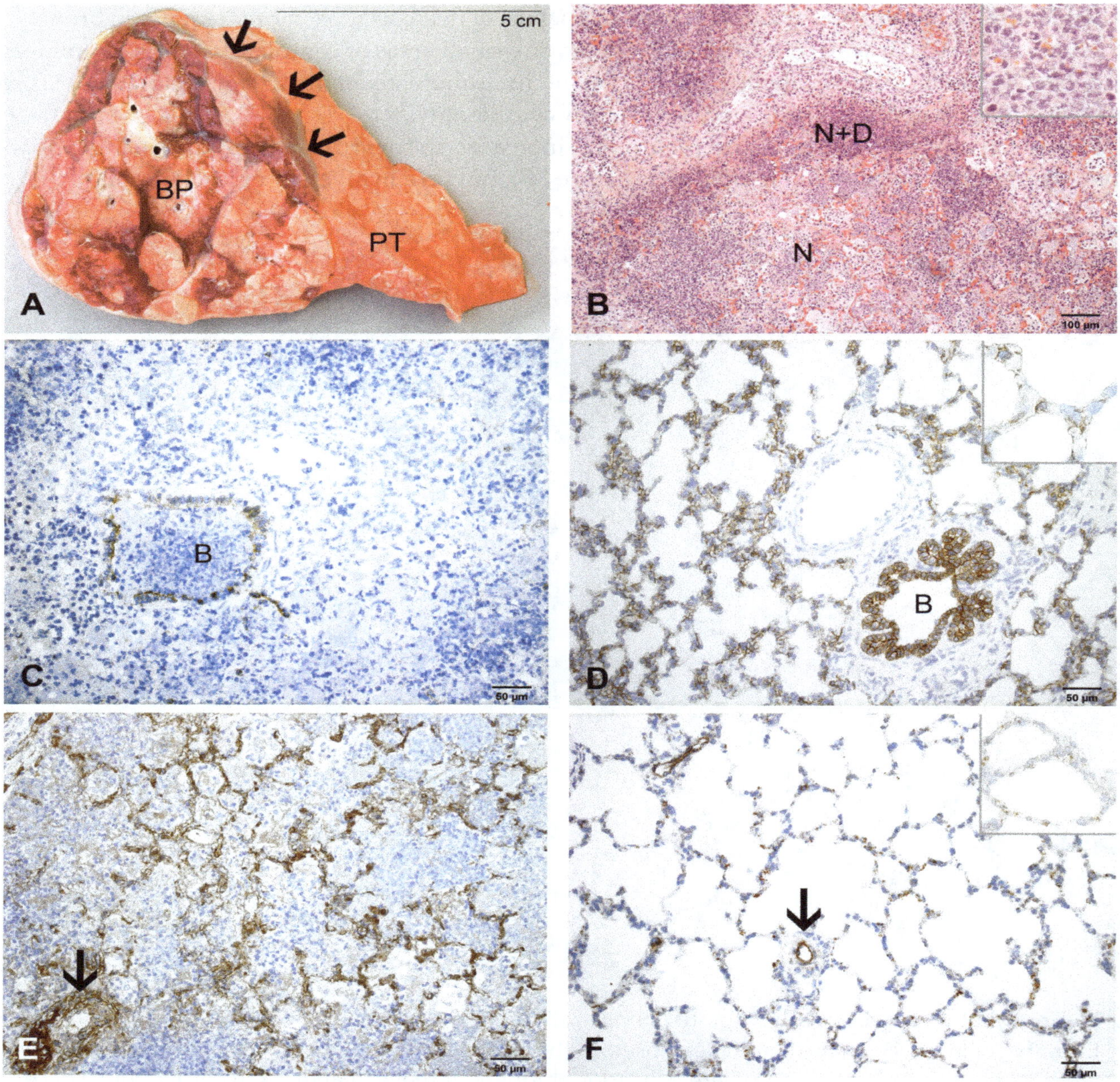

Figure 4. Pulmonary lesions at 4 dpi. (**A**) Section through a basal lobe. The lobular lesion (BP) bulges above the surface of the surrounding pulmonary tissue (PT). The cut surface is drey and marbled grey-red. Interlobular septae and subpleural space are dilated by fibrinous exudate (arrows). (**B**) A large area of necrosis (N) is demarcated by neutrophils and cellular detritus (N+D). Inset: higher magnification of necrosis. HE-stain. (**C**) Epithelial cells are labelled only in segments of the bronchiolar wall (B). There is no labelling of epithelial cells in the surrounding alveoli. IHC, cytokeratin. (**D**) Labelling of epithelial cells in a bronchiolus (B) and surrounding alveoli in the healthy lung of a control calf. Inset: higher magnification of AEC1 in alveolar septae. IHC, cytokeratin. (**E**) Accumulation of fibrin in the wall and perivascular space of an arteriole (arrow). Interalveolar capillaries are dilated by fibrin thrombi (brown). IHC, factor VIII. (**F**) Labeling of factor VIII (brown) is restricted to endothelial cells (arteriole as example, arrow) and thrombocytes in the healthy lung of a control calf. Inset: higher magnification capillaries in alveolar septae. IHC, factor VIII.

2.2.4. At 7 dpi

Gross pulmonary lesions were as described at 4 dpi, but only 14–22% of the pulmonary volume was affected (Figure 1). Pleural lesions had progressed from fibrinous to fibroblastic.

By histology, lesions were characterized by multiple confluent areas of necrosis (Figure 5A). A few weakly cytokeratin-positive cells were present multifocally at the periphery of the necrotic tissue (Figure 5A,B). These epithelial cells were single or formed small aggregates. Airways were filled with macrophages and neutrophils. Compared to 4 dpi, the number of neutrophils was lower and the number of macrophages increased. Moderate infiltrates of lymphocytes and plasma cells were present around bronchi, bronchioles, altered arterioles and in pulmonary tissue adjacent to interlobular septa (Figure 5A). Fibroblasts and delicate collagen fibers had formed in the thickened interlobular septa and subpleural space. Chlamydial inclusions were predominantly present in areas of necrosis (Figure 5C).

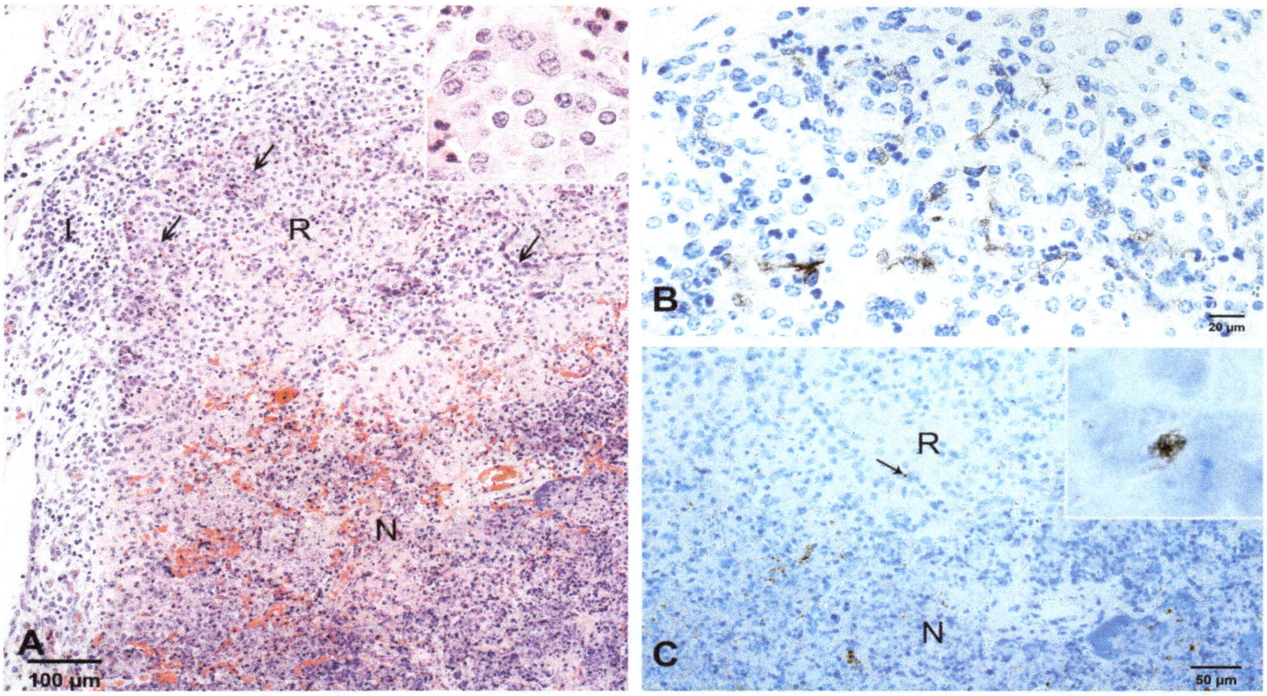

Figure 5. Pulmonary lesions at 7 dpi. (**A**) A few, small groups of epithelial cells (arrows, examples) form a small zone of regeneration (R) at the periphery of a necrosis (N). There is an infiltrate (I) of macrophages, lymphocytes and plasma cells in the adjacent interlobular septum. Inset: higher magnification of a rudimentary alveolar wall. HE-stain. (**B**) Higher magnification of the zone of regeneration. A few cells are weakly positive for cytokeratin (brown). IHC, cytokeratin. (**C**) Chlamydial inclusions (brown) predominate in the necrosis (N) and are rare (arrow) in the zone of regeneration (R). Inset: higher magnification of a chlamydial inclusion in the zoe of regeneration. IHC, chlamydia.

2.2.5. At 10 dpi

Pulmonary lesions were grey, demarcated by hyperemia and firm (Figure 6A). They amounted to 8% in two calves and 11% of pulmonary volume in one calf (Figure 1) Pleural lesions were fibroblastic.

By histology, wide zones of regenerating pulmonary tissue were surrounding areas of necrosis (Figure 6B). The zone of regeneration was characterized by multifocal epithelial cell aggregates forming irregular tubular and alveolar structures (Figure 6C). Epithelial cells had the cuboidal shape of AEC2 and mitotic figures were frequent (Figure 6B inset). Factor VIII-positive endothelial shoots originated from interlobular septa and passed into the zone of regeneration (Figure 6D). Infiltrates of macrophages, lymphocytes and plasma cells were present throughout the zone of regeneration, especially along interlobular septa, and around arterioles, bronchioles and bronchioli (Figure 6A). They formed multifocal lymphoid aggregates. The exudate in bronchioli and bronchi was lined by epithelial cells resulting in bronchiolitis obliterans. A few fibroblasts and delicate collagen fibers were observed in the bronchiolitis obliterans, perivascular space and interalveolar septa. The distribution of chlamydial inclusions was as described at 7 dpi, but their number was lower.

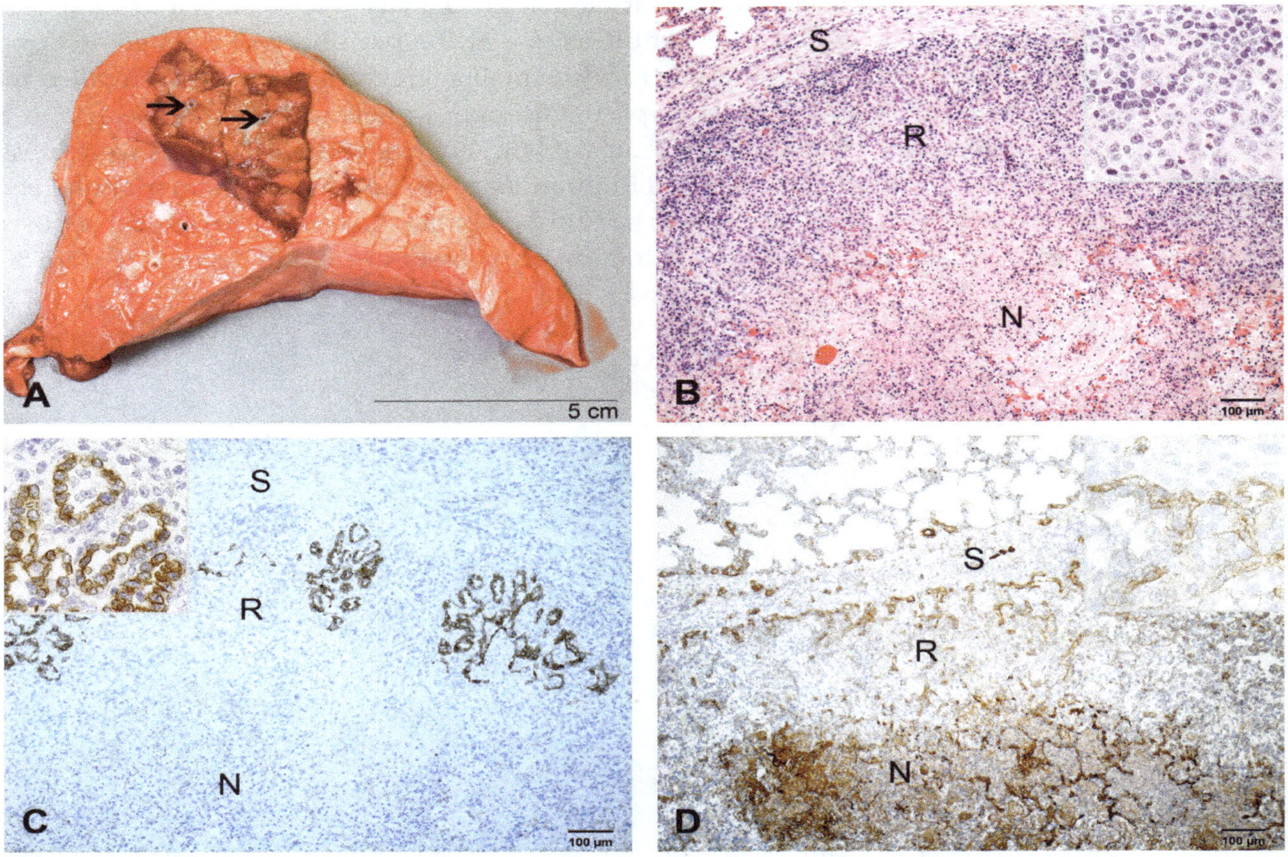

Figure 6. Pulmonary lesions at 10 dpi. (**A**) Section through a basal lobe. The greyish lesion centered round a bronchus (arrow) is demarcated by hyperemia. (**B**) A broad zone of regeneration (R) with multifocal epithelial proliferates surrounds the necrosis (N). Infiltrates of macrophages, lymphocytes and plasma cells are especially prominent next to the interlobular septum (S). Inset: higher magnification of the zone of regeneration. HE-stain. (**C**) Multiple foci of epithelial proliferates (brown) in the zone of regeneration (R) form alveolar structures lined with cuboidal cells. Inset: higher magnification cuboidal epithelial cells. IHC, cytokeratin. (**D**) Capillaries (brown) originating from the interlobular septum (S) pass into the zone of regeneration (R). Fibrinous exudate (brown) is present within the necrosis (N). Inset: higher magnification of capillaries. IHC, factor VIII.

2.2.6. At 14 dpi

Pulmonary lesions were reduced to 3% of pulmonary volume in one and less than 1% in two calves (Figure 1). They were firm, white, poorly demarcated (Figure 7A) and frequently accompanied by fibrous adhesions between pulmonary lobes as well as between pulmonary lobes and thoracic wall.

By histology, lesions were characterized by extensive regeneration of pulmonary tissue and only small foci of necrosis (Figure 7B). In areas of regeneration, cuboidal epithelial cells formed irregular alveolar spaces (Figure 7C). Lesions in airways were organized by bronchiolitis and bronchitis obliterans (Figure 7D). Alveolar spaces were separated by thick interalveolar tissue, which contained capillaries originating from subpleural tissue and interlobular septa, and diffuse infiltrates of macrophages, lymphocytes and plasma cells (Figure 7A,B,D). Organized lymphoid tissue forming tertiary lymphoid tissue in interlobular septa and bronchus-associated lymphoid tissue (BALT) around airways and blood vessels was more abundant than at 10 dpi (Figure 7B). There was no leakage of fibrin through arteriolar walls (Figure 7E). The fibrinous exudate in the wall and around arterioles was replaced by several layers of collagen fibres, which compressed the vascular lumen (Figure 7E,F). An increased amount of collagen fibers was also observed in interalveolar and interlobular septa, and in the bronchiolitis obliterans. Chlamydial inclusions were seen in very few alveolar macrophages.

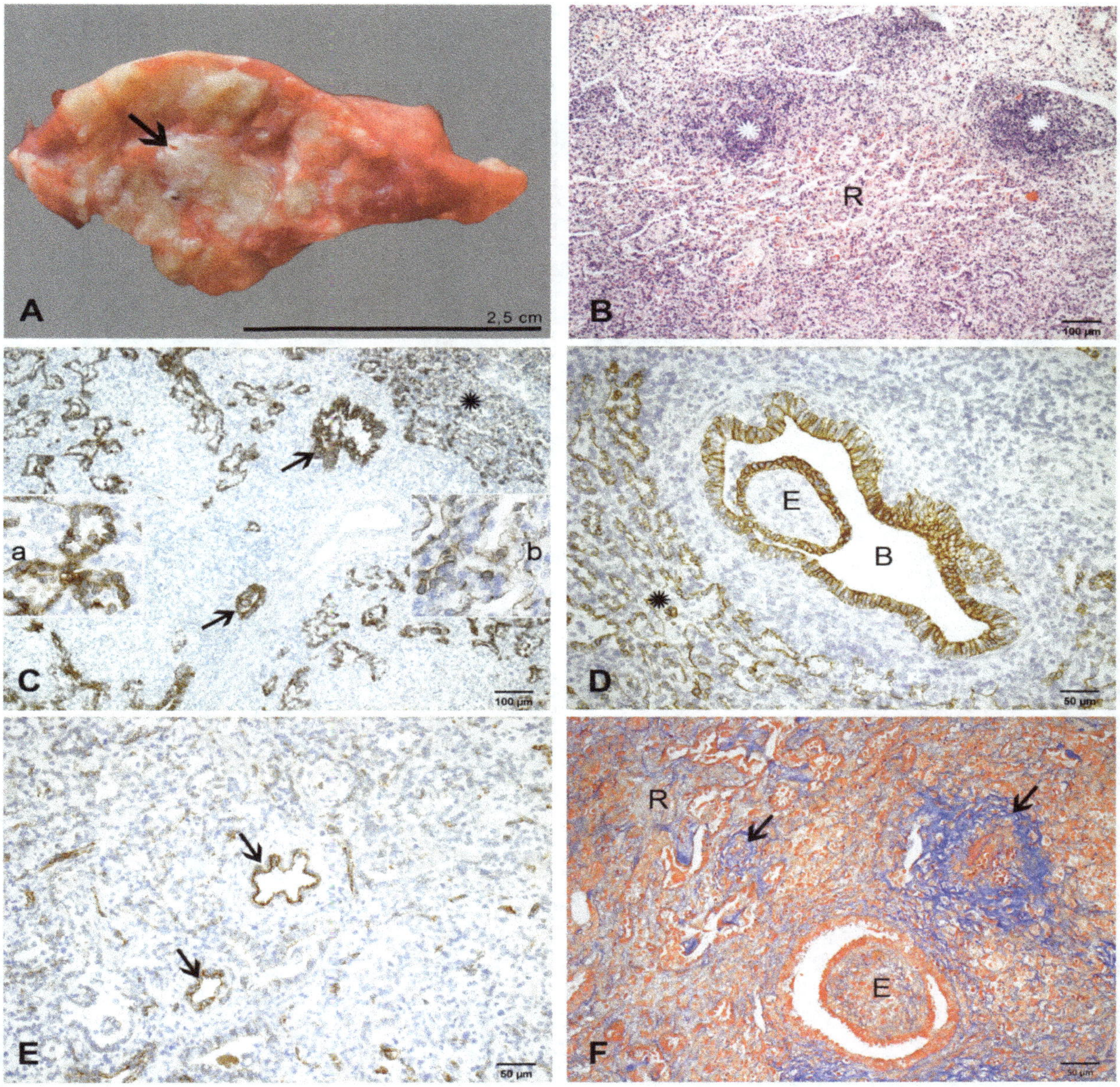

Figure 7. Pulmonary lesions at 14 dpi. (**A**) Section through a middle lobe. The small lesions (white) are centered around a bronchus (arrow) and not well demarcated. (**B**) Extensive regeneration (R) of pulmonary tissue with thick interalveolar septa and narrow alveolar spaces; multifocal organized lymphoid tissue (stars) in the interlobular septum. HE-stain. (**C**) Cuboidal epithelial cells (brown) form irregular alveolar spaces; an area with more progressed regeneration is indicated (star). Bronchiolitis obliterans is seen in most airways (arrows). Inset a: higher magnification of cuboidal epithelial cells forming alveolar spaces. Inset b: higher magnification of delicate, elongated epithelial cells in the area with progressed regeneration. IHC, cytokeratin. (**D**) Higher magnification of more regular alveolar structures lined by type 2 alveolar epithelial cells (star) and the exudate (E) within a bronchiolus (B) lined by cuboidal epithelial cells. IHC, cytokeratin. (**E**) Factor VIII labels endothelial cells in blood vessels (arrows, examples). There is no exudation of fibrin into and through vascular walls. IHC, factor VIII. (**F**) Fibrinous exudate within and around arteriolar walls (arrows) is replaced by collagen fibers (blue). Increased collagen is present in interalveolar septa in the area of regeneration (R) and in the exudate (E) organized by bronchiolitis obliterans. Azan stain.

2.2.7. At 35/37 dpi

Lungs had a normal appearance (Figure 8A). Only a few, very small foci of soft, sunken, dark red pulmonary tissue (2% of total pulmonary volume in one calf and less than 1% in two calves) associated with mild focal fibrous pleuritis were found (Figures 1 and 8B).

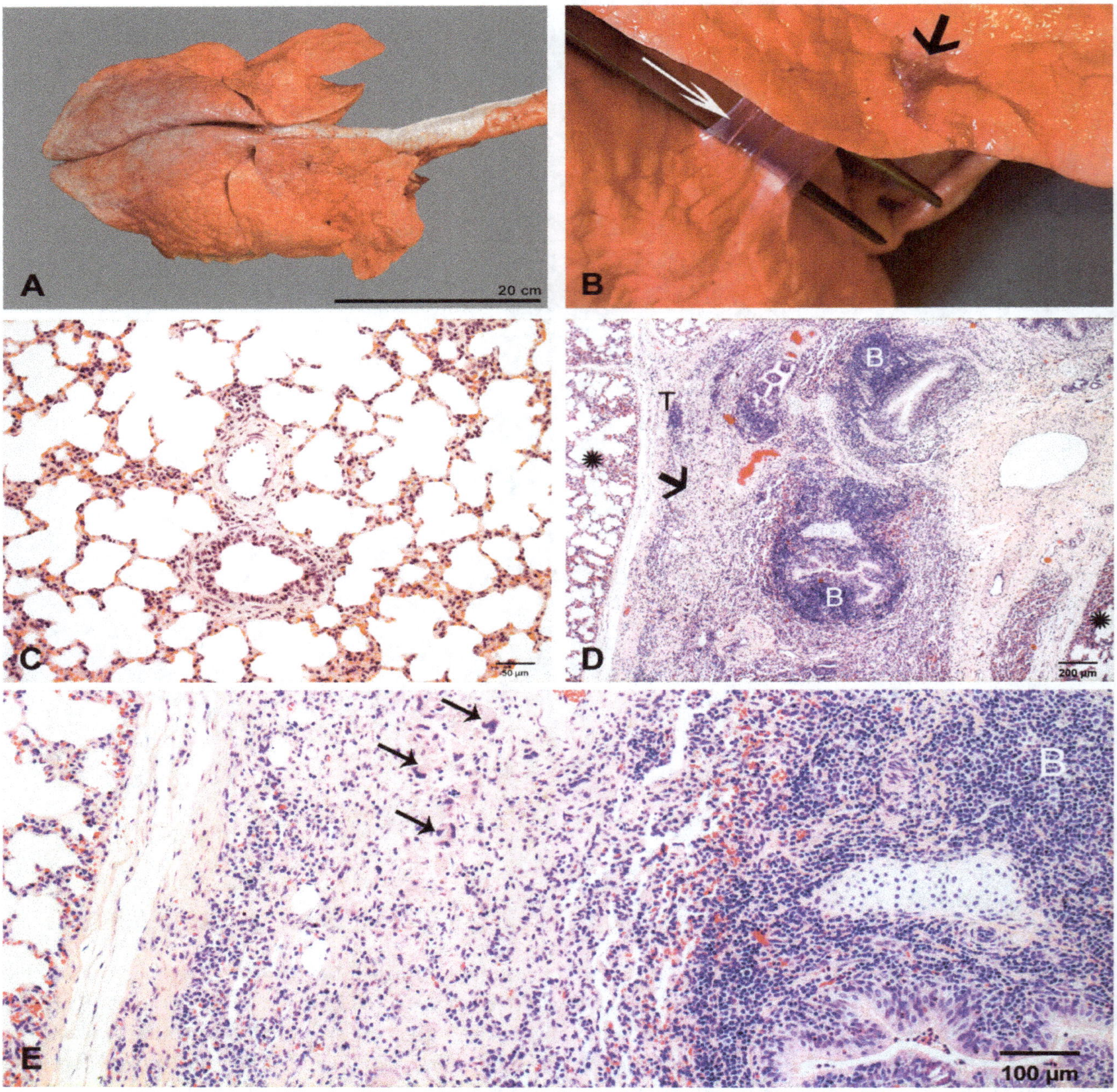

Figure 8. Pulmonary lesions at 35/37 dpi. (**A**) Gross appearance of lung after regeneration. (**B**) Very small lesion in a middle lobe (short arrow) and focal fibrous pleuritis (long arrow) between middle lobe (M) and basal lobe (B). (**C**) Normal pulmonary morphology. HE-stain. (**D**) Small lesion surrounded by normal lung tissue (stars); lesions are characterized by infiltrates of macrophages and multinucleated giant cells (arrow), hyperplastic BALT (B, examples) and tertiary lymphoid tissue (T). HE-stain. (**E**). Higher magnification of the area indicated by the arrow in Figure 8D: infiltrates of macrophages and multinucleated giant cells (arrows, examples), and hyperplastic BALT (B). HE-stain.

By histology, airways, blood vessels and alveolar compartment had completely normal morphology in most of the pulmonary tissue (Figure 8C). BALT and diffuse immune cells had regressed to normal amounts. There were no tertiary lymphoid tissue and no signs of fibrosis.

The small lesions were characterized by infiltrates of macrophages and multinucleated giant cells embedded in vascularized fibrotic tissue (Figure 8D,E). Lymphocytic infiltrates were organized as peribronchial and perivascular BALT, and tertiary lymphoid tissue in the interlobular septa. Chlamydial inclusions were not detected.

3. Discussion

A bovine model of respiratory infection with the zoonotic pathogen *C. psittaci* was previously established [19]. This model has been used to investigate the course of disease, effects on pulmonary functions as well as shedding, transmission and zoonotic potential of *C. psittaci* [20–22]. The infection model was very efficient, since all calves inoculated with the pathogen developed pneumonia, but none of the controls. The model was highly reproducible, and therefore repeatedly used to examine outcomes of different treatment regimens [23,24]. The localization of lesions corresponded to the inoculation sites and was distinct from field infections that have a cranioventral distribution [25]. Thus, the model consistently allows induction of lesions at predetermined sites of the lung.

For this qualitative histological study, groups of 3 of the 21 calves inoculated were necropsied at predetermined days post inoculation. Although the number of animals is low, the validity of observations is supported by the concordance of histological findings and consistent progression patterns. The morphological evaluation of the lung at sequential time points after inoculation revealed the potential of this model to study tissue reactions from initial stages of inflammation to extensive necrosis, up to stepwise organization and regeneration. The reactions observed are matching well with the steps reported as general reactions of pulmonary tissue to an insult [26]: primary lesions are often amplified through inflammatory host reactions. If the host is capable of limiting damage and proliferation of the infectious agent, organization begins. This may result in reparation, resolution or remodeling. Reparation implies repopulation with epithelial cells, but dysfunctional tissue structure. In a remodeled lung, pulmonary tissue is replaced with connective tissue, which is dysfunctional and may cause ectasia and emphysema of adjacent tissue. A successful return to normal structure and function is termed resolution or regeneration.

In the model presented, the initial insult was the intrabronchial inoculation with *C. psittaci*, which has a tropism for epithelial cells [27]. This resulted in a limited infection of AEC1. Infected alveolar epithelial cells have the potential to produce and release cytokines, e.g., the proinflammatory cytokine IL8, which is highly chemotactic for neutrophils, chemokines and growth factors initiating the augmentation [28,29]. Chlamydiae are released during the replication cycle from AEC1 into the alveolar lumen where they get into contact with alveolar macrophages. Bacterial LPS may induce necrosis of alveolar macrophages and release of IL-1α, which lead to a loss of vascular integrity and thus increase the influx of neutrophils from the pulmonary vasculature into the alveoli and airways [30]. Neutrophils display unique migration mechanisms in the lung resulting in particularly high numbers [31]. Inflammatory mediators enhance neutrophil activity and their deleterious effect on endothelium and epithelium [32,33]. The severe exudation and the necrosis of bronchiolar epithelium observed in the calves are most likely due to host reactions and not an effect of chlamydial replication, since no chlamydial inclusions were present in vascular endothelium or airway epithelium.

The massive release of protein-rich exudate and fibrin as seen at 3 dpi and 4 dpi is a common reaction in cattle and has been attributed to an imbalance of pro- and antifibrinolytic factors [34]. Fibrin can further increase vascular permeability, influence the expression of inflammatory mediators and alter migration and proliferation of various cell types [35]. Fibrin thrombi may occlude capillaries and arterioles and thus reduce perfusion; fibrinous exudate within alveoli prevents ventilation. This results in tissue hypoxia and, eventually, necrosis as observed as fibrinonecrotic bronchopneumonia with highest severity at 4 dpi.

While the number of neutrophils continuously declined, the number of macrophages increased during this initial phase. Airway macrophages possess high phagocytic activity to remove debris and exudate, which also included chlamydiae. Processing and presentation of chlamydiae and chlamydial antigens by macrophages may enhance the pathogen-specific immune response. Macrophages also play an important role in the downregulation of immune response and in tissue repair [30,36]. Sloughed epithelial cells, dying neutrophils and microvesicles as encountered in areas of necrosis comprise a rich depot of phosphatidyl serines that can reprogram macrophages from a proinflammatory to an antiinflammatory and prorepair state [9].

In patients with localized destructive processes such as necrotizing pneumonia, which may progress to cavitating lesions, it has been postulated that there is no return to preexisting tissue architecture [37]. In our model, tissue necrosis but no cavitation occurred. Under field conditions, fibrinonecrotic bronchopneumonia in domestic animals rarely resolves completely and sequelae, like sequestra, abscesses, gangrene, fibrosis, scars or chronic pleuritis, are frequent [38]. This may be due to the ability or failure of the host to clear the pathogen and terminate chronic inflammation. After the initial infection of AEC1, chlamydial inclusions were present in continuously decreasing numbers in neutrophils and macrophages. At 14 dpi, they had been almost cleared. From 7 dpi to 14 dpi, the infiltration of lymphocytes representing an adaptive immune response continuously increased [39]. Besides diffuse lymphoid infiltrates, organized structures developed as tertiary lymphoid tissue in the interalveolar septa and as BALT around airways. This local immune reaction was transient and had disappeared at 35/37 dpi.

At the same time, small aggregates of epithelial cells, as first signs of tissue repair, were observed at the edge of necrosis. The pulmonary epithelium does not exhibit a constant turnover, but can respond robustly after injury to replace damaged cells. In the alveolar niche, especially type 2 alveolar epithelial cells (AEC2) have an enormous reparative potential [40–42]. They clonally generate more AEC2 [43]. The cuboidal AEC2 grow, proliferate, follow the basement membrane and secrete basement membrane components, but are inefficient for gas exchange [44].

The multifocal distribution of epithelial cell regenerates at the edge necrosis may be attributable to the fact, that a few AEC2 were retained at these sites and served as starting points [43]. This process may have been supported by remnants of basal membrane, an important scaffold for AEC2 [45]. Recently it was shown that even functionally mature AEC1 could replicate and generate AEC2 [46]. Thus, the delicate epithelial cells observed at 7 dpi might also represent surviving AEC1. Cuboidal epithelial cells interpreted as AEC2 increasingly replaced areas of necrosis. The process started at the periphery and moved towards the center of necrotic tissue leaving only a few small foci of necrosis at 14 dpi. Efficient epithelialization is likely to be crucial for the prevention of pathologic lung remodeling [26].

The cuboidal epithelial cells formed organized alveolar spaces. Maintenance of alveolar units requires complex interactions between various cell types including epithelial cells, endothelial cells, mesenchymal cells, macrophages and other immune cells, and a great variety of mediators [9,47]. Vascularization in areas of re-epithelialization can originate from multipotent mesenchymal stem cells or from blood vessels in adjacent tissue by sprouting. Capillary sprouts originating from the connective tissue of interlobular septa adjacent to areas of necrosis were seen as early as 10 dpi. The sprouting process involves several specialized types of endothelial cells. Vascular endothelial growth factor or inflammatory cytokines induce the formation of tip cells that use filopodia to sense environmental cues, translate these into dynamic processes and express matrix metalloproteinases for invasion [48]. Tip cells use extracellular matrix as a scaffold, provided in this case by the epithelial cells and basement membrane. Stalk cells elongate the sprouting vessels, form the lumen and connect it to the circulation, while phalanx cells stabilize the new vessels and optimize their function [48]. The combination of vascularization and epithelialization contributed to the successful neo-alveolarization observed. The final step in this process is the maturation of cuboidal alveolar epithelial cells to AEC1 and thus functional alveoli [8,40]. This took place between 14 dpi and 37 dpi when the last calves were examined.

The fibrinous exudate and growth factors, e.g., transforming growth factor β, released from inflammatory cells, such as macrophages, and endothelial cells induced immigration of fibroblasts and production of collagen and extracellular matrix. The first fibroblasts and collagen fibers were observed at 7 dpi and distinct fibrosis around arterioles and in the interalveolar septa at 14 dpi. Since there was no permanent or progressive fibrosis in our model, it does not reflect pulmonary fibrosis in humans [37,49], but it is an example that the development of fibrosis can be prevented. The time course of development and resolution of fibrosis in the calves was comparable to that in bleomycin-induced lung fibrosis in mice, where the maximal extent of fibrosis was found at 14 days after a single instillation and subsided after treatment was withdrawn [50].

There was a good correlation between clinical data, deterioration of lung function and pulmonary lesions (Table 1). The more extensive lesions during the initiation phase were associated with systemic signs, e.g., fever, increased respiratory rate and decreased tidal volume. As soon as the volume of pulmonary lesions decreased and organization started, lung function and clinical signs returned to normal values. This occurred before regeneration was complete, because cattle ventilate only about 30% of the total lung volume when breathing spontaneously under resting conditions [51].

In conclusion, the experimental infection of calves with *C. psittaci* allows (1) to dissect the tissue processes involved in the development and resolution of inflammation, lesion development, neo-alveolarization, revascularization, waxing and waning of immune cell infiltrates, and fibrosis in the lung, (2) to correlate clinical with morphological findings and (3) to investigate the influence of treatment regimens on lung regeneration. These qualitative histological data may serve as basis for further in-depth studies using more advanced methods.

4. Materials and Methods

4.1. Animals

Forty-two conventionally raised calves (Holstein-Friesian, male) were included in this study. Animals originated from a farm without history of *Chlamydia*-associated health problems. Before the study, the herd of origin was regularly tested for the presence of Chlamydiae by the National Reference Laboratory for Psittacosis. Calves were purchased at the age of 14–28 days weighing between 42.2 and 71.2 kg. Animals were included in the study after a quarantine period of at least 20 days and confirmation of a clinically healthy status.

Throughout the entire study, animals were reared under standardized conditions (room climate: 18–20 °C) and in accordance with international guidelines for animal welfare. Nutrition included commercial milk replacer and coarse meal. Water and hay were supplied ad libitum. None of the given feed contained antibiotics.

This study was carried out in strict accordance with European and National Law for the Care and Use of Animals. The protocol was approved by the Committee on the Ethics of Animal Experiments and the Protection of Animals of the State of Thuringia, Germany (Permit Number: 04-002/07, 18 December 2007). All experiments were done in a containment of biosafety level 2 under supervision of the authorized institutional Agent for Animal Protection. Bronchoscopy to inoculate the pathogen was strictly performed under general anesthesia. During the entire study, every effort was made to minimize suffering.

4.2. Experimental Design

Twenty-one calves were inoculated with *C. psittaci* and twenty-one calves served as controls. The inoculum was placed at eight defined pulmonary sites by bronchoscope. Each calf underwent daily clinical examination. Groups of three calves were euthanized at 2, 3, 4, 7, 10, 14 and 35 or 37 dpi. At necropsy, distribution and extent of pulmonary lesions were determined and samples collected for histological, immunohistochemical and microbiological investigations.

4.3. Inoculum and Inoculation

C. psittaci strain 02DC15 was isolated at the Friedrich-Loeffler-Institut, Jena, Germany, from an aborted calf fetus in 2002. The isolate was classified as *C. psittaci* genotype A-VS1 by DNA microarray testing and *omp*A gene sequencing [52]. Chlamydiae were propagated in buffalo green monkey kidney cell culture using standard procedures [53]. Frozen stocks of strain 02DC15 were diluted to the required titer in stabilizing SPGA medium and used as inoculum in the present trial.

Calves were inoculated with 10^8 ifu of *C. psittaci* strain 02DC15 in 6 mL stabilizing medium SPGA (containing saccharose, phosphatile substances, glucose and bovine albumin) [54]. Control calves received the same amount of SPGA containing buffalo green monkey kidney cells.

The inoculation by bronchoscope has been described in detail [19,55]. In brief, non-fed calves were anesthetized with xylazin (0.2 mg/kg body weight, Rompun 2%, Bayer Vital GmbH, Leverkusen, Germany) and ketamine (1.7 ± 0.3 mg/kg body weight, Ursotamin, Serumwerk Bernburg AG, Bernburg, Germany). A flexible video endoscope (Veterinary Video-Endoscope PV-SG 22–140, Karl Storz GmbH and Co.KG, Germany) was inserted through the oral cavity and 0.5–1.5 mL of inoculum were placed at eight defined pulmonary sites (Figure 9).

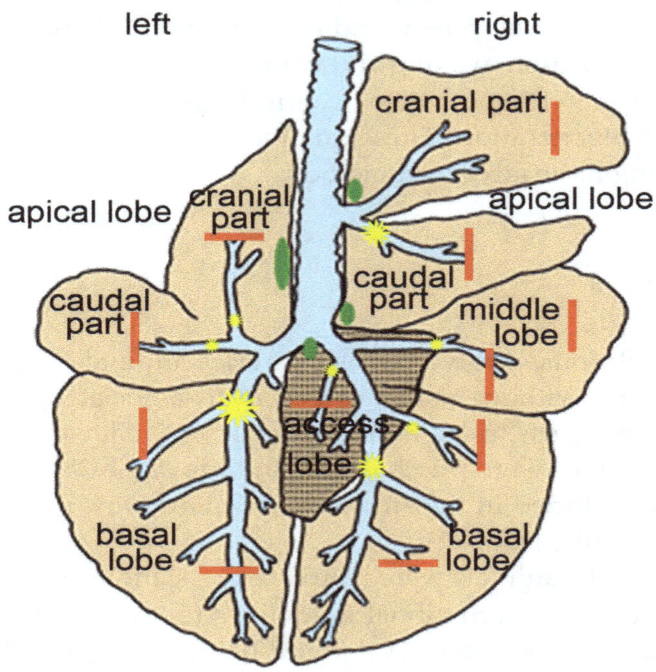

Figure 9. Schematic drawing of bovine lung. Inoculation sites are indicated as yellow stars (small—0.5 mL, middle-sized—1.0 mL and large—1.5 mL), sampling sites as red bars and and regional lymph nodes in green.

4.4. Clinical Scoring and Pulmonary Function Testing

Clinical observations were recorded twice daily and included feed intake, rectal temperature, respiratory rate and the presence or absence of clinical signs of diarrhea or respiratory disease. In addition, the appearance of oral mucosa, conjunctivae, skin, hair and dyspnea were assessed daily, and the heart rate was counted. Extremities, umbilicus and mandibular lymph nodes were palpated and inducement of cough was tested. Results were summarized using a 49-point clinical score consisting of subscores for general condition (maximum 8 points), respiratory system (maximum 17 points), cardiovascular system (maximum 13 points) and other organ systems (maximum 11 points) as described [19].

Pulmonary function testing was performed using the impulse oscillometry system (IOS) as described elsewhere [22].

4.5. Necropsy, Gross Pathology and Tissue Samples

Always three calves inoculated with chlamydiae and three controls were euthanized at 2, 3, 4, 7, 10, 14 and 35/37 dpi. In deep anesthesia (pentobarbital-sodium, 770 ± 123 mg/10 kg body weight, intravenously, Release, WdT eG, Garbsen, Germany), the trachea was exposed and large clamps were placed distal to the larynx to prevent contamination of the airways by blood or gastric contents. Subsequently, animals were sacrificed by exsanguination. The lung was removed and macroscopic lesions were recorded. To determine the total percentage of pulmonary lesions, the percentage of lesions was subjectively assessed for each lobe and multiplied by the relative percentage of the respective pulmonary lobe of the total lung volume. The volumes had been determined in 18 age-matched calves prior to this study and were measured as displacement of water. For this, the total lung volume was determined; then the different lobes were dissected, the main bronchi closed and their volume measured. On average, the left cranial and caudal apical lobes contributed 5%, the left caudal lobe 34%, the right cranial apical lobe 5%, the right caudal apical lobe 7%, the middle lobe 8%, the right caudal lobe 35% and the accessory lobe 1% to the total lung volume (Figure 9).

Samples were collected from each lung lobe (Figure 9) and fixed in 3.5% neutral buffered formalin. Sites with macroscopic lesions were preferentially sampled. Then a complete necropsy was performed.

4.6. Histopathology

Formalin-fixed tissues were embedded in paraffin after 24 h. Formalin-fixed paraffin-embedded (FFPE) tissue sections were stained with hematoxylin and eosin to evaluate lesions. Consecutive sections were stained with azan to demonstrate collagen fibers and by PAS-reaction for glycogen-rich material.

4.7. Immunohistochemistry

Consecutive FFPE tissue sections were used to label chlamydiae, epithelial cells and blood vessels by the indirect immunoperoxidase method. As primary antibodies, the anti-chlamydial-LPS antibody ACI-P500 (Progen, Heidelberg, Germany), anti-cytokeratin antibody MNF116 (Dako Denmark, Glostrup, Denmark) and anti-factor VIII polyclonal antiserum (Dako Denmark, Glostrup, Denmark) were used. Peroxidase-labeled sheep anti-mouse IgG (NA 931, GE Healthcare Europe GmbH, Freiburg, Germany) served as secondary antibody for the monoclonal antibodies and peroxidase-labeled goat anti-rabbit IgG for the polyclonal antiserum. Sections were digested with 0.05% proteinase K (Merck, Darmstadt, Germany) for antigen retrieval. Diaminobenzidine was used as chromogen.

4.8. Exclusion of Co-Infections

The herd of origin was known to be free of bovine herpes virus 1 and bovine virus diarrhea/mucosal disease virus. Routine microbiological screening revealed that all animals were negative for *Salmonella* infections (fecal swabs) and relevant enteric parasites (fecal smears). To verify relevant respiratory co-pathogens, the presence of *Mycoplasma, Pasteurella* or *Mannheimia* spp. was evaluated in nasal swabs taken immediately before challenge and before necropsy as well as in lung tissue samples obtained during necropsy. Neither *Mannheimia haemolytica* nor *Mycoplasma bovis* was detected in any sample. *Pasteurella multocida* and *Mycoplasma bovirhinis* were detected in nasal swabs, but never in any lung tissue sample. Serological findings confirmed that animals did not acquire infections with respiratory viruses relevant in bovines (i.e., bovine respiratory syncytial virus, parainfluenza 3 virus or adenovirus type 3).

Author Contributions: Conceptualization, E.M.L.-T. and P.R.; Formal analysis, J.L.; Funding acquisition, K.S. and P.R; Investigation, E.M.L.-T., J.L., C.O. and P.R.; Methodology, E.M.L.-T., J.L., C.O., K.S. and P.R.; Project administration, K.S. and P.R.; Resources, E.M.L.-T., K.S. and P.R.; Supervision, E.M.L.-T.; Visualization, E.M.L.-T. and J.L.; Writing—original draft, E.M.L.-T.; Writing—review and editing, J.L., C.O., K.S. and P.R.. All authors have read and agreed to the published version of the manuscript.

Acknowledgments: The authors are very grateful to Annelie Langenberg, Sylke Stahlberg, Ines Lemser, and all colleagues of the technical staff of the animal house for their excellent assistance while performing the in vivo phase of this study. We thank Sabine Scharf, Christine Grajetzki and Simone Bettermann for excellent technical assistance in preparation of the inocula, PCR and related techniques. Furthermore, we wish to express our gratitude to Kerstin Heidrich, Sabine Lied, Monika Godat for skillful technical assistance in the ex vivo phase, and Wolfram Maginot for excellent photographic support. Help in microbiological testing given by Ulrich Methner and Silke Keiling, Martin Heller and Susann Bahrmann, Mandy Elschner, Astrid Rassbach and Katja Fischer is gratefully acknowledged.

Abbreviations

AEC1	type 1 alveolar epithelial cells
AEC2	type 2 alveolar epithelial cells
BALT	bronchus-associated lymphoid tissue
C.	chlamydia
CAP	community acquired pneumonia
dpi	days after inoculation
FFPE	formalin-fixed paraffin embedded tissue
ifu	inclusion-forming units
IL	interleukin

References

1. Marshall, D.C.; Goodson, R.J.; Xu, Y.; Komorowski, M.; Shalhoub, J.; Maruthappu, M.; Salciccioli, J.D. Trends in mortality from pneumonia in the Europe union: A temporal analysis of the European detailed mortality database between 2001 and 2014. *Resp. Res.* **2018**, *19*, 81. [CrossRef]
2. Welte, T.; Torres, A.; Nathwani, D. Clinical and economic burden of community-acquired pneumonia among adults in Europe. *Thorax* **2012**, *67*, 71–79. [CrossRef]
3. Cillóniz, C.; Torres, A.; Niederman, M.; van der Eerden, M.; Chalmers, J.; Welte, T.; Blasi, F. Community-acquired pneumonia related to intracellular pathogens. *Intensive Care Med.* **2016**, *42*, 1374–1386. [CrossRef]
4. Torres, A.; Blasi, F.; Peetermans, W.E.; Viegi, G.; Welte, T. The aetiology and antibiotic management of community-acquired pneumonia in adults in Europe: A literature review. *Eur. J. Clin. Microbiol. Infect. Dis.* **2014**, *33*, 1065–1079. [CrossRef]
5. Wubbel, L.; Muniz, L.; Ahmed, A.; Trujillo, M.; Carubelli, C.; Mccoig, C.; Abramo, T.; Leinonen, M.; McCracken, G.H., Jr. Etiology and treatment of community-acquired pneumonia in ambulatory children. *Pediatr. Infect. Dis. J.* **1999**, *43*, 876–881. [CrossRef] [PubMed]
6. Dumke, R.; Schnee, C.; Pletz, M.W.; Rupp, J.; Jacobs, E.; Sachse, K.; Rohde, G.; CAPNETZ Study Group. Mycoplasma pneumoniae and Chlamydia spp. infection in community-acquired pneumonia, Germany, 2011–2012. *Emerg. Infect. Dis.* **2015**, *21*, 426–434. [CrossRef] [PubMed]
7. Spoorenberg, S.M.C.; Bos, W.J.W.; van Hannen, E.J.; Dijkstra, F.; Heddema, E.R.; van Velzen-Blad, H.; Heijligenberg, R.; Grutters, J.C.; de Jongh, B.M.; Ovidius Study Group. *Chlamydia psittaci*: A relevant cause of community-acquired pneumonia in two Dutch hospitals. *Neth. J. Med.* **2016**, 75–81.
8. Herriges, M.; Morrisey, E.E. Lung development: Orchestrating the generation and regeneration of a complex organ. *Development* **2014**, *141*, 502–513. [CrossRef]
9. Zemans, R.L.; Henson, P.M.; Henson, J.E.; Janssen, W.J. Conceptual approaches to lung injury and repair. *Ann. Am. Thorac. Soc.* **2015**, *12*, S9–S15. [CrossRef]
10. Slauson, D.O.; Hahn, F.F. Criteria for development of animal models of diseases of the respiratory system. *Am. J. Pathol.* **1980**, *101*, 103–122.
11. Bonniaud, P.; Fabre, A.; Frossard, N.; Guignabert, C.; Inman, M.; Kuebler, W.M.; Maes, T.; Shi, W.; Stampfli, M.; Uhlig, S.; et al. Optimising experimental research in respiratory diseases: An ERS statement. *Eur. Respir. J.* **2018**, *51*, 1702133. [CrossRef] [PubMed]
12. Ireland, J.J.; Roberts, R.M.; Palmer, G.H.; Bauman, D.E.; Bazer, F.W. A commentary on domestic animals as

dual-purpose models that benefit agricultural and biomedical research. *J. Anim. Sci.* **2008**, *86*, 2797–2805. [CrossRef] [PubMed]

13. Tsaia, Y.-F.; Kub, Y.-H. Necrotizing pneumonia: A rare complication of pneumonia requiring special consideration. *Curr. Opin. Pulm. Med.* **2012**, *1*, 246–252. [CrossRef] [PubMed]
14. Krutikov, M.; Rahman, A.; Tiberi, S. Necrotizing pneumonia (aetiology, clinical features and management). *Curr. Opin. Pulm. Med.* **2019**, *25*, 225–232. [CrossRef] [PubMed]
15. Hilton, B.; Tavare, A.N.; Creer, D. Necrotising pneumonia caused by non-PVL Staphylococcus aureus with 2-year follow-up. *BMJ Case Rep.* **2017**. Published Online First: 28.11.2017, bcr-2017-221779. [CrossRef]
16. Sawicki, G.S.; Lu, F.L.; Valim, C.; Cleveland, R.H.; Colin, A.A. Necrotising pneumonia is an increasingly detected complication of pneumonia in children. *Eur. Respir. J.* **2008**, *31*, 1285–1291. [CrossRef]
17. Alifano, M.; Lorut, C.; Lefebvre, A.; Khattar, L.; Damotte, D.; Huchon, G.; Regnard, J.-F.; Rabbat, A. Necrotizing pneumonia in adults: Multidisciplinary management. *Intens. Care Med.* **2011**, *37*, 1888–1889. [CrossRef]
18. Koivula, I.; Stén, M.; Mäkelä, P.H. Prognosis after community-acquired pneumonia in the elderly: A population-based 12-year follow-up study. *Arch. Intern. Med.* **1999**, *159*, 1550–1555. [CrossRef]
19. Reinhold, P.; Ostermann, C.; Liebler-Tenorio, E.; Berndt, A.; Vogel, A.; Lambertz, J.; Rothe, M.; Rüttger, A.; Schubert, E.; Sachse, K. A bovine model of respiratory Chlamydia psittaci infection: Challenge dose titration. *PLoS ONE* **2012**, *7*, e30125. [CrossRef]
20. Ostermann, C.; Schroedl, W.; Schubert, E.; Sachse, K.; Reinhold, P. Dose-dependent effects of *Chlamydia psittaci* infection on pulmonary gas exchange, innate immunity and acute-phase reaction in a bovine respiratory model. *Vet. J.* **2013**, *196*, 351–359. [CrossRef]
21. Ostermann, C.; Rüttger, A.; Schubert, E.; Schrödl, W.; Sachse, K.; Reinhold, P. Infection, disease, and transmission dynamics in calves after experimental and natural challenge with a bovine *Chlamydia psittaci* isolate. *PLoS ONE* **2013**, *8*, e64066. [CrossRef] [PubMed]
22. Ostermann, C.; Linde, S.; Siegling-Vlitakis, C.; Reinhold, P. Evaluation of pulmonary dysfunctions and acid–base imbalances induced by *Chlamydia psittaci* in a bovine model of respiratory infection. *Multidiscip. Respir. Med.* **2014**, *9*, 10. [CrossRef] [PubMed]
23. Prohl, A.; Lohr, M.; Ostermann, C.; Liebler-Tenorio, E.; Berndt, A.; Schroedl, W.; Rothe, M.; Schubert, E.; Sachse, K.; Reinhold, P. Enrofloxacin and macrolides alone or in combination with rifampicin as antimicrobial treatment in a bovine model of acute *Chlamydia psittaci* infection. *PLoS ONE* **2015**, *10*, e0119736. [CrossRef] [PubMed]
24. Prohl, A.; Lohr, M.; Ostermann, C.; Liebler-Tenorio, E.; Berndt, A.; Schroedl, W.; Rothe, M.; Schubert, E.; Sachse, K.; Reinhold, P. Evaluation of antimicrobial treatment in a bovine model of acute *Chlamydia psittaci* infection: Tetracycline versus tetracycline plus rifampicin. *FEMS Pathog. Dis.* **2015**, *73*, 1–12.
25. Panciera, R.J.; Confer, A.W. Pathogenesis and pathology of bovine pneumonia. *Vet. Clin. North. Am. Food Anim. Pract.* **2010**, *26*, 191–214. [CrossRef]
26. Beers, M.F.; Morrisey, E.E. The three R's of lung health and disease: Repair, remodeling, and regeneration. *J. Clin. Investig.* **2011**, *121*, 2065–2073. [CrossRef]
27. Virok, D.P.; Nelson, D.E.; Whitmire, W.M.; Crane, D.D.; Goheen, M.M.; Caldwell, H.D. Chlamydial infection induces pathobiotype-specific protein tyrosine phosphorylation in epithelial cells. *Infect. Immun.* **2005**, *73*, 1939–1946. [CrossRef]
28. Rasmussen, S.J.; Eckmann, L.; Quayle, A.J.; Shen, L.; Zhang, Y.-X.; Anderson, D.J.; Fierer, J.; Stephens, R.S.; Kagnoff, M.F. Secretion of proinflammatory cytokines by epithelial cells in response to chlamydia infection suggests a central role for epithelial cells in chlamydial pathogenesis. *J. Clin. Investig.* **1997**, *99*, 77–87. [CrossRef]
29. Jahn, H.-U.; Krüll, M.; Wuppermann, F.N.; Klucken, A.C.; Rosseau, S.; Seybold, J.; Hegemann, J.H.; Jantos, C.A.; Suttorp, N. Infection and activation of airway epithelial cells by *Chlamydia pneumoniae*. *J. Infect. Dis.* **2000**, *182*, 1678–1687. [CrossRef]
30. Vanella, K.M.; Wynn, T.A. Mechanism of organ injury and repair by macrophages. *Annu. Rev. Physiol.* **2017**, *79*, 593–617. [CrossRef]
31. Kovtun, A.; Messerer, D.A.C.; Scharffetter-Kochanek, K.; Huber-Lang, M.; Ignatius, A. Neutrophils in tissue trauma of the Skin, bone, and lung: Two sides of the same coin. *J. Immunol. Res.* **2018**, *2018*, 8173983. [CrossRef] [PubMed]

32. Carden, D.; Xiao, F.; Moak, C.; Willis, B.H.; Robinson-Jackson, S.; Alexander, S. Neutrophil elastase promotes lung microvascular injury and proteolysis of endothelial cadherins. *Am. J. Physiol.* **1998**, *275*, H385–H392. [CrossRef] [PubMed]
33. Ginzberg, H.H.; Cherapanov, V.; Dong, Q.; Cantin, A.; McCulloch, C.A.G.; Shannon, P.T.; Downey, G.P. Neutrophil-mediated epithelial injury during transmigration: Role of elastase. *Am. J. Physiol. Gastrointest. Liver Physiol.* **2001**, *281*, G705–G717. [CrossRef]
34. Car, B.D.; Suyemoto, M.M.; Neilsen, N.R.; Slauson, D.O. The role of leukocytes in the pathogenesis of fibrin deposition in bovine acute lung injury. *Am. J. Pathol.* **1991**, *138*, 1191–1198. [PubMed]
35. Wygrecka, M.; Jablonska, E.; Guenther, A.; Preissner, K.T.; Markart, P. Current view on alveolar coagulation and fibrinolysis in acute inflammatory and chronic interstitial lung diseases. *Thromb. Haemost.* **2008**, *99*, 494–501. [PubMed]
36. Puttur, F.; Gregory, L.G.; Lloyd, C.M. Airway macrophages as the guardians of tissue repair in the lung. *Immunol. Cell. Biol.* **2019**, *97*, 246–257. [CrossRef] [PubMed]
37. Wallace, W.A.; Fitch, P.M.; Simpson, A.J.; Howie, S.E. Inflammation-associated remodelling and fibrosis in the lung - a process and an end point. *Int. J. Exp. Pathol.* **2007**, *88*, 103–110. [CrossRef]
38. Lopez, A. Respiratory System. In *Pathologic Basis of Veterinary Disease*, 4th ed.; McGavin, M.D., Zachary, J.F., Eds.; Mosby Elsevier: St. Louis, MO, USA, 2007; pp. 509–513.
39. Roan, N.R.; Starnbach, M.N. Immune-mediated control of chlamydia infection. *Cell. Microbiol.* **2008**, *10*, 9–19. [CrossRef]
40. Evans, M.J.; Cabral, L.J.; Stephens, R.J.; Freeman, G. Transformation of alveolar type 2 cells to type 1 cells following exposure to NO_2. *Exp. Mol. Pathol.* **1975**, *22*, 142–150. [CrossRef]
41. Chen, F.; Fine, A. Stem cells in lung injury and repair. *Am. J. Pathol.* **2016**, *186*, 2544–2550. [CrossRef]
42. Tata, P.R.; Rajagopal, J. Plasticity in the lung: Making and breaking cell identity. *Development* **2017**, *144*, 755–766. [CrossRef] [PubMed]
43. Barkauskas, C.E.; Cronce, M.J.; Rackley, C.R.; Bowie, E.J.; Keene, D.R.; Stripp, B.R.; Randell, S.H.; Noble, P.W.; Hogan, B.L. Type 2 alveolar cells are stem cells in adult lung. *J. Clin. Investig.* **2013**, *123*, 3025–3036. [CrossRef] [PubMed]
44. Fang, K.C. Mesenchymal regulation of alveolar repair in pulmonary fibrosis. *Am. J. Respir. Cell. Mol. Biol.* **2000**, *23*, 142–145. [CrossRef] [PubMed]
45. Vracko, R. Basal lamina scaffold-anatomy and significance for maintenance of orderly tissue structure. *Am. J. Pathol.* **1974**, *77*, 314–346. [PubMed]
46. Jain, R.; Barkauskas, C.E.; Takeda, N.; Bowie, E.J.; Aghajanian, H.; Wang, Q.; Padmanabhan, A.; Manderfield, L.J.; Gupta, M.; Li, D.; et al. Plasticity of Hopx(+) type I alveolar cells to regenerate type II cells in the lung. *Nat. Commun.* **2015**, *6*, 6727. [CrossRef] [PubMed]
47. Rodríguez-Castillo, J.A.; Pérez, D.B.; Ntokou, A.; Seeger, W.; Morty, R.E.; Ahlbrecht, K. Understanding alveolarization to induce lung regeneration. *BMC Respir. Res.* **2018**, *19*, 148. [CrossRef]
48. De Smet, F.; Segura, I.; De Bock, K.; Hohensinner, P.J.; Carmeliet, P. Mechanisms of vessel branching: Filopodia on endothelial tip cells lead the way. *Arterioscler. Thromb. Vasc. Biol.* **2009**, *29*, 639–649. [CrossRef]
49. Chua, F.; Gauldie, J.; Laurent, G.J. Pulmonary fibrosis: Searching for model answers. *Am. J. Respir. Cell. Mol. Biol.* **2005**, *33*, 9–13. [CrossRef]
50. Izbicki, G.; Segel, M.J.; Christensen, T.G.; Conner, M.W.; Breuer, R. Time course of bleomycin-induced lung fibrosis. *Int. J. Exp. Pathol.* **2002**, *83*, 111–119. [CrossRef]
51. Veit, H.P.; Farrell, R.L. The anatomy and physiology of the bovine respiratory system relating to pulmonary disease. *Cornell Vet.* **1978**, *68*, 555–581.
52. Sachse, K.; Laroucau, K.; Vorimore, F.; Magnino, S.; Feige, J.; Müller, W.; Kube, S.; Hotzel, H.; Schubert, E.; Slickers, P.; et al. DNA microarray-based genotyping of *Chlamydophila psittaci* strains from culture and clinical samples. *Vet. Microbiol.* **2009**, *135*, 22–30. [CrossRef] [PubMed]
53. Goellner, S.; Schubert, E.; Liebler-Tenorio, E.; Hotzel, H.; Saluz, H.P.; Sachse, K. Transcriptional response patterns of *Chlamydophila psittaci* in different in vitro models of persistent infection. *Infect. Immun.* **2006**, *74*, 4801–4808. [CrossRef] [PubMed]
54. Bovarick, M.R.; Miller, J.C.; Snyder, J.C. The influence of certain salts, amino acids, sugars, and proteins on

the stability of rickettsiae. *J. Bacteriol.* **1950**, *59*, 509–522. [CrossRef]
55. Prohl, A.; Ostermann, C.; Lohr, M.; Reinhold, P. The bovine lung in biomedical research: Visually guided bronchoscopy, intrabronchial inoculation and in vivo sampling techniques. *J. Vis. Exp.* **2014**, *89*, e51557. [CrossRef]

14

Mechanisms of ATII-to-ATI Cell Differentiation during Lung Regeneration

Mohit Aspal [1] **and Rachel L. Zemans** [2,3,*]

[1] College of Literature, Science and the Arts, University of Michigan, Ann Arbor, MI 48109, USA; aspalmoh@umich.edu

[2] Division of Pulmonary and Critical Care Medicine, Department of Internal Medicine, University of Michigan, 109 Zina Pitcher Place, Ann Arbor, MI 48109-2200, USA

[3] Program in Cellular and Molecular Biology, University of Michigan, Ann Arbor, MI 48109, USA

* Correspondence: zemansr@med.umich.edu

Abstract: The alveolar epithelium consists of (ATI) and type II (ATII) cells. ATI cells cover the majority of the alveolar surface due to their thin, elongated shape and are largely responsible for barrier function and gas exchange. During lung injury, ATI cells are susceptible to injury, including cell death. Under some circumstances, ATII cells also die. To regenerate lost epithelial cells, ATII cells serve as progenitor cells. They proliferate to create new ATII cells and then differentiate into ATI cells. Regeneration of ATI cells is critical to restore normal barrier and gas exchange function. Although the signaling pathways by which ATII cells proliferate have been explored, the mechanisms of ATII-to-ATI cell differentiation have not been well studied until recently. New studies have uncovered signaling pathways that mediate ATII-to-ATI differentiation. Bone morphogenetic protein (BMP) signaling inhibits ATII proliferation and promotes differentiation. Wnt/β-catenin and ETS variant transcription factor 5 (Etv5) signaling promote proliferation and inhibit differentiation. Delta-like 1 homolog (Dlk1) leads to a precisely timed inhibition of Notch signaling in later stages of alveolar repair, activating differentiation. Yes-associated protein/Transcriptional coactivator with PDZ-binding motif (YAP/TAZ) signaling appears to promote both proliferation and differentiation. We recently identified a novel transitional cell state through which ATII cells pass as they differentiate into ATI cells, and this has been validated by others in various models of lung injury. This intermediate cell state is characterized by the activation of Transforming growth factor beta (TGFβ) and other pathways, and some evidence suggests that TGFβ signaling induces and maintains this state. While the abovementioned signaling pathways have all been shown to be involved in ATII-to-ATI cell differentiation during lung regeneration, there is much that remains to be understood. The up- and down-stream signaling events by which these pathways are activated and by which they induce ATI cell differentiation are unknown. In addition, it is still unknown how the various mechanistic steps from each pathway interact with one another to control differentiation. Based on these recent studies that identified major signaling pathways driving ATII-to-ATI differentiation during alveolar regeneration, additional studies can be devised to understand the interaction between these pathways as they work in a coordinated manner to regulate differentiation. Moreover, the knowledge from these studies may eventually be used to develop new clinical treatments that accelerate epithelial cell regeneration in individuals with excessive lung damage, such as patients with the Acute Respiratory Distress Syndrome (ARDS), pulmonary fibrosis, and emphysema.

Keywords: alveolar epithelium; lung injury; lung regeneration

---

1. Introduction

There are two types of cells in the alveolar epithelium: large, flattened alveolar type I (ATI) cells that cover 95%–98% of the alveolar surface and permit gas exchange and cuboidal alveolar type II (ATII) cells that are the progenitor cells responsible for regenerating ATI and ATII cells during homeostasis and after injury [1–3]. The lung epithelium serves as a barrier that protects the body from airborne pathogens and prevents leakage of bodily fluids into the airspaces. In the event of epithelial cell death, such as during infection or after exposure to cigarette smoke, the barrier is compromised. During homeostasis, alveolar epithelial cells have a long but limited lifespan [1]. After the death of an occasional alveolar epithelial cell, barrier function is maintained by adequate levels of ATII cell proliferation and differentiation to replace the lost cells. During lung injury, excessive epithelial cell death results in impaired barrier function. ATI cells are particularly susceptible to injury, but ATII cells can die in cases of severe or certain types of injury.

It has long been known that ATII cells are the principal progenitor responsible for regenerating the injured alveolar epithelium [1,4–6], although it is increasingly recognized that other progenitors can be mobilized under certain circumstances [7–9]. ATII cells proliferate to replace lost cells, and once sufficient cell numbers have been restored, some differentiate into ATI cells to restore normal alveolar structure. Since ATI cells are largely responsible for barrier function and gas exchange, the regeneration of ATI cells is absolutely critical to restore normal lung function. Signaling pathways that promote ATII cell proliferation have been identified by us and others and include keratinocyte growth factor (KGF), hepatocyte growth factor (HGF), epidermal growth factor (EGF), Wnt/β-catenin, forkhead box protein M1 (FoxM1), and others [10–20]. Although we have some understanding of the mechanisms that drive ATII cell proliferation, the signaling pathways that drive ATII-to-ATI cell differentiation have remained elusive. Recently, in large part due to the emergence of lineage tracing technology [21], several studies have uncovered various signaling pathways shown to be involved in this differentiation step: Wnt/β-catenin, Notch, YAP/TAZ, BMP, and TGFβ. Here, we discuss this recent work and the contribution these studies have made to advance our understanding of lung regeneration. We also briefly discuss future research questions that can be examined based on the strong foundation established by this handful of studies. For example, the various signaling pathways identified to regulate ATI cell differentiation undoubtedly interact with one another in a coordinated manner to control differentiation. However, the way they interact—whether they operate upstream, downstream, or parallel to one another—is still unknown. In addition, future studies will be necessary to confirm the extent to which these pathways, identified in mouse models of regeneration, are active in the human lung. Strengthened understanding of the mechanisms involved in ATII-to-ATI cell differentiation ultimately may lead to development of new clinical treatments that accelerate lung repair in individuals with excessive lung damage, such as patients with Acute Respiratory Distress Syndrome (ARDS), pulmonary fibrosis, and emphysema.

2. Wnt/β-Catenin Signaling

We previously reported that inhibition of Wnt/β-catenin signaling prevented ATII cell proliferation during regeneration after lung injury [13]. More recently, elegant studies using lineage tracing and inducible ATII cell-specific gene deficient mice have confirmed that Wnt/β-catenin signaling is critical for ATII cell proliferation after lung injury in multiple models [14,15]. Interestingly, these studies also identified a small subset of ATII cells that function as alveolar stem cells during homeostasis. These stem cells are responsible for maintaining ATII cells during homeostatic turnover and do so in a Wnt/β-catenin-dependent manner. Moreover, during homeostasis, adjacent PDGFRα+ fibroblasts are the source of secreted Wnts, which maintain the ATII cells and are thus considered to be the niche of the ATII stem cells. Wnt signaling is required not only for ATII cell proliferation but also for maintenance of the ATII cell phenotype, as knockout of β-catenin induces differentiation into ATI cells. Following lung injury, the larger population of ATII cells that is mobilized to proliferate themselves produce Wnts, stimulating proliferation via autocrine signaling even in ATII cells outside the niche [14]. Presumably, the Wnt signaling that maintains the ATII cell phenotype during homeostasis also does so during ATII cell proliferation during regeneration and must be downregulated to permit ATII-to-ATI differentiation.

3. Notch Signaling

Notch signaling has been strongly implicated in proliferation and differentiation in many organs. After embryonic tissue development, such as the development of the lung epithelium, the expression of the Notch ligand delta-like 1 homolog (Dlk1) disappears, returning only in some adult tissues undergoing regeneration. A recent landmark study uncovered the role of Notch, specifically Dlk1, in alveolar regeneration. In acute lung injury, temporal regulation of Notch signaling by Dlk1 was shown to have a role in alveolar repair, promoting ATII-to-ATI differentiation. In *Pseudomonas aeruginosa*-induced mice lung injury model, Dlk1 leads to a precisely timed inhibition of Notch signaling in later stages of alveolar repair, which activates differentiation [22]. The regenerative role of Dlk1 in alveolar differentiation was supported by several experimental studies. Experiments using inducible ATII cell-specific *Dlk1* mutant mice, lineage-tracing studies, RNA-seq, Notch reporter and ATII-specific constitutively active Notch mice revealed that Notch signaling is initially activated in ATII cells during the proliferation phase, but that later, Notch signaling is downregulated by Dlk1 as ATII cells differentiate into ATI cells [22]. This high-to-low Notch switch was essential for ATII cell differentiation into ATI cells. In ATII cell-specific *Dlk1* conditional knockout mice, high Notch activation is sustained. This results in delayed ATI cell differentiation and the accumulation of an intermediate cell population of alveolar epithelial cells that expressed low levels of both ATI and ATII cell markers. This phenotype was partially rescued by Notch inhibition [22]. In conclusion, Notch signaling is activated during the proliferation phase of alveolar regeneration but is later deactivated due to Dlk1 upregulation, promoting ATII-to-ATI cell differentiation. However, a key remaining unknown is how Dlk1 expression is regulated. If Dlk1 upregulation is a critical signal for inducing ATI cell differentiation, understanding the factors upstream of Dlk1 expression will be key for understanding the overall regulation of ATII-to-ATI cell differentiation.

4. BMP/SMAD Signaling

Bone morphogenetic protein (BMP) signaling in mammalian systems has been shown to play a variety of complex roles in proliferation and differentiation in many organs. Recently, a seminal study demonstrated that dynamic changes in BMP signaling play a critical role in alveolar regeneration [23]. BMP signaling is active in the vast majority of ATII and ATI cells during homeostasis. During regeneration, BMP signaling is downregulated during ATII cell proliferation and then upregulated during ATI cell differentiation. This activation and deactivation of BMP signaling is attributable to dynamic expression of BMP ligands, receptors, and antagonists. Moreover, using both pharmacologic and genetic approaches in cultured alveolar organoids and mice, the investigators demonstrated that BMP inhibits ATII cell proliferation and promotes ATII-to-ATI cell differentiation. Interestingly, the fibroblasts that constitute the ATII cell niche also display a reduction in BMP signaling during ATII cell proliferation, with a rebound during ATII-to-ATI cell differentiation. BMP gain of function in the fibroblasts had no effect on fibroblast proliferation but similarly inhibited ATII cell proliferation [23]. Taken together, these data suggest that during homeostasis, active BMP signaling maintains ATII cell quiescence; during regeneration, deactivation of BMP signaling promotes ATII cell proliferation, whereas reactivation of BMP signaling promotes ATI cell differentiation. This finding establishes a strong foundation upon which future questions may be addressed: What is the mechanism by which BMP signaling inhibits ATII cell proliferation? Does it directly inhibit the cell cycle or does it prime ATII cells to be less responsive to known mitogens such as KGF, HGF, Wnt, and EGF? Similarly, how does BMP signaling induce ATI cell differentiation? More generally, the observations that BMP signaling simultaneously inhibits proliferation and drives differentiation suggests that proliferation may not be a necessary prerequisite for differentiation. Finally, the mechanisms by which BMP signaling in fibroblasts limits their ability to promote ATII cell proliferation are unknown at this time.

5. Yap/Taz Signaling

YAP and TAZ are important transcription coactivators in the Hippo signaling pathway known to be involved in embryonic development, homeostasis, and tissue regeneration after injury. An elegant recent study has shown YAP/TAZ to play a crucial role in ATII-to-ATI differentiation in alveolar repair [24]. In the Streptococcus pneumoniae model of lung injury, YAP and TAZ expression and nuclear localization increased in ATII cells after lung injury. Moreover, ATII cell specific Yap/Taz knockout mice displayed impaired ATII cell proliferation and ATII-to-ATI cell differentiation during regeneration. These mice also developed fibrotic lesions, consistent with the widely accepted view that impaired epithelial regeneration begets fibrosis. The expression of several genes known to promote cell proliferation and differentiation, including FGFs, Wnts, EGFR, and BMP4, were reduced in YAP/TAZ deficient ATII cells, although it is as of yet unknown whether these genes mediate the role of YAP/TAZ signaling in ATII cell proliferation and differentiation. Another study used alveolar organoid cultures and the bleomycin model of lung injury to demonstrate the role of TAZ signaling in ATII-to-ATI cell differentiation [25]. In this study, TAZ nuclear localization was observed in ATI but not ATII cells. Moreover, pharmacologic inhibitors and TAZ knockout prevented ATII-to-ATI cell differentiation in organoids. In the bleomycin lung injury model, conditional deletion of TAZ in ATII cells also led to reduced ATI cell regeneration and, as in the S. pneumoniae model, resulted in greater fibrosis. Interestingly, the ATII cell-specific YAP/TAZ knockout mice exhibited prolonged inflammation, apparently due to an inability to upregulate Inhibitor-of-NFκB, alpha (IκBα), a repressor of Nuclear-Factor κB (NFκB). Chromatin immunoprecipitation (ChIP) experiments in an alveolar epithelial cell line suggested that IκBα is a direct YAP/TAZ target gene. Moreover, Yap/Taz knockdown inhibited, whereas Yap/TAZ overexpression increased, IκBα. Moreover, IκBα overexpression attenuated the prolonged inflammation, delay in alveolar regeneration, and fibrosis observed in YAP/TAZ knockout mice. In contrast to the S. pneumoniae model, there was no defect in proliferation of TAZ KO ATII cells. A third study using the pneumonectomy model of compensatory lung growth revealed that YAP signaling is activated in ATII cells and ATII cell specific deletion of YAP inhibited ATII cell proliferation and ATII-to-ATI cell differentiation [26]. YAP inhibition also decreases proliferation during homeostasis [27]. However, despite its role in ATII-to-ATI cell differentiation during regeneration [24–26] and development [25], it appears that this pathway is dispensable for normal ATI cell turnover during lung homeostasis.

6. Recruited Macrophages

During alveolar regeneration in many models, the lung monocyte/macrophage population expands. Monocyte-derived macrophages are recruited from the circulation, and resident alveolar macrophages proliferate [28–30]. Some of these macrophages contribute to epithelial injury [31], but some are likely to contribute to repair. A landmark study showed that preventing the recruitment of monocyte-derived macrophages via genetic deletion of the monocyte chemokine receptor CCR2 impaired ATII cell proliferation and ATII-to-ATI cell differentiation [32]. The recruited macrophages displayed an M2-like gene expression signature, consistent with their reparative phenotype. Knockout of the receptor that skews macrophages towards an M2 phenotype, IL4RA, resulted in impaired regeneration. Additional experimentation suggested that IL13 derived from ILC2s may contribute to M2 polarization during lung regeneration. Taken together, these data suggest a critical role for recruited M2 macrophages in alveolar regeneration. Although the full panel of mediators that macrophages secrete to induce alveolar regeneration remains to be determined, a couple of studies have elucidated a role for macrophage-derived mediators in ATII cell proliferation. One elegant study several years ago suggested that macrophage-derived TNFα stimulates ATII cell production of Granulocyte-macrophage colony-stimulating factor (GM-CSF), which induces ATII cell proliferation via autocrine signaling [33]. A more recent study suggested that macrophage TFF2 signaling induced expression of Wnts, which promote ATII cell proliferation [34].

7. Cdc42

In a series of studies, Nan Tang et al. demonstrated that mechanical tension induced by pneumonectomy results in actin polymerization and spreading of regenerating ATII cells [26]. Under these circumstances, ATII cell-specific deletion of Cell division control protein 42 homolog (Cdc42) inhibited ATII cell proliferation and actin polymerization [26,35]. Moreover, Cdc42 deficient ATII cells fail to differentiate into ATI cells [35]. In fact, the investigators observed that new alveoli failed to form after pneumonectomy, resulting in an enlargement of existing alveoli. Eventually, these mice developed fibrosis, linking a failure of ATI cell regeneration to fibrosis.

8. Etv5 Signaling

The ETS family transcription factor ETV5, previously implicated in lung development [36], was recently shown to be necessary for ATII cell proliferation and the maintenance of ATII cell identity in the adult lung. ETV5 deficiency induced ATII-to-ATI cell differentiation both in vitro and during homeostasis in vivo [37]. In the bleomycin model of lung injury, Etv5 deficiency resulted in impaired ATII cell proliferation with enhanced ATII-to-ATI cell differentiation. Etv5 deficiency also reduced ATII cell proliferation in the Kras model of lung cancer. ChIP-seq identified Etv5 binding sites in the promoters of ATI and ATII cell genes but the specific genes that were enriched and whether the regulation of gene expression is direct is unknown.

9. TGFβ

To identify additional candidate signaling pathways that may regulate ATII-to-ATI cell differentiation, we performed single cell RNA sequencing on lineage tagged ATII cells during regeneration in the LPS model of lung injury [38]. We identified three transitional cell states: (1) proliferating ATII cells indicated by high expression of cell cycle markers such as *mKi67* and *Pcna*, (2) an intermediate cell state characterized by high expression of markers of cell cycle arrest such as p15 and p53 as well as downregulation of ATII cell markers and modest upregulation of ATI cell markers, and (3) differentiating ATII cells characterized by further upregulation of ATI cell markers than approaches that of mature ATI cells. Other groups subsequently identified a similar intermediate cell state in various models of regeneration [35,39–41], strongly suggesting that the mechanisms of regeneration are conserved regardless of the type of initial injury. Further interrogation of the gene expression profiles of these transitional cell states, including pathway analysis, revealed activation of specific pathways. Specifically, TGFβ signaling was low in the proliferating cells, highly upregulated in the intermediate cells state, and then downregulated in differentiating cells. Additional in vitro experiments suggested that TGFβ signaling is necessary to induce proliferating cells to exit the cell cycle but subsequent downregulation of TGFβ may promote differentiation. However, the role of TGFβ in alveolar regeneration in vivo and the function of the many other pathways identified by the scRNAseq studies requires additional investigation. The pathogenesis of pulmonary fibrosis is widely believed to arise from ineffectual regeneration of the alveolar epithelium after injury, although the specific regenerative defect has been unknown. Since pulmonary fibrosis is characterized by hyperplasia of alveolar epithelial cells with a morphology that is transitional between ATII and ATI cells and is driven by unchecked TGFβ activation, we hypothesized that the specific regenerative defect driving fibrosis may be an arrest in the ATII-ATI intermediate state. We confirmed the persistence of this intermediate state in both the bleomycin mouse model of pulmonary fibrosis and in human pulmonary fibrosis [42].

10. Limitations

Despite the recent progress made in studies of ATII-to-ATI differentiation, several experimental limitations must be discussed. One experimental constraint stems from the difficulty of isolating the differentiation stage in in vivo models of regeneration. As mentioned, ATII cell proliferation typically precedes ATII-to-ATI cell differentiation. In most of the studies discussed above, gene deletion was induced prior to injury, thus, any effect observed on the rate of differentiation may be confounded by an effect on the preceding proliferation phase. In other words, if gene knockout impairs both proliferation and differentiation, it may be hard to discern whether this gene plays a direct role in differentiation or whether the impaired differentiation is a consequence of impaired proliferation. Of course, this assumes that ATII-to-ATI cell differentiation requires a preceding round of replication; the extent to which ATII-to-ATI cell differentiation might occur with a preceding round of replication is unknown.

Another limitation lies in the methods for quantification of proliferation and differentiation. Many commonly used models of lung injury are characterized by quite mild ATI cell loss and regeneration. The percent of ATI cells that are regenerated by ATII cells at the end of regeneration is approximately 3%–4% [20,21]. This is presumably the percent of ATI cells that were lost during injury (unless non-ATII cell progenitors differentiate into ATI cells). Given the low degree of ATI cell injury and regeneration, it is difficult to study the effects of interventions such as gene knockout or drugs. Highly accurate and high throughput techniques are necessary to discern a decrease in ATI cell differentiation below an already low level. In more severe injury models, the degree of ATI cell loss and regeneration may be slightly higher but is typically accompanied by loss of ATII cells, which is the cell type of interest, and this can lead to the mobilization of alternate progenitors [8,9], further confounding interpretation. A final issue relates to the quantitation of proliferation and differentiation in an unbiased manner. The above discussed studies use many different methods to quantify proliferation and differentiation. Many studies assess ATII cell proliferation by counting cell profiles per high power field or by the number of cells detectable by flow cytometry after lung digest, methods that are subject to bias [43]. Most studies quantitate ATII-to-ATI cell differentiation using images captured by fluorescent microscopy of tissue stained for a membrane ATI cell protein. The resolution of fluorescent microscopy, even confocal, is low enough that individual ATI cells cannot be counted. To overcome this limitation, many researchers measure the surface area of the labeled cells as they appear in cross section. Differentiation is then quantitated as the percent of total ATI cells that are lineage labeled. This is a reasonable approach if the denominator, the total ATI cells, remains constant, which may or not be the case in inflammatory lung injury but is not the case during compensatory regrowth after pneumonectomy in which new septa are created. Use of flow cytometry to count ATI cell number, which has been used, is likely to be quite inaccurate due to the difficulty recovering intact ATI cells after lung injury. Although counting ATII or ATI cell number [43] and measuring the actual surface area of ATI cells [21] by stereology may be the most unbiased approach available, this method requires specialized expertise and is tedious. Ideally, investigators in the field would use a common methodology that is accurate but also high throughput enough to detect small differences. In the meantime, it is important that investigators understand and recognize the biases inherent to the approaches they use.

11. Future Directions

In summary, based on solid studies, it appears that YAP/TAZ, Cdc42, Notch, BMP, TGFβ, and Etv5 signaling pathways are involved in the regulation of ATII-to-ATI cell differentiation during alveolar regeneration. In the future, additional research should be done to better understand this regulation. First, in most cases, the upstream stimuli that activate these pathways are unknown. In the case of the pneumonectomy model, mechanical tension is the trigger for Cdc42 and YAP activation, but it is unknown what might activate YAP/TAZ signaling in other models of lung injury. As discussed above, the signals that induce Dlk1 upregulation should ultimately be investigated and a unified picture of how these signals integrate with the other pathways involved will emerge. Kras activates Etv5 in lung cancer but it remains to be determined whether this is the critical stimulus in lung injury. In lung injury, the critical limiting step for TGFβ signaling may be at the level of activation of the ligand from its inactive form by integrins [44], but what induces that process is still unknown. The triggers for BMP and Notch signaling remain unclear. Moreover, although these key pathways have been identified, the mechanisms by which they induce ATI cell differentiation are unknown. Many of these pathways cells change in transcription, but it is unknown whether ATI cell markers are direct transcriptional targets or whether other target genes trigger additional signaling pathways that ultimately induce differentiation. Additionally, as alluded to, ATI cell differentiation entails extensive changes in both gene expression and cell morphology. The mechanisms by which the identified molecular signals regulate these changes in gene expression and cell morphology in a coordinated manner remains to be determined.

In addition, although there is now strengthened understanding of the other individual pathway mechanisms, the sequence of these signals—whether pathways are downstream, upstream, or parallel relative to one another—is still largely unknown. As more work is done, it will become clear how these various pathways interact with each other in a coordinated manner to drive differentiation. Taken together, the work of Nan Tang et al. demonstrates that Cdc42 is upstream of YAP signaling [26,35]. YAP/TAZ signaling is known to negatively regulate Wnt/β-catenin signaling [25], and Wnt/β-catenin prevents ATI cell differentiation; thus, it is possible that one mechanism by which YAP/TAZ drives ATI cell differentiation is via β-catenin inhibition.

It is interesting that several of the transcriptional pathways identified, β-catenin, TGFβ, and Etv5, actually inhibit differentiation and must be withdrawn to permit differentiation. Whether there is a common factor, e.g., epigenetic, that synchronizes the downregulation of these pathways, thus driving ATI cell differentiation, could be explored. Moreover, this suggests, as some have noted, that differentiation may be the default process, with active signaling required to maintain the progenitor state. This notion is supported by the concept of the ATII cell niche maintaining the ATII cell phenotype, with removal from the niche resulting in ATI cell differentiation [1,14]. Consistent with this notion is the well-established observation that ATII cells isolated from the organism differentiate into ATI cells by default in culture without specific and aggressive interventions to maintain the ATII cell phenotype [45–48].

Future studies that explore mechanisms of cell-cell crosstalk in the context of alveolar epithelial cell differentiation are warranted. In this regard, the demonstration that recruited monocyte-derived macrophages play a critical role was a seminal finding. The mediators that M2 macrophages produce, which stimulate ATII cell proliferation and/or differentiation, are yet to be determined. In addition, although this study did not find a role for T and B cells, it is highly possible that other immune cell populations are also involved. Other studies have identified prominent roles of immune cells in ATII cell proliferation [49,50]; whether they also regulate ATII-to-ATI cell differentiation should be explored. The mediators used by macrophages or other immune cells to drive ATII-to-ATI cell differentiation and whether these may be some of the known mediators discussed above should be investigated. Fibroblasts were identified to be a source of BMP during regeneration [23] and a source of Wnts during homeostasis [14,15]. The cellular source of Notch and TGFβ ligands could be studied, as could the mechanisms that trigger these cells to produce these ligands. In summary, future studies should investigate the initiation of the signaling pathways identified to regulate ATI cell differentiation, and whether cell communication is coordinated via juxtacrine, paracrine, or autocrine signals.

Future translation of these studies into human tissues and subjects is also warranted. Ineffective alveolar regeneration is thought to underlie the pathogenesis of acute and chronic lung diseases. Once the mechanisms of normal alveolar regeneration are understood, we must begin to understand how these go awry during the pathogenesis of lung disease. We and others recently uncovered a novel transitional state occurring during ATII-to-ATI cell differentiation, with evidence to suggest that persistence of this state occurs in human pulmonary fibrosis [35,39,42]. However, additional studies to understand why this transitional state persists, how this leads to fibrosis, and whether and how the exit from this transitional state towards terminal differentiation impacts fibrosis must be performed. In addition, the ways in which the pathways now implicated in physiologic ATI cell differentiation, Notch, YAP/TAZ, etc. may become hijacked during the development of chronic lung disease should be investigated. Biorepositories of fixed human diseased lung tissue are a critical resource. Banked frozen human ATII cells can be cultured in standard two-dimensional cultures [47,51] or in three-dimensional organoids [52]. In addition, the culture of precision-cut human lung will allow examination of ATII cell behavior in its native state in the alveolus [53]. Ultimately, drugs that target the individual pathways or common convergent pathways may be used as clinical treatments to promote epithelial repair and prevent lung disease in instances of excessive lung damage.

12. Conclusions

We know that in the lung, ATII epithelial progenitors are recruited during alveolar regeneration to replace lost ATI—and sometimes ATII—cells. Although we understand that the process of alveolar regeneration occurs in proliferation and differentiation stages, our understanding of the mechanisms of differentiation is still in its infancy. Recent studies have significantly advanced our understanding of some signaling mechanisms shown to be involved in ATII-to-ATI differentiation. Signaling pathways shown to play a role in ATII-to-ATI cell differentiation include BMP, Notch, TGFβ, β-catenin, Etv5, Cdc42, and Yap/Taz (Figure 1). Cells present in the alveolus that appear to contribute to ATI cell differentiation include fibroblasts and monocyte-derived macrophages.

These various signaling pathways have all been shown to be involved in alveolar regeneration, with various mechanistic steps from each pathway likely interacting with one another to control differentiation. These investigations establish the foundation for further studies in this field. Using this understanding of the signaling pathways behind ATII-to-ATI differentiation during alveolar repair, similar studies can be devised to understand the interaction between these various mechanisms in coordination to control differentiation. Additionally, a strengthened understanding of these molecular pathways involved in differentiation may lead to development of new clinical treatments that accelerate lung repair in individuals with excessive lung damage.

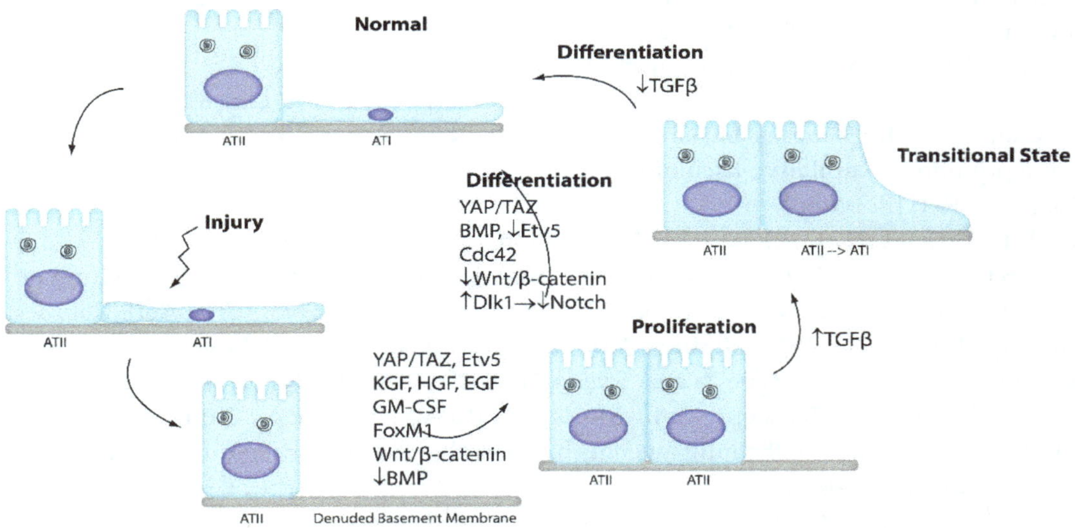

Figure 1. The alveolar epithelium consists of ATI and ATII cells. ATI cells are very susceptible to injury. ATII cells regenerate ATI cells. ATII cells proliferate and then differentiate into ATI cells. Many pathways have been identified that promote ATII cell proliferation: KGF [16], HGF [17,54], EGF [19,20], GM-CSF [33], FoxM1 [10], Wnt/β-catenin [13–15], Etv5 [37], and YAP/TAZ [24,26], whereas downregulation of BMP signaling induces proliferation [23]. Recent studies suggest that multiple pathways are also involved in ATII-to-ATI cell differentiation: YAP/TAZ [24,26], Cdc42 [35], and BMP [23] promote differentiation, whereas Wnt/β-catenin [14,15], Etv5 [37], and Notch [22] maintain the ATII cell phenotype. We recently identified a novel transitional state through which ATII cells pass as they differentiate into ATI cells [38]. Our data suggested that TGFβ promotes cell cycle exit and entry into the transitional state, whereas TGFβ downregulation permits terminal differentiation. Further studies are necessary to confirm these findings and elucidate how these pathways intersect in a coordinated manner to regulate ATII-to-ATI cell differentiation.

References

1. Barkauskas, C.E.; Cronce, M.J.; Rackley, C.R.; Bowie, E.J.; Keene, D.R.; Stripp, B.R.; Randell, S.H.; Noble, P.W.; Hogan, B.L. Type 2 alveolar cells are stem cells in adult lung. *J. Clin. Investig* **2013**, *123*, 3025–3036. [CrossRef] [PubMed]
2. Dobbs, L.G.; Johnson, M.D.; Vanderbilt, J.; Allen, L.; Gonzalez, R. The great big alveolar TI cell: Evolving concepts and paradigms. *Cell Physiol. Biochem.* **2010**, *25*, 55–62. [CrossRef] [PubMed]
3. Schneider, J.P.; Wrede, C.; Hegermann, J.; Weibel, E.R.; Mühlfeld, C.; Ochs, M. On the Topological Complexity of Human Alveolar Epithelial Type 1 Cells. *Am. J Respir Crit. Care Med.* **2019**, *199*, 1153–1156. [CrossRef] [PubMed]
4. Evans, M.J.; Cabral, L.J.; Stephens, R.J.; Freeman, G. Transformation of alveolar type 2 cells to type 1 cells following exposure to NO2. *Exp. Mol. Pathol.* **1975**, *22*, 142–150. [CrossRef]
5. Evans, M.J.; Dekker, N.P.; Cabral-Anderson, L.J.; Freeman, G. Quantitation of damage to the alveolar epithelium by means of type 2 cell proliferation. *Am. Rev. Respir Dis.* **1978**, *118*, 787–790. [CrossRef]
6. Evans, M.J.; Cabral, L.J.; Stephens, R.J.; Freeman, G. Renewal of alveolar epithelium in the rat following exposure to NO2. *Am. J. Pathol.* **1973**, *70*, 175–198.
7. Kathiriya, J.J.; Brumwell, A.N.; Jackson, J.R.; Tang, X.; Chapman, H.A. Distinct Airway Epithelial Stem Cells Hide among Club Cells but Mobilize to Promote Alveolar Regeneration. *Cell Stem Cell* **2020**, *26*, 346–358. [CrossRef]
8. Vaughan, A.E.; Brumwell, A.N.; Xi, Y.; Gotts, J.E.; Brownfield, D.G.; Treutlein, B.; Tan, K.; Tan, V.; Liu, F.C.; Looney, M.R.; et al. Lineage-negative progenitors mobilize to regenerate lung epithelium after major injury. *Nature* **2015**, *517*, 621–625. [CrossRef]
9. Rock, J.R.; Barkauskas, C.E.; Cronce, M.J.; Xue, Y.; Harris, J.R.; Liang, J.; Noble, P.W.; Hogan, B.L. Multiple stromal populations contribute to pulmonary fibrosis without evidence for epithelial to mesenchymal transition. *Proc. Natl. Acad. Sci. USA* **2011**, *108*, E1475–E1483. [CrossRef]
10. Liu, Y.; Sadikot, R.T.; Adami, G.R.; Kalinichenko, V.V.; Pendyala, S.; Natarajan, V.; Zhao, Y.Y.; Malik, A.B. FoxM1 mediates the progenitor function of type II epithelial cells in repairing alveolar injury induced by Pseudomonas aeruginosa. *J. Exp. Med.* **2011**, *208*, 1473–1484. [CrossRef]
11. Mock, J.R.; Dial, C.F.; D'Alessio, F.R.; Doerschuk, C.M. Foxp3+ Regulatory T Cell Expression Of Keratinocyte Growth Factor During Acute Lung Injury Resolution. *Am. J. Respir Crit. Care Med.* **2016**, *193*, A6143.
12. Rafii, S.; Cao, Z.; Lis, R.; Siempos, I.I.; Chavez, D.; Shido, K.; Rabbany, S.Y.; Ding, B.S. Platelet-derived SDF-1 primes the pulmonary capillary vascular niche to drive lung alveolar regeneration. *Nat. Cell Biol.* **2015**, *17*, 123–136. [CrossRef] [PubMed]
13. Zemans, R.L.; Briones, N.; Campbell, M.; McClendon, J.; Young, S.K.; Suzuki, T.; Yang, I.V.; De Langhe, S.; Reynolds, S.D.; Mason, R.J.; et al. Neutrophil transmigration triggers repair of the lung epithelium via beta-catenin signaling. *Proc. Natl. Acad. Sci. USA* **2011**, *108*, 15990–15995. [CrossRef] [PubMed]
14. Nabhan, A.N.; Brownfield, D.G.; Harbury, P.B.; Krasnow, M.A.; Desai, T.J. Single-cell Wnt signaling niches maintain stemness of alveolar type 2 cells. *Science* **2018**, *359*, 1118–1123. [CrossRef] [PubMed]
15. Zacharias, W.J.; Frank, D.B.; Zepp, J.A.; Morley, M.P.; Alkhaleel, F.A.; Kong, J.; Zhou, S.; Cantu, E.; Morrisey, E.E. Regeneration of the lung alveolus by an evolutionarily conserved epithelial progenitor. *Nature* **2018**, *555*, 251–255. [CrossRef]
16. Panos, R.J.; Rubin, J.S.; Csaky, K.G.; Aaronson, S.A.; Mason, R.J. Keratinocyte growth factor and hepatocyte growth factor/scatter factor are heparin-binding growth factors for alveolar type II cells in fibroblast-conditioned medium. *J. Clin. Invest.* **1993**, *92*, 969–977. [CrossRef]
17. Mason, R.J.; Leslie, C.C.; McCormick-Shannon, K.; Deterding, R.R.; Nakamura, T.; Rubin, J.S.; Shannon, J.M. Hepatocyte growth factor is a growth factor for rat alveolar type II cells. *Am. J. Respir Cell Mol. Biol.* **1994**, *11*, 561–567. [CrossRef]
18. Fehrenbach, H.; Kasper, M.; Tschernig, T.; Pan, T.; Schuh, D.; Shannon, J.M.; Muller, M.; Mason, R.J. Keratinocyte growth factor-induced hyperplasia of rat alveolar type II cells in vivo is resolved by differentiation into type I cells and by apoptosis. *Eur. Respir J.* **1999**, *14*, 534–544. [CrossRef]
19. Ding, B.S.; Nolan, D.J.; Guo, P.; Babazadeh, A.O.; Cao, Z.; Rosenwaks, Z.; Crystal, R.G.; Simons, M.; Sato, T.N.; Worgall, S.; et al. Endothelial-derived angiocrine signals induce and sustain regenerative lung alveolarization. *Cell* **2011** *147*, 539–553. [CrossRef]

20. Desai, T.J.; Brownfield, D.G.; Krasnow, M.A. Alveolar progenitor and stem cells in lung development, renewal and cancer. *Nature* **2014**, *507*, 190–194. [CrossRef]
21. Jansing, N.L.; McClendon, J.; Henson, P.M.; Tuder, R.M.; Hyde, D.M.; Zemans, R.L. Unbiased Quantitation of ATII to ATI Cell Transdifferentiation During Repair After Lung Injury in Mice. *Am. J. Respir Cell Mol. Biol.* **2017**, *57*, 519–526. [CrossRef] [PubMed]
22. Finn, J.; Sottoriva, K.; Pajcini, K.V.; Kitajewski, J.K.; Chen, C.; Zhang, W.; Malik, A.B.; Liu, Y. Dlk1-Mediated Temporal Regulation of Notch Signaling Is Required for Differentiation of Alveolar Type II to Type I Cells during Repair. *Cell Rep.* **2019**, *26*, 2942–2954. [CrossRef] [PubMed]
23. Chung, M.I.; Bujnis, M.; Barkauskas, C.E.; Kobayashi, Y.; Hogan, B.L.M. Niche-mediated BMP/SMAD signaling regulates lung alveolar stem cell proliferation and differentiation. *Development* **2018**, *145*, dev163014. [CrossRef] [PubMed]
24. LaCanna, R.; Liccardo, D.; Zhang, P.; Tragesser, L.; Wang, Y.; Cao, T.; Chapman, H.A.; Morrisey, E.E.; Shen, H.; Koch, W.J.; et al. Yap/Taz regulate alveolar regeneration and resolution of lung inflammation. *J. Clin. Invest.* **2019**, *130*, 2107–2122. [CrossRef]
25. Sun, T.; Huang, Z.; Zhang, H.; Posner, C.; Jia, G.; Ramalingam, T.R.; Xu, M.; Brightbill, H.; Egen, J.G.; Dey, A.; et al. TAZ is required for lung alveolar epithelial cell differentiation after injury. *JCI Insigh* **2019**, *5*. [CrossRef]
26. Liu, Z.; Wu, H.; Jiang, K.; Wang, Y.; Zhang, W.; Chu, Q.; Li, J.; Huang, H.; Cai, T.; Ji, H.; et al. MAPK-Mediated YAP Activation Controls Mechanical-Tension-Induced Pulmonary Alveolar Regeneration. *Cell Rep.* **2016**, *16*, 1810–1819. [CrossRef]
27. Zhou, B.; Flodby, P.; Luo, J.; Castillo, D.R.; Liu, Y.; Yu, F.X.; McConnell, A.; Varghese, B.; Li, G.; Chimge, N.O.; et al. Claudin-18-mediated YAP activity regulates lung stem and progenitor cell homeostasis and tumorigenesis. *J. Clin. Invest.* **2018**, *128*, 970–984. [CrossRef]
28. Mould, K.J.; Jackson, N.D.; Henson, P.M.; Seibold, M.; Janssen, W.J. Single cell RNA sequencing identifies unique inflammatory airspace macrophage subsets. *JCI Insight.* **2019**, *4*, e126556. [CrossRef]
29. Misharin, A.V.; Morales-Nebreda, L.; Reyfman, P.A.; Cuda, C.M.; Walter, J.M.; McQuattie-Pimentel, A.C.; Chen, C.I.; Anekalla, K.R.; Joshi, N.; Williams, K.J.N.; et al. Monocyte-derived alveolar macrophages drive lung fibrosis and persist in the lung over the life span. *J. Exp. Med.* **2017**, *214*, 2387–2404. [CrossRef]
30. Moore, B.B.; Paine, R.; Christensen, P.J.; Moore, T.A.; Sitterding, S.; Ngan, R.; Wilke, C.A.; Kuziel, W.A.; Toews, G.B. Protection from pulmonary fibrosis in the absence of CCR2 signaling. *J. Immunol.* **2001**, *167*, 4368–4377. [CrossRef]
31. Herold, S.; Steinmueller, M.; von Wulffen, W.; Cakarova, L.; Pinto, R.; Pleschka, S.; Mack, M.; Kuziel, W.A.; Corazza, N.; Brunner, T.; et al. Lung epithelial apoptosis in influenza virus pneumonia: the role of macrophage-expressed TNF-related apoptosis-inducing ligand. *J. Exp. Med.* **2008**, *205*, 3065–3077. [CrossRef] [PubMed]
32. Lechner, A.J.; Driver, I.H.; Lee, J.; Conroy, C.M.; Nagle, A.; Locksley, R.M.; Rock, J.R. Recruited Monocytes and Type 2 Immunity Promote Lung Regeneration following Pneumonectomy. *Cell Stem Cell* **2017**, *21*, 120–134. [CrossRef] [PubMed]
33. Cakarova, L.; Marsh, L.M.; Wilhelm, J.; Mayer, K.; Grimminger, F.; Seeger, W.; Lohmeyer, J.; Herold, S. Macrophage tumor necrosis factor-alpha induces epithelial expression of granulocyte-macrophage colony-stimulating factor: impact on alveolar epithelial repair. *Am. J. Respir Crit. Care Med.* **2009**, *180*, 521–532. [CrossRef] [PubMed]
34. Hung, L.-Y.; Sen, D.; Oniskey, T.K.; Katzen, J.; Cohen, N.A.; Vaughan, A.E.; Nieves, W.; Urisman, A.; Beers, M.F.; Krummel, M.F.; et al. Macrophages promote epithelial proliferation following infectious and non-infectious lung injury through a Trefoil factor 2-dependent mechanism. *Mucosal Immunology* **2019**, *12*, 64–76. [CrossRef] [PubMed]
35. Wu, H.; Yu, Y.; Huang, H.; Hu, Y.; Fu, S.; Wang, Z.; Shi, M.; Zhao, X.; Yuan, J.; Li, J.; et al. Progressive Pulmonary Fibrosis Is Caused by Elevated Mechanical Tension on Alveolar Stem Cells. *Cell* **2020**, *180*, 107–121. [CrossRef] [PubMed]
36. Liu, Y.; Jiang, H.; Crawford, H.C.; Hogan, B.L. Role for ETS domain transcription factors Pea3/Erm in mouse lung development. *Dev. Biol.* **2003**, *261*, 10–24. [CrossRef]
37. Zhang, Z.; Newton, K.; Kummerfeld, S.K.; Webster, J.; Kirkpatrick, D.S.; Phu, L.; Eastham-Anderson, J.; Liu, J.; Lee, W.P.; Wu, J.; et al. Transcription factor Etv5 is essential for the maintenance of alveolar type II cells. *Proc. Natl. Acad. Sci. USA* **2017**, *114*, 3903–3908. [CrossRef]

38. Riemondy, K.A.; Jansing, N.L.; Jiang, P.; Redente, E.F.; Gillen, A.E.; Fu, R.; Miller, A.J.; Spence, J.R.; Gerber, A.N.; Hesselberth, J.R.; et al. Single cell RNA sequencing identifies TGFβ as a key regenerative cue following LPS-induced lung injury. *JCI Insight.* **2019**, *4*, 123637. [CrossRef]
39. Strunz, M.; Simon, L.M.; Ansari, M.; Mattner, L.F.; Angelidis, I.; Mayr, C.H.; Kathiriya, J.; Yee, M.; Ogar, P.; Sengupta, A.; et al. Longitudinal single cell transcriptomics reveals Krt8+ alveolar epithelial progenitors in lung regeneration. *bioRxiv* **2019**. [CrossRef]
40. Kobayashi, Y.; Tata, A.; Konkimalla, A.; Katsura, H.; Lee, R.F.; Ou, J.; Banovich, N.E.; Kropski, J.A.; Tata, P.R. Persistence of a novel regeneration-associated transitional cell state in pulmonary fibrosis. *biorxiv* **2020**. [CrossRef]
41. Joshi, N.; Watanabe, S.; Verma, R.; Jablonski, R.P.; Chen, C.I.; Cheresh, P.; Markov, N.S.; Reyfman, P.A.; McQuattie-Pimentel, A.C.; Sichizya, L.; et al. A spatially restricted fibrotic niche in pulmonary fibrosis is sustained by M-CSF/M-CSFR signalling in monocyte-derived alveolar macrophages. *Eur. Respir J.* **2020**, *55*, 1900646. [CrossRef] [PubMed]
42. Jiang, P.; Gil de Rubio, R.; Hrycaj, S.M.; Gurczynski, S.J.; Riemondy, K.A.; Moore, B.B.; Omary, M.B.; Ridge, K.M.; Zemans, R.L. Ineffectual AEC2-to-AEC1 Differentiation in IPF: Persistence of KRT8. *Am. J. Respir Crit. Care Med.* **2020**. [CrossRef] [PubMed]
43. Jansing, N.L.; Patel, N.; McClendon, J.; Redente, E.F.; Henson, P.M.; Tuder, R.M.; Hyde, D.M.; Nyengaard, J.R.; Zemans, R.L. Flow Cytometry Underestimates and Planimetry Overestimates Alveolar Epithelial Type 2 Cell Expansion after Lung Injury. *Am. J. Respir Crit. Care Med.* **2018**, *198*, 390–392. [CrossRef] [PubMed]
44. Munger, J.S.; Huang, X.; Kawakatsu, H.; Griffiths, M.J.; Dalton, S.L.; Wu, J.; Pittet, J.F.; Kaminski, N.; Garat, C.; Matthay, M.A.; et al. The integrin alpha v beta 6 binds and activates latent TGF beta 1: a mechanism for regulating pulmonary inflammation and fibrosis. *Cell* **1999**, *96*, 319–328. [CrossRef]
45. Borok, Z.; Danto, S.I.; Lubman, R.L.; Cao, Y.; Williams, M.C.; Crandall, E.D. Modulation of t1alpha expression with alveolar epithelial cell phenotype in vitro. *Am. J. Physiol.* **1998**, *275*, L155–L164.
46. Marconett, C.N.; Zhou, B.; Rieger, M.E.; Selamat, S.A.; Dubourd, M.; Fang, X.; Lynch, S.K.; Stueve, T.R.; Siegmund, K.D.; Berman, B.P.; et al. Integrated transcriptomic and epigenomic analysis of primary human lung epithelial cell differentiation. *PLoS Genet* **2013**, *9*, e1003513. [CrossRef]
47. Wang, J.; Edeen, K.; Manzer, R.; Chang, Y.; Wang, S.; Chen, X.; Funk, C.J.; Cosgrove, G.P.; Fang, X.; Mason, R.J. Differentiated human alveolar epithelial cells and reversibility of their phenotype in vitro. *Am. J. Respir Cell Mol. Biol.* **2007**, *36*, 661–668. [CrossRef]
48. Correll, K.A.; Edeen, K.E.; Zemans, R.L.; Redente, E.F.; Serban, K.A.; Curran-Everett, D.; Edelman, B.L.; Mikels-Vigdal, A.; Mason, R.J. Transitional human alveolar type II epithelial cells suppress extracellular matrix and growth factor gene expression in lung fibroblasts. *Am. J. Physiol. Lung Cell Mol. Physiol.* **2019**, *317*, L283–L294. [CrossRef]
49. Mock, J.R.; Garibaldi, B.T.; Aggarwal, N.R.; Jenkins, J.; Limjunyawong, N.; Singer, B.D.; Chau, E.; Rabold, R.; Files, D.C.; Sidhaye, V.; et al. Foxp3+ regulatory T cells promote lung epithelial proliferation. *Mucosal Immunol.* **2014**, *7*, 1440–1451. [CrossRef]
50. Dial, C.F.; Tune, M.K.; Doerschuk, C.M.; Mock, J.R. Foxp3+ Regulatory T Cell Expression of Keratinocyte Growth Factor Enhances Lung Epithelial Proliferation. *Am. J. Respir Cell Mol. Biol.* **2017**, *57*, 162–173. [CrossRef]
51. Kosmider, B.; Messier, E.M.; Janssen, W.J.; Nahreini, P.; Wang, J.; Hartshorn, K.L.; Mason, R.J. Nrf2 protects human alveolar epithelial cells against injury induced by influenza A virus. *Respir Res.* **2012**, *13*, 43. [CrossRef] [PubMed]
52. Zacharias, W.J.; Morrisey, E.E. Isolation and culture of human alveolar epithelial progenitor cells. *Protoc. Exch.* **2018**. [CrossRef]
53. Alsafadi, H.N.; Uhl, F.E.; Pineda, R.H.; Bailey, K.E.; Rojas, M.; Wagner, D.E.; Königshoff, M. Applications and Approaches for 3D Precision-cut Lung Slices: Disease Modeling and Drug Discovery. *Am. J. Respir Cell Mol. Biol.* **2020**. [CrossRef] [PubMed]
54. Leslie, C.C.; McCormick-Shannon, K.; Shannon, J.M.; Garrick, B.; Damm, D.; Abraham, J.A.; Mason, R.J. Heparin-binding EGF-like growth factor is a mitogen for rat alveolar type II cells. *Am. J. Respir Cell Mol. Biol.* **1997**, *16*, 379–387. [CrossRef] [PubMed]

Permissions

All chapters in this book were first published by MDPI; hereby published with permission under the Creative Commons Attribution License or equivalent. Every chapter published in this book has been scrutinized by our experts. Their significance has been extensively debated. The topics covered herein carry significant findings which will fuel the growth of the discipline. They may even be implemented as practical applications or may be referred to as a beginning point for another development.

The contributors of this book come from diverse backgrounds, making this book a truly international effort. This book will bring forth new frontiers with its revolutionizing research information and detailed analysis of the nascent developments around the world.

We would like to thank all the contributing authors for lending their expertise to make the book truly unique. They have played a crucial role in the development of this book. Without their invaluable contributions this book wouldn't have been possible. They have made vital efforts to compile up to date information on the varied aspects of this subject to make this book a valuable addition to the collection of many professionals and students.

This book was conceptualized with the vision of imparting up-to-date information and advanced data in this field. To ensure the same, a matchless editorial board was set up. Every individual on the board went through rigorous rounds of assessment to prove their worth. After which they invested a large part of their time researching and compiling the most relevant data for our readers.

The editorial board has been involved in producing this book since its inception. They have spent rigorous hours researching and exploring the diverse topics which have resulted in the successful publishing of this book. They have passed on their knowledge of decades through this book. To expedite this challenging task, the publisher supported the team at every step. A small team of assistant editors was also appointed to further simplify the editing procedure and attain best results for the readers.

Apart from the editorial board, the designing team has also invested a significant amount of their time in understanding the subject and creating the most relevant covers. They scrutinized every image to scout for the most suitable representation of the subject and create an appropriate cover for the book.

The publishing team has been an ardent support to the editorial, designing and production team. Their endless efforts to recruit the best for this project, has resulted in the accomplishment of this book. They are a veteran in the field of academics and their pool of knowledge is as vast as their experience in printing. Their expertise and guidance has proved useful at every step. Their uncompromising quality standards have made this book an exceptional effort. Their encouragement from time to time has been an inspiration for everyone.

The publisher and the editorial board hope that this book will prove to be a valuable piece of knowledge for researchers, students, practitioners and scholars across the globe.

List of Contributors

Katharina M. Quell, Kuheli Dutta, Ülkü R. Korkmaz and Larissa Nogueira de Almeida
Institute for Systemic Inflammation Research, University of Lübeck, 23538 Lübeck, Germany

Tillman Vollbrandt
Cell Analysis Core Facility, University of Lübeck, 23538 Lübeck, Germany

Peter König
Institute of Anatomy, University of Lübeck, 23538 Lübeck, Germany
Airway Research Center North, Member of the German Center for Lung Research (DZL), 23538 Lübeck, Germany

Ian Lewkowich
Division of Immunobiology, Cincinnati Children's Hospital, Cincinnati, OH 45229, USA
Department of Pediatrics, University of Cincinnati, Cincinnati, OH 45229, USA

George S. Deepe, Jr.
College of Medicine, University of Cincinnati, Cincinnati, OH 45229, USA

Admar Verschoor
Department of Infectious Diseases and Microbiology, University of Lübeck, 23538 Lübeck, Germany

Jörg Köhl
Institute for Systemic Inflammation Research, University of Lübeck, 23538 Lübeck, Germany
Airway Research Center North, Member of the German Center for Lung Research (DZL), 23538 Lübeck, Germany
Division of Immunobiology, Cincinnati Children's Hospital, Cincinnati, OH 45229, USA

Yves Laumonnier
Institute for Systemic Inflammation Research, University of Lübeck, 23538 Lübeck, Germany
Airway Research Center North, Member of the German Center for Lung Research (DZL), 23538 Lübeck, Germany

Eva Delbrel, Abdoulaye Soumare, Dominique Marchant and Emilie Boncoeur
Université Paris 13, Sorbonne Paris Cité, Laboratoire 'Hypoxie & Poumon' (Inserm U1272), F-93017 Bobigny, France

Yurdagül Uzunhan, Thomas Gille and Carole Planès
Université Paris 13, Sorbonne Paris Cité, Laboratoire 'Hypoxie & Poumon' (Inserm U1272), F-93017 Bobigny, France
Assistance Publique Hôpitaux de Paris (APHP), Hôpital Avicenne, F-93017 Bobigny, France

Julia Hollenbach
Institute of Functional and Applied Anatomy, Hannover Medical School, 30625 Hannover, Germany

Christian Mühlfeld and Julia Schipke
Institute of Functional and Applied Anatomy, Hannover Medical School, 30625 Hannover, Germany
Biomedical Research in Endstage and Obstructive Lung Disease Hannover (BREATH), Member of the German Center for Lung Research (DZL), 30625 Hannover, Germany
Cluster of Excellence REBIRTH (From Regenerative Biology to Reconstructive Therapy), 30625 Hannover, Germany

Vitalii Kryvenko, Susanne Herold and István Vadász
Department of Internal Medicine, Justus Liebig University, Universities of Giessen and Marburg Lung Center (UGMLC), Member of the German Center for Lung Research (DZL), 35392 Giessen, Germany
The Cardio-Pulmonary Institute (CPI), 35392 Giessen, Germany

Miriam Wessendorf
Department of Internal Medicine, Justus Liebig University, Universities of Giessen and Marburg Lung Center (UGMLC), Member of the German Center for Lung Research (DZL), 35392 Giessen, Germany

Rory E. Morty and Werner Seeger
Department of Internal Medicine, Justus Liebig University, Universities of Giessen and Marburg Lung Center (UGMLC), Member of the German Center for Lung Research (DZL), 35392 Giessen, Germany
The Cardio-Pulmonary Institute (CPI), 35392 Giessen, Germany
Department of Lung Development and Remodeling, Max Planck Institute for Heart and Lung Research, 61231 Bad Nauheim, Germany

Olga Vagin
Department of Physiology, David Geffen School of Medicine, University of California at Los Angeles, Los Angeles, CA 90095, USA
Veterans Administration Greater Los Angeles Healthcare System, Los Angeles, CA 90073, USA

Laura A. Dada and Jacob I. Sznajder
Division of Pulmonary and Critical Care Medicine, Feinberg School of Medicine, Northwestern University, Chicago, IL 60611, USA

Nina Rühl and Karolin Albert
Institute of Functional and Applied Anatomy, Hannover Medical School, Hannover 30625, Germany

Elena Lopez-Rodriguez and Matthias Ochs
Institute of Functional and Applied Anatomy, Hannover Medical School, Hannover 30625, Germany
Biomedical Research in Endstage and Obstructive Lung Diseases (BREATH), Member of the German Centerfor Lung Research (DLZ), Hannover 30625, Germany
REBIRTH, Cluster of Excellence, Hannover 30625, Germany
Institute of Vegetative Anatomy, Charite, Berlin 10117, Germany

Bradford J Smith
Department of Bioengineering, University of Colorado Denver, Denver, CO 80045, USA

Timothy E Weaver
Division of Pulmonary Biology, University of Cincinnati College of Medicine, Cincinnati, OH 45221, USA

Lars Knudsen
Institute of Functional and Applied Anatomy, Hannover Medical School, Hannover 30625, Germany
Biomedical Research in Endstage and Obstructive Lung Diseases (BREATH), Member of the German Centerfor Lung Research (DLZ), Hannover 30625, Germany
REBIRTH, Cluster of Excellence, Hannover 30625, Germany

Jan Philipp Schneider
Institute of Functional and Applied Anatomy, Hannover Medical School, Carl-Neuberg-Straße 1, 30625 Hannover, Germany
Biomedical Research in Endstage and Obstructive Lung Disease Hannover (BREATH), Member of the German Center for Lung Research (DZL), Hannover Medical School, Carl-Neuberg-Straße 1, 30625 Hannover, Germany

Christoph Wrede and Christian Mühlfeld
Institute of Functional and Applied Anatomy, Hannover Medical School, Carl-Neuberg-Straße 1, 30625 Hannover, Germany
Biomedical Research in Endstage and Obstructive Lung Disease Hannover (BREATH), Member of the German Center for Lung Research (DZL), Hannover Medical School, Carl-Neuberg-Straße 1, 30625 Hannover, Germany
Research Core Unit Electron Microscopy, Hannover Medical School, Carl-Neuberg-Straße 1, 30625 Hannover, Germany

Kwang-Jin Kim
Will Rogers Institute Pulmonary Research Center and Hastings Center for Pulmonary Research, Keck School of Medicine, University of Southern California, Los Angeles, CA 90033-0906, USA
Division of Pulmonary, Critical Care and Sleep Medicine, Department of Medicine, Keck School of Medicine, University of Southern California, Los Angeles, CA 90033-0906, USA
Department of Physiology and Neuroscience, Keck School of Medicine, University of Southern California, Los Angeles, CA 90089-9037, USA
Department of Pharmacology and Pharmaceutical Sciences, School of Pharmacy, University of Southern California, Los Angeles, CA 90089-9121, USA
Department of Biomedical Engineering, Viterbi School of Engineering, University of Southern California, Los Angeles, CA 90089-1111, USA

Constantinos Sioutas
Sonny Astani Department of Civil and Environmental Engineering, Viterbi School of Engineering, University of Southern California, Los Angeles, CA 90089-2531, USA

Edward D. Crandall
Will Rogers Institute Pulmonary Research Center and Hastings Center for Pulmonary Research, Keck School of Medicine, University of Southern California, Los Angeles, CA 90033-0906, USA
Division of Pulmonary, Critical Care and Sleep Medicine, Department of Medicine, Keck School of Medicine, University of Southern California, Los Angeles, CA 90033-0906, USA
Department of Pathology, Keck School of Medicine, University of Southern California, Los Angeles, CA 90033-9092, USA
Mork Family Department of Chemical Engineering and Materials Science, Viterbi School of Engineering, University of Southern California, Los Angeles, CA 90089-1211, USA

Arnold Sipos
Will Rogers Institute Pulmonary Research Center and Hastings Center for Pulmonary Research, Keck School of Medicine, University of Southern California, Los Angeles, CA 90033-0906, USA
Division of Pulmonary, Critical Care and Sleep Medicine, Department of Medicine, Keck School of Medicine, University of Southern California, Los Angeles, CA 90033-0906, USA

Tanyalak Parimon, Changfu Yao and Paul W Noble
Division of Pulmonary and Critical Care Medicine, Department of Medicine, Women's Guild Lung Institute, Cedars-Sinai Medical Center, Los Angeles, CA 90048, USA

Barry R Stripp and Peter Chen
Division of Pulmonary and Critical Care Medicine, Department of Medicine, Women's Guild Lung Institute, Cedars-Sinai Medical Center, Los Angeles, CA 90048, USA
Department of Biomedical Sciences, Cedars-Sinai Medical Center, Los Angeles, CA 90048, USA

Karl-Philipp Wesslau, Anabel Stein, Michael Kasper and Kathrin Barth
Institute of Anatomy, Dresden University of Technology, D-01307 Dresden, Germany

Matthias Ochs
Institute of Functional Anatomy, Charité-Universitätsmedizin Berlin, 10117 Berlin, Germany
German Center for Lung Research (DZL), 10117 Berlin, Germany

Jan Hegermann
Research Core Unit Electron Microscopy and Institute of Functional and Applied Anatomy, Hannover Medical School, 30625 Hannover, Germany

Sara Timm
Core Facility Electron Microscopy, Charité-Universitätsmedizin Berlin, 10117 Berlin, Germany

Geraldine Nouailles
Department of Infectious Diseases and Respiratory Medicine, and Division of Pulmonary Inflammation, Charité-Universitätsmedizin Berlin, 10117 Berlin, Germany

Jasmin Matuszak and Szandor Simmons
Institute of Physiology, Charité-Universitätsmedizin Berlin, 10117 Berlin, Germany

Martin Witzenrath
German Center for Lung Research (DZL), 10117 Berlin, Germany
Department of Infectious Diseases and Respiratory Medicine, and Division of Pulmonary Inflammation, Charité-Universitätsmedizin Berlin, 10117 Berlin, Germany

Wolfgang M. Kuebler
German Center for Lung Research (DZL), 10117 Berlin, Germany
Institute of Physiology, Charité-Universitätsmedizin Berlin, 10117 Berlin, Germany

Johanna Christine Jansing, Christian Mühlfeld and Christina Brandenberger
Institute of Functional and Applied Anatomy, Hannover Medical School, 30625 Hannover, Germany
Biomedical Research in Endstage and Obstructive Lung Disease Hannover (BREATH), Member of the German Center for Lung Research (DZL), 30625 Hannover, Germany

Jan Fiedler and Thomas Thum
Institute of Molecular and Translational Therapeutic Strategies, Hannover Medical School, 30625 Hannover, Germany
REBIRTH Center for Translational Regenerative Medicine, 30625 Hannover, Germany

Andreas Pich
Institute of Toxicology, Hannover Medical School, 30625 Hannover, Germany

Janika Viereck
Institute of Molecular and Translational Therapeutic Strategies, Hannover Medical School, 30625 Hannover, Germany

Heimo Mairbäurl
Translational Lung Research Center (TLRC), part of the German Center for Lung Research (DZL), University of Heidelberg, 69120 Heidelberg, Germany

Christoph Dehnert
Medbase Checkup Center, 8400 Zürich, Switzerland

Franziska Macholz, Daniel Dankl and Marc M. Berger
Department of Anesthesiology, Perioperative and General Critical Care Medicine, University Hospital Salzburg, 5020 Salzburg, Austria

Mahdi Sareban
University Institute of Sports Medicine, Prevention and Rehabilitation, and Research Institute of Molecular Sports Medicine and Rehabilitation, Paracelsus Medical University, 5020 Salzburg, Austria

Elisabeth M. Liebler-Tenorio, Carola Ostermann and Petra Reinhold
Institute for Molecular Pathogenesis, Friedrich-Loeffler-Institut, Federal Research Institute for Animal Health, Naumburgerstr. 96a, 07743 Jena, Germany

Jacqueline Lambertz
Institute for Molecular Pathogenesis, Friedrich-Loeffler-Institut, Federal Research Institute for Animal Health, Naumburgerstr. 96a, 07743 Jena, Germany
Chemisches und Veterinäruntersuchungsamt Rhein-Ruhr-Wupper (CVUA-RRW), Deutscher Ring 100, 47798 Krefeld, Germany

Konrad Sachse
Institute for Molecular Pathogenesis, Friedrich-Loeffler-Institut, Federal Research Institute for Animal Health, Naumburgerstr. 96a, 07743 Jena, Germany
Institute of Bioinformatics, Friedrich-Schiller-Universität Jena, Leutragraben 1, 07743 Jena, Germany

Mohit Aspal
College of Literature, Science and the Arts, University of Michigan, Ann Arbor, MI 48109, USA

Rachel L. Zemans
Division of Pulmonary and Critical Care Medicine, Department of Internal Medicine, University of Michigan, 109 Zina Pitcher Place, Ann Arbor, MI 48109-2200, USA
Program in Cellular and Molecular Biology, University of Michigan, Ann Arbor, MI 48109, USA

Index